MEDICINE AND MEMORY IN TIBET

STUDIES ON ETHNIC GROUPS IN CHINA

Stevan Harrell, Editor

MEDICINE AND MEMORY IN TIBET

Amchi Physicians in an Age of Reform

THERESIA HOFER

UNIVERSITY OF WASHINGTON PRESS
Seattle

Printed and bound in the United States of America
Composed in Minion, typeface designed by Robert Slimbach
COVER PHOTOGRAPH: Moxibustion applied to
a patient's head. Photo by Meinrad Hofer.
22 21 20 19 18 5 4 3 2 1

UNIVERSITY OF WASHINGTON PRESS
www.washington.edu/uwpress

LIBRARY OF CONGRESS CATALOGING-IN-PUBLICATION DATA
Names: Hofer, Theresia, author.
Title: Medicine and memory in Tibet : Amchi physicians in an age of reform / Theresia Hofer.
Description: Seattle : University of Washington Press, 2018. | Series: Studies on ethnic groups in China | Includes bibliographical references and index.
Identifiers: LCCN 2017029406 (print) | LCCN 2017028012 (ebook) | ISBN 9780295742984 (hardcover : acid-free paper) | ISBN 9780295742991 (paperback : acid-free paper) | ISBN 9780295743004 (ebook)
Subjects: LCSH: Medicine, Tibetan—History—20th century. | Medicine, Tibetan—History—21st century. | Physicians—China—Tibet Autonomous Region—History. | Memory—Social aspects—China—Tibet Autonomous Region—History. | Social networks—China—Tibet Autonomous Region—History. | Ethnicity—China—Tibet Autonomous Region—History. | Social change—China—Tibet Autonomous Region—History. | Tibet Autonomous Region (China)—Social conditions. | Tibet Autonomous Region (China)—Relations—China. | China—Relations—China—Tibet Autonomous Region.
Classification: LCC R603.T5 H65 2018 (ebook) | LCC R603.T5 (print) | DDC 610.951/5-dc23
LC record available at https://lccn.loc.gov/2017029406

CONTENTS

FOREWORD

Research conducted in Tibet is precious in any age, since that land is not easily accessible even in the best of times. Today, as access becomes ever more difficult—especially for foreign researchers—analysis based on research on the ground is invaluable. Theresia Hofer had both the enterprising spirit and good fortune to be able to conduct "officially official" research in 2003 and "officially unofficial" research in 2006–7 while studying Tibetan language at Tibet University and serving as a consultant with a medical project conducted by the Swiss Red Cross.

Research carried out in areas of the Tibet Autonomous Region remote from the capital city of Lhasa is doubly precious, partly because rural areas are difficult to reach and partly because there is little material available on many areas. Hofer has the linguistic skills and deep cultural knowledge to be able to interview and collect documents in Shigatse Town and in Ngamring and Lhatse Counties, and her personal acquaintance with several rural, urban, and monastic physicians gave her entry to observe how they cared for their patients.

Research on medicine in Tibet is rare, since Tibetan medicine is less familiar to outsiders than the Chinese or Ayurvedic systems. Research on medicine as it is practiced among the common people is especially valuable, since there is almost no documentation in languages other than Tibetan and since age-old practices passed down within local family traditions are in danger of disappearing, even as the Chinese regime governing Tibet promotes preservation and "modernization" of the traditions of the Mentsikhang (Institute of Medicine and Astrology) and Tibetan medicine hospitals.

The Medical Houses explored in this book are houses both in the physical sense of structures where a doctor holds consultations and prescribes and prepares medications and in the metaphorical sense of enduring social groups, based primarily on kinship ties, that pass on the texts and clinical expertise on which diagnosis and treatment are based. Hofer became acquainted with the members of several of these houses, located mostly in rural areas, listened to their house histories and personal stories, examined their treasured medical texts with them, and sat in on their consultations.

And what a story these houses have to tell! Like so many stories about Tibet and Tibetans, it begins with an idealized past before the 1959 revolt against Chinese rule, when the doctors practiced their art without political interference; then moves to their suppression and personal suffering in the early years of the Cultural Revolution beginning in 1966; continues to their cautious revival beginning in the 1970s, even before Chinese Communist Party leader Hu Yaobang's famous visit to Tibet in 1980; and finally brings us to their immersion in the whirlwind of modernization that began to overtake the region after the turn of the millennium.

We are not sure just what has happened to western Tibet's Medical Houses since the Lhasa demonstrations of 2008. The Chinese regime has continually tightened policies, increased surveillance and "patriotic education," and reduced opportunities for Tibetan-language learning, while at the same time pursuing reckless economic development, developing hydroelectric power and mining, promoting immigration (though mostly to Lhasa) by the Han (China's ethnic majority), and encouraging tourism not just to see the breathtaking scenery but to learn an official, bowdlerized version of Tibetan culture minus the "problematic" parts of the religion—that is, the connection between religion and the state. Will the children of the Medical Houses carry on their knowledge and practice? Whatever the future holds, Theresia Hofer has given us an insightful account of what they were like and how they endured through years of revolution and reform, hinting that they may well adapt and flourish in the current age of renewed repression.

—STEVAN HARRELL

SUMMER SOLSTICE, 2017

ACKNOWLEDGMENTS

My most heartfelt thanks go to the Tibetan research participants in Tsang for so willingly and generously sharing their lives, medical work, and memories with me, jointly seeking clarity, and providing their hospitality. Although many names used in this book are pseudonyms, my appreciation and respect for each individual remains the same. I am particularly grateful to the late Yonten Tsering and his wife Yeshe Lhamo in Shigatse, and to Ngawang Dorjé and his family in Lhasa, for letting me become a part of their families and for teaching me so much. All interpretations and conclusions drawn from the research are solely my own, as are any errors.

In Lhasa, Shigatse Town, and Beijing, too, I received indispensable help with my research and enjoyed the friendship of many people who influenced this book in subtle but important ways, and to whom I am deeply grateful. They include Rinzin, the late Tsering Gyalpo, Nyima Tsering, Nyima Lhamo, Penpa Tsering, Tashi Norbu, Tsering Dikey, Jigmé, Dawa, Leigh Miller, Jason Sangster, Kabir Heimsath, Maria Luisa Nodari, Ruth and Flaviu Huber, Ursula Rechberg, Dawn Collins, and Mingji Cuomo in Lhasa; Thomas Aebi, Leo Näscher, Lobsang, Jake, Adrun, Mike, Sabriye and Paul, and Putri and Yulha in Shigatse; and Professor Thubten Phuntsog, Wang Liu, and Zhen Yan in Beijing. I would also like to acknowledge my hosts and teachers at Tibet University for providing me with a long-term visa and residence permit and for allowing me to progress as a student of the Tibetan language, while continuing to be a researcher. The fieldwork and visits since 2006 would not have been the same without the friendship and intermittent translation assistance of Peyang, whom I admire for her strength of character and for inspiring hope when hope seems impossible.

Over the past decade I have been blessed to meet and work with a remarkable group of colleagues and friends who share a passion for and deep commitment to the study of Tibetan medicine in the contemporary world: Vincanne Adams, Calum Blaikie, Alessandro Boesi, Sienna R. Craig, Frances Garrett, Barbara Gerke, Denise Glover, Janet Gyatso, Stephan Kloos, Alex McKay, Colin Millard, Nianggajia, Audrey Prost, Geoffrey Samuel, Mona Schrempf, Katharina Sabernig, Martin Saxer, Herbert Schwabl, Tawni Tidwell, Stacey Van Vleet and Ronit Yoeli-Tlalim, among others. I have also benefited greatly from colleagues working in social anthropology and modern history of the greater Himalayan and Tibetan region, and here my thanks go in particular to Robbie Barnett, Hildegard Diemberger, Françoise Robin, Isabelle Henrion-Dourcy, Ken Bauer, Mark Turin, and Sara Shneiderman. Hildegard Diemberger, Guntram Hazod, Andre Gingrich, Ernst Steinkellner, and Charles Ramble were early supporters, and I am especially grateful for their guidance with my first research and language efforts in the region. Many people along the way have helped me sharpen my argument and clarify the presentation of materials. I specifically thank Sienna Craig, Barbara Gerke, Sara Shneiderman, Alex McKay, Heidi Fjeld, Dikke Lindskog, Michael Stanley-Baker, Shigehisa Kuriyama, and Martin Saxer for taking the time for discussion, comments, and in some cases corrections and help with the content, shape, and structure of the book, and to Ann Jones for all her support of my work. Though any inaccuracies and shortcomings are all my own, this book owes a great deal to my colleagues. I am also grateful to those colleagues who have been working in NGOs in Tibet, foremost the Swiss Red Cross and its international collaboration department for giving me access to internal reports and encouraging exchange and research with the beneficiaries of their programs in Tsang.

At University College London, I was extremely fortunate to work under the able guidance of Vivienne Lo, with assistance from Hildegard Diemberger from Cambridge. In London I benefited from Tibetan language training at SOAS, thanks to Ulrich Pagel. Feedback and encouragement by Geoffrey Samuel and Guy Attewell were crucial in my early thinking about this book. At the University of Oslo (UiO), Heidi Fjeld has been most helpful and resourceful, helping to shape the book and my life in manifold ways. Other colleagues, friends, and students associated with Oslo's Tibet-Norway Network of University Collaboration also opened spaces for discussing Tibetan issues and immediately made me feel at home. Special thanks go to Hanna Havnevik for all she has done to support the network and Tibetan studies in Oslo, and to Astrid Hovden, Per Kværne, and Inger Vasstveit for the wonderful company and friendship. I also benefited from working with the MA and PhD students from Tibetan universities based in Oslo during my stay. The practical course in Tibetan medicine that I took at the Milan New Yuthok Institute for Tibetan Medicine, taught by Dr Pasang Yonten Arya, clarified many practical aspects of this complex healing tradition. I am grateful for Dr. Pasang's lucid explanations and up-to-date interpretations of often obscure aspects of Tibetan medical writing, and to my colleagues on the course.

Virginia Woolf aptly said that a woman must have money and a room of her own if she is to write. Although meant for the writing of fiction, this surely also applies to the crafting of ethnography. I am very grateful for having gained the freedom and the time to write, through financial means, writing spaces, and the loving support of family and friends.

I am grateful to the Nansen Foundation for providing the small research grant that brought me to UiO in the first place, to the European Commission's Marie Curie-Skłodowska Fellowship (Grant 303139), held at UiO between 2012 and 2014, and the Wellcome Trust Research Fellowship (Grant 104523) held at the Universities of Oxford and Bristol. And what rooms of my own I had! Heartfelt thanks to my hosts and colleagues at the Section for Medical Anthropology and Medical History at UiO's Institute of Health and Society and especially to the Risdal Otnes family and Heidi for letting me use their "little red cabin" in Skåbu for extended stints of writing in the spring, summer, and autumn of 2014 and to Ingeborg Magerøy and family for lending their beloved Mossero cabin, also in Skåbu, to a "perfectly strange Austrian" in the summer of 2015.

As for the family members and friends who sustained me through the research and writing, thanks go to my parents, Maria and Winfried Hofer; my guardian spirit Jutta; the incredible Ingrid, Adelheid, and Rotraud; my sister Mechthild, Konrad, and the girls; my brother Meinrad, as well as Esther and their Sander boy; Lucy Powell; the Rapela clan, including Mechu, Jonas and Fausto, and Mariana and Manuel; Heidi, Dikke, and their families; Richard Barnett; the extended Vidnes family in Oslo; Hilary and

Jon; Edward, Sarah, and the girls; and most of all to Thea Vidnes and our own girls.

I am also very grateful to Lorri Hagman, executive editor at the University of Washington Press, for her sustained interest in this book and our long-term collaboration, which has been so enjoyable. Studies on Ethnic Groups in China series editor Stevan Harrell has been a great developmental editor, and I am grateful for all the critical feedback and comments he provided upon first and subsequent readings, and for his foreword. I am also thankful to the external reviewers of the manuscript for this book, for their tremendous input and constructive feedback. Thanks also to copyeditor Elizabeth Berg, to designer Katrina Noble, and to my brother Meinrad Hofer, for allowing me to use his images and for finalizing the maps.

NOTE ON TERMINOLOGY AND ROMANIZATION

This book uses a system of romanization for Tibetan names and terms that largely follows the Tibetan and Himalayan Library's Simplified Phonetic Transcription of Standard Tibetan devised by David Germano and Nicolas Tounadre.[1] Exceptions to following this system are words already commonly used internationally, such as Sowa Rigpa (not Sowa Rikpa) for *Gso ba rig pa* (Science of Healing) and Shigatse (not Zhikatsé) for Gzhis ka rtse (the capital of Shigatse Prefecture). For specialists, I provide exact transliterations of Tibetan terms in the glossary, following Wylie (1959). For Tibetan-authored works, I romanize the author's name in the text and the notes, and list their works in the bibliography, where I provide the authors' name and the details of the Tibetan reference in full using Wylie's system, so that specialists can track down these works. Tibetan and Chinese book titles are provided in English translation in the text, with the exception of the main Tibetan medical text, *Four Treatises*, which I also refer to as the *Gyüshi*. I tend not to translate Tibetan names for illnesses, as this would entail a loss of their "semantic network" (Good 1977) and would inaccurately render their meaning in specific contexts through lexical English or biomedical equivalents. I also do not translate Tibetan names of medicines and medical ingredients, as European-derived identification and classification of individual Tibetan materia medica is largely unsatisfactory.

Tibetan does not mark plural and singular in the spelling of nouns. I therefore indicate the English plural at the end of Tibetan terms with an unitalicized "s" or, where appropriate, no plural ending at all, such as *amchi*s or *amchi* for doctors. Again, exceptions are commonly used Tibetan terms, such as thankas and lamas, which are anglicized and thus not italic. I capitalize Sowa Rigpa and similar proper nouns, such as Ayurveda. Chinese terms are provided in pinyin, the official People's Republic of China (PRC) mode of transliteration. All prices are given in Chinese Yuan Renminbi (CNY). At the time of research, ¥10 was worth approximately US$1.3. Terms are Tibetan unless indicated otherwise for Chinese (C) or Sanskrit (Skt).

Tibet has had shifting and often disputed political, geographical, ethnographic, and linguistic definitions. I use *central Tibet* to refer to regions of Ü (the Lhasa area) and Tsang (western central Tibet), and *western Tibet* (mainly Ngari) and *eastern Tibet* to refer to the regions of Amdo and Kham. *Tibet* includes all the areas inside the borders of China where Tibetans are a substantial portion of the population, such as in various Tibetan autonomous prefectures and counties in the Tibet Autonomous Region (TAR) and neighboring Qinghai, Sichuan, Gansu, and Yunnan Provinces. This is mainly for simplicity's sake and accords with most of my Tibetan interlocutors' understanding of what and who is a part of "Tibet" and how this contrasts with what in their view is "China." When Tibetans speak about the non-Tibetan areas of China, they use the term Gyanag (Tib. "China"). However, when speaking or writing Chinese, the term *neidi* (C. "interior") is also commonly used among Tibetans, in many publications translated as "mainland China." I use "China proper" or the "interior" as translation for *neidi*, but "China" for the Tibetan Gyanag. The Tibet Autonomous Region is the current name for a part of Tibet that was under the control and administration of the Lhasa government, at least between 1913 and 1951 (see map 1). Within it lies Tsang, the traditional term for a part of central Tibet that is now administered as Shigatse Prefecture—I use these interchangeably (see map 2). For counties (Tib. *dzong*; C. *xian*) I use "county." Under Communist administration, counties have been subdivided into districts, or *xiang*, and I translate these as "townships."

ABBREVIATIONS

CCP	Chinese Communist Party
CMS	Cooperative Medical Services
GMP	Good Manufacturing Practices
NCMS	New Cooperative Medical Services
PRC	People's Republic of China
SEM	Socialist Education Movement
SRC	Swiss Red Cross
TAR	Tibet Autonomous Region
TASS	Tibetan Academy of Social Sciences
TCM	Traditional Chinese Medicine
TDF	Tibet Development Fund
TTM	Traditional Tibetan Medicine

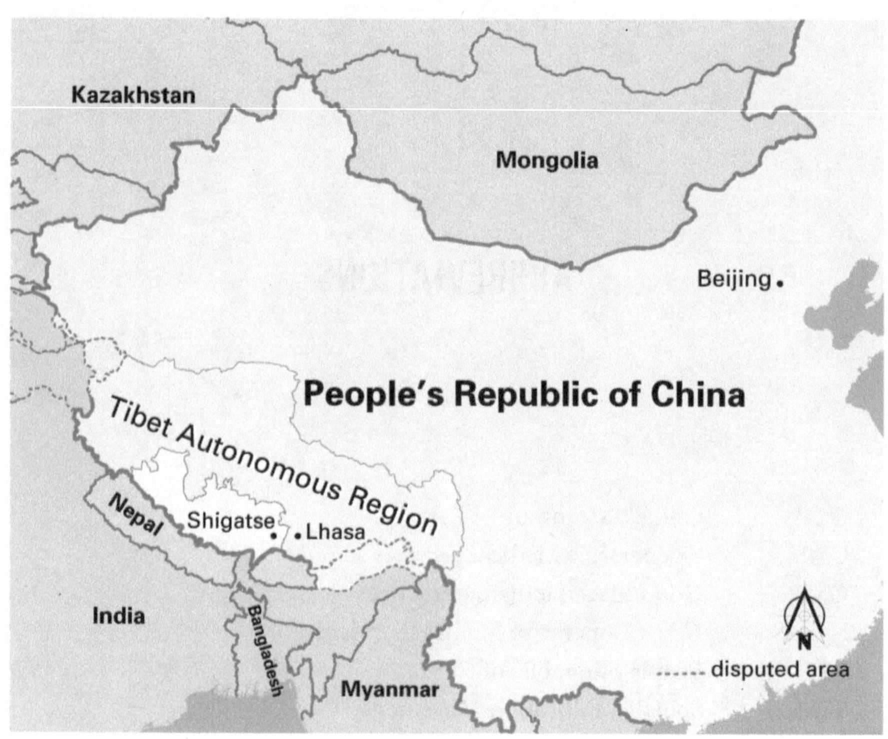

MAP 1. The Tibet Autonomous Region (TAR) within the People's Republic of China. Lhasa is the TAR's regional capital and Shigatse the second-largest town.

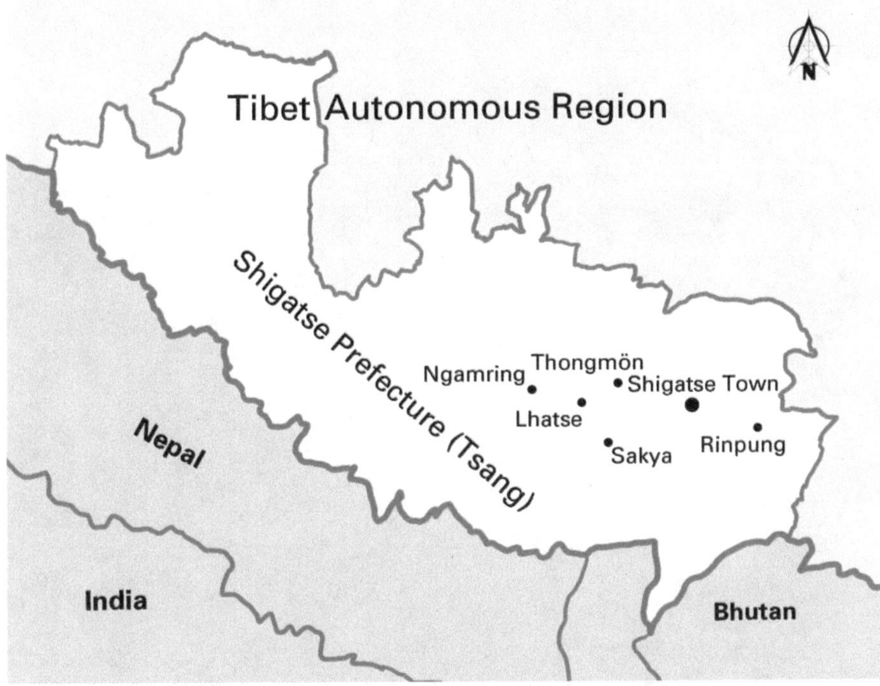

MAP 2. The locations of Shigatse Town and Ngamring, Lhatse, Rinpung, Sakya, and Thongmön Counties within Shigatse Prefecture (TAR), where the fieldwork for this book took place.

INTRODUCTION

UNDER a clear autumn sky, Amchi Yonten Tsering and I were chatting in his Shigatse courtyard in the morning sun when the first patient of the day knocked on the front door. An elderly monk was let inside, accompanied by a younger colleague. We exchanged a few words and found out they were from nearby Tashilhunpo Monastery, the seat of the reincarnated line of the Panchen Lama and today the home to some four hundred monks. The sixty-seven-year-old doctor Yonten Tsering suggested going inside the house to "look at illness" (*natsa taya*), his way of referring to a medical consultation.

"What ails you?" he asked the monk, by then seated in the family living room.

"My heart [*nying*]. I am told I have high blood pressure [*trakshé tobo*]."

The doctor reached for his manual sphygmomanometer to take the monk's blood pressure. He noted the result in his case records before going on to feel the patient's pulse on both wrists with three fingers at the *tsön*, *ken*, and *chak* points, pressing differently over the radial arteries on each. This was one of my favorite moments in consultations: when practitioners seemingly disappeared into themselves and their patient, picking up subtle but sure signs from within the body that elude those untrained in their recognition and interpretation. Yonten Tsering inspected the monk's eyes and tongue, then pressed on the crown of his head, a location used to test for pains related to the wind *nyépa* (or force) in the body. Yonten Tsering interpreted the monk's evident discomfort at this as a critical sign of the underlying condition. After a few more questions, the resultant diagnosis voiced to the patient was *lungné*, a "wind disorder." "But," the doctor assured him, "it is not too bad, and the medicines will help you." He instructed the monk to continue with the Tibetan medicines he was already taking, adding to those three from the *amchi*'s own stock. These, he explained, should be taken for forty-five days and be complemented with the external therapy of *hormen*. The latter consisted of a small cotton bag containing partially crushed nutmeg, caraway seeds, and roasted barley flour (*tsampa*), which was to be applied on certain points on the body. Yonten Tsering gave homemade samples to the younger monk, instructing him to make more and warm the *hormen* bags in hot oil or butter, then massage and press them onto several points on the body of the elderly monk every evening: one on the top vertebrae of his back, one on the sternum, and two others on the head. Seamlessly, the medical encounter then shifted into convivial conversation over cups of tea that Yonten Tsering's wife, Yeshe Lhamo, had served us. A bit over half an hour after they had first arrived, the monks left without any money having changed hands. Then I turned to Yonten Tsering with my questions.

KEY QUESTIONS AND TOPICS

This book offers the first full-length ethnography of Tibetan medical practitioners in central Tibet working outside the well-documented Tibetan medical institutions in Lhasa, including the Mentsikhang, Tibetan Medical College, and TAR Tibetan Pharmaceutical Factory. I recount and analyze their medical work and personal trajectory over the past decades, taking readers to the various places where Tibetan medical doctors, also known as *amchi*,[1] like Yonten Tsering, lived and worked, mainly in rural settings in Tsang and in Shigatse Town. The region of Tsang, which comprises much of western and central Tibet, was administered prior to the 1950s by the Tashilhunpo Labrang, the seat of the Panchen Lama in Shigatse Town. Together with Ü, or the "center" (i.e., the eastern parts of central Tibet), Ü-Tsang had been ruled by the Dalai Lamas since the mid-seventeenth century and enjoyed de facto independence from 1913 to 1951.[2] After the occupation of central Tibet by the People's Republic of China in 1951 and upon the formation of the Tibet Autonomous Region (TAR) in 1965, Tsang became a part of this province and the TAR one of five provinces of the People's Republic of China (PRC) with major Tibetan populations. While Tsang has remained an important political and geographical unit in central Tibet, it is now administered under Shigatse Prefecture, still with Shigatse Town as its capital but with most political matters decided in Lhasa or Beijing (see map 1).

Tibetan medicine as practiced by local doctors in Tsang has been both interconnected with and separate from Tibetan medicine as portrayed in official textbooks and previous anthropological work. This study departs in four major ways from extant ethnographies and available scholarship on the twentieth-century history of Tibetan medicine.

First, it offers accounts of *amchi* who were not part of the Tibetan state-supported medical structures that were incorporated during the 1950s into the new PRC socialist health care system, even if some of them later joined it. It specifically inquires into these practitioners' experiences and negotiation of socioeconomic and medical reforms. This allows the reader to trace events and narratives of the Communist socioeconomic reforms from a substantially different perspective: that of people who by choice or by force remained outside the official health care system as they worked on the margins (geographical and otherwise) of the Tibetan and, subsequently, the PRC state. So far, for reasons of difficult research access and the power of state institutions in the writing and representation of history, these perspectives have been absent from most local, national, or foreign accounts.

Second, it draws on the evolving literature addressing memory and oral history in socialist and postsocialist contexts as well as some of the wider literature theorizing the intersections of anthropology and history, and of current lived realities and their recent, often violent, past. The book analyzes marginal *amchi*s' accounts not only in terms of the opportunity they offer to expand and question the central institutional and nationalist accounts, but also to actively and critically inquire into the social and political dynamics and processes that influence and determine all memory and history.

Third, by consistently addressing gender, I tackle the lack of understanding of gender in Tibetan medicine in the period under discussion. This volume offers analytical tools that allow inclusion of more women in the study of Tibetan medicine and comparison of their lives and work with those of men, fostering a more nuanced appreciation of how the reforms impacted men and women in different ways. It thus speaks to a different subaltern history of Tibetan experience.

Fourth, this work demonstrates how *amchi*s outside the major state-sponsored institutions have continued to contribute in significant ways to the survival and continued transformation of Tibetan medicine into the present day. Through their negotiation of and agency within the often harsh and violent reforms and a delicate maneuver within the new regime, Tibetan medicine began to be revitalized in the early 1970s. Some aspects of classical literature were republished and swiftly refashioned to serve the needs of the state as well as the *amchi*s' patients. This transformation took place much earlier than in other domains of Tibetan culture and made Tibetan medicine an important health care resource for Tibetans throughout the 1980s and 1990s, and one of the strongholds of Tibetan culture, language, and local economy in contemporary China.

BASIC ELEMENTS OF TIBETAN MEDICINE

Tibetan medicine is not a continuous, unchanging entity, either in terms of who practices it or in the way it is theorized and applied. There is, however, a set of core principles and practices that have weathered the storms of historical change and the continuous adaptation of Tibetan medicine. Some of these principles were still drawn on and variously interpreted by the people I worked with in Tsang.

Many of the theoretical and empirical principles of Sowa Rigpa—Tibetan for science or art of healing[3]—are founded upon Buddhist philosophy translated into a theory that understands the human body, mind, and spirit as a continuous interaction between macrocosm and microcosm. This takes place mainly through the interplay of the "five elements," or *jungwa nga*, and most significantly, the *nyépa sum*. The *nyépa sum* are *lung* or wind, *tripa* or bile, and *béken* or phlegm. In Tibetan, *nyépa*, much like the Indian *doṣa* (Maas 2007/8), literally means "fault." However, a common translation has been "humor" (Gyatso 2005/6),[4] which is problematic mainly because in Tibetan medical theory the *nyépa sum* are directly linked to the three poisons (*duksum*)—desire (related to wind), anger (related to bile), and ignorance (related to phlegm)—which form the core of Buddhist philosophy and morality and in Sanskrit are referred to as *kleśa*. Taking this together with a broader idea of the *nyépa* in Tibetan medicine, and to preserve the multivalent meaning of the Tibetan term, I use the Tibetan term here, or the "three forces."

The five elements—earth (*sa*), water (*chu*), fire (*mé*), air/wind (*lung*), and space (*namkha*)—form the basis of the three *nyépa*, air and space forming *lung*, fire forming *tripa*, and earth and water forming *béken*. Similar to the five agents or five phases of Chinese medicine (which include wood and metal instead of air and space), the five elements are cosmophysical elements in constant flux, immanent in the universe and fundamentally of the same nature inside and outside of the body. In Sowa Rigpa theory, health of the body/mind/spirit and human physiology is described as a state of balance among the five elements and hence the *nyépa*. If such balance is lost and a person falls ill, the *amchi* makes a diagnosis using the three principal diagnostic methods of *ta rek dri*. The first of these is a visual examination of the patient—in particular, the inspection of urine and the tongue, as well as general observation of body shape and color. The second is the palpation of the pulse, and the third is the questioning of the patient (Meyer 1995: 132–35).

Although all illness is ultimately attributed to imbalance of the *nyépa* (in essence the five elements), this does not prevent *amchi* from having a sophisticated understanding of human anatomy, physiology, and various kinds of channels (Garrett and Adams 2008; Meyer 1995; Parfionovich, Dorje, and Meyer 1992), as well as names for hundreds of specific disorders. *Amchi* deal with such discrete afflictions as wounds, swellings, or demonic attacks, as well as diseases related more directly to all three, two, or one of the *nyépa sum*. Treatments in Sowa Rigpa vary and may include behavioral and dietary change, the use of medicines in the form of powders and pills, or external treatments such as massage, bloodletting, and moxibustion. Ritual, prayer, the ingestion of blessed pills, the burning of incense, and the wearing of amulets are also potential therapeutic resources, and Tibetans, like most other human beings, arrange their lives in light of broader cosmological and philosophical considerations.

The *Four Treatises* is the core text of Tibetan medicine, thought by many Tibetan doctors to have been taught by the Medicine Buddha (Sangyé Menla; see figures I.1 and I.2). There has been much debate on the authorship of this work, which dates to the twelfth century (Yang Ga 2014) and

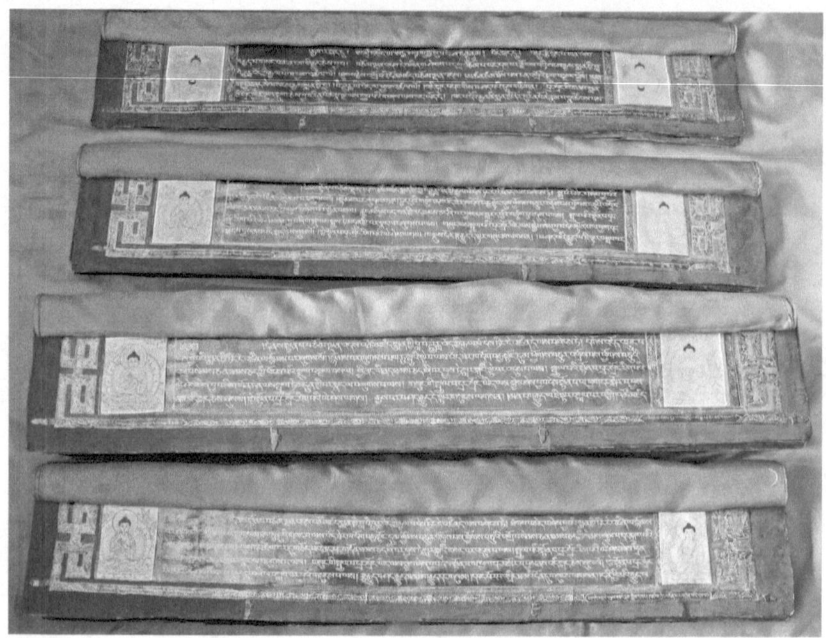

FIGURE I.1. An ornamental copy of the *Four Treatises* held at the Lhasa Mentsikhang, 2006. Photo by the author.

contains fundamental theories of medicine, descriptions of practical application, and instructions on ethics for practitioners. It takes the form of a series of questions and answers between the sages Yilekyé and Rikpé Yeshé—a format similar to other classics of Asian medicine. Its divisions, the *Root Treatise* (*Tsagyü*), the *Explanatory Treatise* (*Shégyü*), the *Oral Instruction Treatise* (*Menngakgyü*), and the *Last Treatise* (*Chimagyü*), are all still studied by medical students today and memorized to varying degrees, usually with the least emphasis on the *Oral Instruction Treatise*, which is the largest of the four volumes. From the fourteenth century onward a number of commentaries have been written on the *Four Treatises*, most often referred to as *drelpa*.[5] In the seventeenth century a set of medical paintings or thankas (*thang kha*) were created under the auspices of Desi Sangyé Gyatso, which provide a visual illustration of much of Sowa Rigpa theory and practice.[6] Many influences from outside Tibet have at various stages been incorporated into the repertoire of Tibetan medicine, and practitioners continue to use the *Four Treatises* and its commentaries as well as new methods.

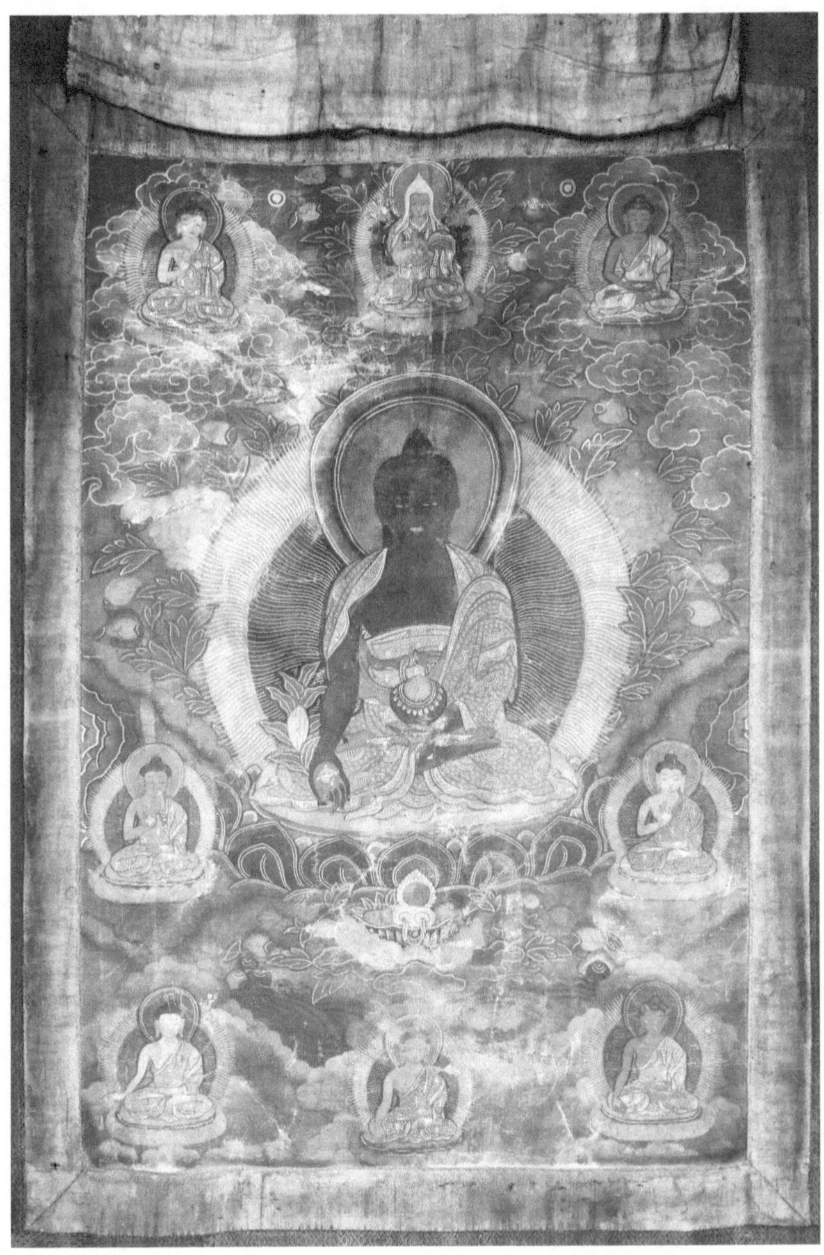

FIGURE I.2. Medicine Buddha thanka in a monastery in Ngamring, 2007. Photo by Meinrad Hofer.

TRANSFORMATIONS OF TIBETAN MEDICINE

There is little doubt that the way Tibetan medicine is practiced in contemporary Tibet has been greatly affected by the various reforms that followed the occupation and integration of Tibet into the People's Republic of China. How these transformations have been depicted and represented, we can state with certainty, has been influenced, like the broader historiography of modern Tibet, by the agendas of the opposing governments of Tibet: that of Tibet proper (within the People's Republic of China) on the one hand and Tibet in Exile (the Government in Exile based in Dharamsala) on the other. Their stances, as befits their political interests, are usually on opposite ends of the spectrum. The key players in the writing of Tibetan medical histories since the 1950s have included Chinese scholars and current and former Tibetan staff of the two foremost institutions of Tibetan medicine: the Lhasa Mentsikhang inside Tibet and this institution's exile manifestation, the Men-Tsee-Khang, established in 1961 in Dharamsala (Hofer 2011d: 101–37).[7] Their accounts have also played a key role in the dominant academic narrative on Tibetan medicine in this period.

Pioneering work by the anthropologist Craig Janes (1995) has been crucial for understanding major events in the twentieth-century history of Tibetan medicine inside what is now the People's Republic of China. It is focused mainly on the central Tibetan region of Ü-Tsang, the area that we consider here, by contrast to the eastern Tibetan regions of Kham and Amdo. Based on political histories, interviews with TAR officials and senior doctors at the Lhasa Mentsikhang and one of its branch hospitals, as well as extensive fieldwork, Janes analyzed the history of Tibetan medicine in the twentieth century according to five broad historical periods (1995: 12–22).

Between 1913 and 1951, during the de facto independence of central Tibet (including Ü, Tsang, and Ngari, all more or less firmly under the control of the Lhasa government), professional, elite Tibetan medical practice expanded through the establishment and teaching activities of the Mentsikhang, the Institute of Medicine and Astrology in Lhasa, founded in 1916. In contrast to the monastic medical college in Lhasa, the Chakpori (established in 1696), the Mentsikhang's mission was to recruit students not only from among the monks but also from the lay aristocracy and the Tibetan army. In the 1920s, thanks to support from the then head of the ecclesiastical branch of the government, physician Jampa Tupwang, and the Thirteenth Dalai Lama as head of the Tibetan Ganden Phodrang government, this institute spearheaded reforms such as a child health campaign based on indigenous medical and astrological ideas and practices. In this period, privately trained and practicing lineage physicians, who according to Janes were associated with the secular aristocracy in Tibet, provided treatment in villages and pastoral communities. Other professionals practiced medicine as a sideline and gained from it a small income.

The decade from 1950 to 1959 was the only one in which Tibetan and Chinese Communist governing structures coexisted in Lhasa, and Janes describes this as a phase of "consolidation" of Tibetan medicine. Due to the "united front" policy of the time—a Communist strategy to win over Tibetan and other ethnic minorities' elites and make them favorably inclined toward socialism, communism, and PRC nation building—Mentsikhang staff encountered a certain respect from incoming Chinese cadres, who through their engagement with the Mentsikhang aimed to show support for the health care offered there as well as demonstrate the new regime's respect for the Tibetan nationality (C. *minzu*). The ethnic identification project was in full swing at that time, and large cohorts of ethnologists and cadres had been employed to define ethnic groups in China, so that they could be successfully integrated and controlled as part of the PRC.[8]

The period from 1959 to 1966 was, according to Janes, "a time of cautious growth," even though the second most important medical institute in Lhasa, Chakpori, was destroyed in 1959 and many of the government-employed doctors imprisoned. After a decisive meeting in 1961, the Mentsikhang gained full-scale financial and logistical support from the Communist authorities in Lhasa. Under the leadership of Jampa Trinlé, who as an early Tibetan CCP member was well versed in working the new system, the institution diversified the outpatient care it had already begun to streamline in the 1950s. The institution was now organized into several departments and in 1963 began to train students again, which had been its core mission up to 1959. Mentsikhang staff were sent out to provide medical care in rural areas surrounding Lhasa. However, at the height of the Socialist Education Movement (SEM, 1963–66), teachers were less respected and students and teachers were "sent down" to the countryside (C. *xia xiang*), to engage in farm labor alongside the masses.

China's Great Proletarian Cultural Revolution (1966–76) included a nationwide purge of so-called counterrevolutionaries, who were thought to infect the literary, artistic, and scholarly elites in particular. Along with other established cultural and scientific institutions, the Mentsikhang was attacked by Red Guards, its scholars and staff dispersed and struggled against. All students and most staff from the Mentsikhang were ordered to rural areas to work on the land. Meanwhile, much of the institution's library and many Buddhist statues and paintings were destroyed by Red Guards, as well as almost all remaining Tibetan medical doctors' homes and monasteries. According to Janes, "By 1973 Tibetan medicine as an institution had virtually disappeared" but at the same time began to be recognized for its potential to provide health care in rural areas.

Janes characterizes the period after 1980 as one of Tibetan medicine's "legitimization and expansion," as, following Mao's death in 1976, Deng Xiaoping ushered in nationwide open-door policies, which in due time led to a relaxation of central government attitudes toward traditional culture and religion. Doctors who had been "sent down to the countryside" in the previous decade were invited to work in the official healthcare system. Some were retrained due to poor standards of medical education in the earlier decade, and the teaching of new cohorts of students began. Some severely punished doctors were officially rehabilitated. These developments were accompanied by increased (and ongoing) infrastructural investments in the hospital, college, and pharmaceutical factory of the Mentsikhang.

After the publication of Janes's article in 1995, his works have included more recent developments, such as the start of the privatization and commodification of Tibetan medicine as economic liberalization initiatives from the mid-1990s gained momentum (Janes 1999a, 2002; discussed in chapters 5 and 6).

Janes's original article provided a rough outline of developments that shaped Tibetan medicine mainly at the Lhasa Mentsikhang, the central Tibetan medical institution in Tibet, in the context of developments in modern China. The article served as a historical introduction to his analysis of Tibetan medicine's contemporary role in health care for Tibetans at that institute and its branch in Tsethang, near Lhasa. Nevertheless, researchers of Tibetan medicine consider it a key reference, not only for how Tibetan medicine fared at the Lhasa Mentsikhang but, by extrapolation, for Tibetan medicine's overall trajectory under socialist reforms in central Tibet and other Tibetan areas of the PRC. While the Mentsikhang was undergoing these changes, more complex things were happening among Tibetan medical practitioners in places where the influence of the central Tibetan medical institutions was limited.

Little is known about how Tibetan medicine practitioners outside the government-backed institute fared during the implementation of reforms and how their role contrasted with that of practitioners of Chinese medicine in the rural PRC. Even in accounts that deal specifically with noninstitutional *amchi*, there is little in-depth information.[9] Memories of the past and current work of a small group of *amchi* studying and working outside the central Tibetan and later Chinese-funded government institutions in Lhasa form the subject matter of this book. Together, these *amchis*' memories and practices demonstrate how the historiography of Tibetan medicine since the 1950s has been hijacked by the central institutions of Tibetan medicine and state-appointed writers.

My approach takes inspiration from the subaltern studies movement, which since the 1980s has stimulated new approaches in the social sciences and humanities. It prioritizes perspectives from nonelite groups and aims to "rescue" history from the "nation," which typically produces singular narratives from a position of centralized, often colonial, power and hegemony.[10] This text thus also remedies somewhat the stark absence of subaltern scholarship in Tibetan studies (P. Hansen 2003), as much as it adds to recently emerging work on the diverse and often uneasy relation of marginal areas and people in the Chinese Tibetosphere with its various centers of political, religious, or sociocultural power and influence.[11]

MARGINS AND CENTERS OF TIBETAN MEDICINE

The three generations of *amchi* from Tsang represented here were born between the 1930s and the 1990s. Some of them are now in their eighties, others in their midtwenties, and some of my elderly interlocutors have passed away since completion of this research. Despite their internal differences and the ways their practices have changed over time, they share one characteristic: they have all been marginally involved with or influenced in their work by the "center." The center here is primarily defined as the Mentsikhang in Lhasa, the foremost central Tibetan medical institution of the first half of the twentieth century. Since the Mentsikhang was part of the secular branch of the Tibetan government, it was integrated into the new PRC bureaucracy but never completely shut down, even during the harshest reforms. After the 1980s it expanded into three branches concerned with training Tibetan doctors (the Tibetan Medical College), doing clinical work (the Mentsikhang out- and inpatient wards), and producing Tibetan medicines (the TAR Tibetan Pharmaceutical Factory). For a century this institution has shaped practitioners' training, as well as clinical and pharmaceutical standards, and in the PRC it is often seen as Tibetan medicine's traditional flagship institute. It has attracted considerable attention from anthropologists focusing on medical work at the outpatient department (Janes 1995, 1999a, 1999b, 2002), the women's department (Adams 2000), so-called integrated medicine (Adams and Li 2008), the first double-blind clinical control trial of a Tibetan drug (Craig 2012, 2013), and medicine production (Saxer 2013; Adams and Craig 2008).

Mentsikhang and Tibetan Medical College teachers and professors have written authoritative histories of their institutions and biographies of famous doctors, often associated with these establishments (Trinlé 2000, 2006). They have also produced textbooks on which college students are examined, which report mainly on the history of the Mentsikhang and are highly inflected by political rhetoric (e.g., Trinlé 2004).

In contrast to such practitioners, the *amchi* described here were trained either in their own families, at a nearby monastery or nunnery, or by an itinerant teacher. With few exceptions, they have not trained or worked in Lhasa.

Since any government policy, either of the Tibetan or the PRC government, is first implemented at the Mentsikhang in Lhasa, the institution can be seen as a barometer of legitimacy for the kinds of practices and ideas that either of the two governments saw as worthwhile to their respective political projects. Since practitioners on the margins fell largely outside the sphere of influence of the Mentsikhang, they were outside the direct control of the Mentsikhang or any other central organ of the state through the 1950s. They came under the orbit of the PRC state only during the period of intensified reforms that began in the 1960s, when the center and central politics and policies became more influential than ever. At that time, for the *amchi* I worked with, the center was no longer a vague, distant entity, with a few tax collectors and administrators making their appearance. It began to enter the most private affairs of the home and the Medical House, and the everyday routines and organization of monasteries and nunneries. At first the new authorities showed little concern over Tibetan medical practice per se but much concern over the *amchi* practitioners' class status. They also worried that Tibetan medicine was tied to religion, in Marxist parlance an opiate that dulled people's perception of their exploitation. And yet, at least partly, it was seen as scientific, and hence selected practitioners were allowed to work with Sowa Rigpa.

Despite the differences in social status, government involvement, and the physical and geographical terrain in which medical work took place, margins and centers are not conceived of here as neatly bounded and oppositional spheres of practice or historical trajectories. Rather, this larger framework is a tool for exploring the dynamics of medicosocial practice on the margins, how norms and shifting legitimacy and authority from the center were conveyed to and negotiated there, and whether and how they differed. These margins have at times influenced medical practice at the center.

Margins and centers of Tibetan medicine in the 1940s and 1950s in central Tibet prior to the reforms can be considered in terms of a "galactic polity," a framework developed for South Asian states by the anthropologist Stanley Tambiah (1976, 1985), later adapted for the Tibetan context (Samuel 1993: 62). Anthropologist Geoffrey Samuel holds that Lhasa was an important political and also religious center in Ü-Tsang, yet several other major regional centers also existed, for instance Sakya and Shigatse, in the region traditionally known as Tsang. Shigatse was the base of the Tashilhunpo Labrang and Monastery and historically the home of the reincarnated line of the Panchen Lamas, second only to the Dalai Lamas, while Sakya was home to one of the schools of Tibetan Buddhism, as well as the seat of its political leaders.

Family medical practitioners and medical houses as well as monastically trained *amchi* in monasteries and nunneries in Tsang were often connected to and influenced by these regional monastic, medical, and political centers; the practitioners and institutes of the Mentsikhang and Chakpori in Lhasa were largely inconsequential to the way Tibetan medicine was practiced there. Most of my fieldwork was carried out in Ngamring County, supplemented by work in Shigatse Town and selected places in Lhatse, Rinpung, Sakya, and Thongmön Counties (see map 2).

There was also a great difference in the social roles and lived lives of *amchi* on the margins and at the center. While rural *amchi* were intimately embedded in the social order of Tibetan village life, Mentsikhang and Chakpori graduates often served government functions, for instance serving as personal physician to the Dalai Lama or other religious or political hierarchs, or working as lay doctors in the newly formed Tibetan army.

Central, regional, and dispersed sociopolitical, religious, and medical authorities were called into question when Communist reforms began in earnest in central Tibet and Tsang in 1959–60. During the in-between phase of the 1950s, when Tibetan and CCP governing structures existed side by side for some time, Beijing had arisen as a new and distant, yet ever more politically powerful, center for Tibet and Tibetans. The capital did not yet exert any major influence where most Tibetan *amchi* worked, in the Medical Houses, monasteries, and nunneries. Government medical teams from China proper were sent to Lhasa and larger towns in Tsang, but no formal medical infrastructure had been established. That began to change as biomedical clinics were built in county seats during the early 1960s. At the same time indigenous medical work was slowly delegitimized with the increasing socioeconomic reforms, class struggle, and finally direct attacks by the Red Guards.

The China-wide barefoot doctor campaign began to reach marginal areas in the early 1970s, and the influence of central state medical authority reached a new pervasiveness in rural Tibetan areas, a result of Mao's stress on rural areas in medical work and linking the barefoot doctors' work to the communal Cooperative Medical Services (CMS). Yet, in contrast to the policy in China, the barefoot doctors did not include Tibetan medical compounds or remedies on the system's own terms, but only advocated some Tibetan materia medica for use in Chinese medical remedies. From Mao's death in 1976 until the early 1990s, a slightly more advanced health care infrastructure was put in place, in which Tibetan medicine was officially relegitimized at the county and township levels but only as an adjunct to biomedical services. From 1994 onward, under TAR party secretary Chen Kuiyan, economic liberalization took hold in the TAR (Barnett 2003). At this point the state began to absolve itself of responsibility for the "health of the masses" on the margins. This trend and the increasing difficulties encountered by rural populations in affording health care have been only slightly curbed by the implementation of a new insurance scheme in 2003, the New Cooperative Medical Services (NCMS), which partially subsidizes state biomedical care but not Tibetan medicines. Various *amchi* have innovated to meet the challenges of providing rural primary health care, particularly the rising prices for Tibetan medicine in a competitive market-driven environment. Elderly doctors travel to remote villages on a regular basis to offer free health care, and the Tashilhunpo Medical Clinic continues to produce its own medicine to keep prices down, espousing a moral economy to meet the crisis of medicine. More recently, practitioners move within, across, and between centers and margins, reflecting major infrastructural developments that have taken place in rural Tsang and Tibetan areas more broadly (Yeh 2013; Fisher 2013).

MEMORY, ETHNOGRAPHY, HISTORICITY

Befitting their social positions and lives in often-remote villages in Tsang, *amchi*s and others remember the past quite differently from the way it is written in official historiography of Lhasa. The memories of Yonten Tsering, for example, are not written records but recollections and stories told in everyday life, shared with his patients, his students, and myself. I compare his recollections with those of other *amchi*, their families, and other members of the community, who—despite having a status in Tibet's pre-1959 society similar to that Yonten Tsering—were often less fortunate and experienced more pronounced violence and forced social transformations. How should we understand such differing accounts? And in what ways do the social and political realities surrounding these stories and memories influence them? Were they used strategically? How do they compare with official accounts?

Anthropologist Michel-Rolph Trouillot's ideas about history are useful for considering such contradictions. He posits that there are "two sides of historicity": the "sociohistorical process" and the "narrative construction about that process" (1995: 22–29). By focusing on the process and conditions of the production of narratives, we can uncover how the two sides of historicity overlap and thus discover the differential exercise of power that makes some narratives possible while silencing others (25). The Chinese saying that "history is written by the victors" sums up at least some of Trouillot's observations, and both optics are pertinent.

In *China's Tibetan Medicine*, Zhen Yan and Cai Jingfeng of the China Institute for History of Medicine, Beijing Academy of Chinese Medical Sciences, write:

> In 1951, Tibet was liberated peacefully. Since then, the history of Tibetan medicine has written a new chapter. Although there was a glorious past in the ancient period with marvelous achievements, in a society based on feudal-slavery as was Tibet, all the attainments in science and technology, including medical science, were the property of the ruling class, who were also the beneficiaries, while the poor had no access to the medical arts.
>
> After 1951, conditions changed a lot. Radical changes occurred in Tibetan medicine, whose goal became to serve the vast masses. The old medical institutions underwent thorough change.
>
> As an integral part of Chinese medical treasures, Tibetan medicine was well inherited and developed. (2005: 33–34).

Jampa Trinlé, longtime director of the Mentsikhang in Lhasa, writes in a college textbook for Tibetan medical students widely available in Lhasa bookshops:

> In the Iron Rabbit year, 1951, Tibet was peacefully liberated. Particularly, since the 3rd session of the 11th local assembly, Communists and all representatives in government respectfully recognized the Tibetan medical science as a very important shiny jewel of the medical treasure house of China [*mes rgyal*]. In order to continue the practice, to explore, to collect and to develop the traditional Tibetan medical science, the representatives drafted a series of resolutions on the system of Tibetan medical science and approved it as the way forward for all related activities. (Trinlé 2004: 133)

In contrast to these writings from within the PRC, Tibetans in exile describe the phase after the occupation of Tibet as a catastrophe for Sowa Rigpa institutions and medical practitioners. According to the foreword to a recent English translation of the *Four Treatises*,

> Tibetan medicine, as a whole, flourished in all aspects until the devastating Chinese invasion of Tibet in 1959 [*sic*]. After the Chinese annexation,

> Tibetan medicine and all other aspects of Tibetan culture and religion were immeasurably affected. The *Chagpori* Medical School in Lhasa was completely destroyed by the Chinese during the Tibetan uprising against Chinese domination in 1959. Vast quantities of medical literature were burned and practitioners of Tibetan medicine were tortured, imprisoned, and persecuted. Thousands of Tibetans, some of them physicians, followed His Holiness the Fourteenth Dalai Lama into exile in 1959. In exile, Tibetan medicine first spread in India and Nepal, and then gradually to the West. (Men-Tsee-Khang 2008: xiv)

These examples represent the vastly opposing political stances on Tibet taken by the PRC state and the exile government. Narratives from ordinary Tibetan medical doctors not only make our understanding of the history and practices of Tibetan medicine more complete but also demonstrate the political purpose of the official histories and, equally important, that of its numerous silences and acts of forgetting.

While state discourses, such as those reverberating in the writing of the late Jampa Trinlé or Chinese writers Zhen Yan and Cai Jingfeng, draw largely on the *episteme* of a Marxist evolutionary history, the memories of the doctors I worked with derive from *epistemes* that intimately connected to their everyday lives and their communities in Tsang. The latter are expressed in memories, going beyond the mere spoken word. Recent scholarship in anthropology that theorizes the intersection of ethnography with history, for example, is useful for broadening the kinds of links people make among pasts, presents, and futures (Hirsch and Steward 2005). Other relevant forms of the *amchis*' engagement with the past are visible in aspects of material and immaterial culture and through the embodiment of the past in medical practice, such as the doctors' "looking at illness" and the preparation of medicines.

Individual and collective memories expressed in conversations and interviews are revealing, such as the way one *amchi* from a high-class family repeatedly praised the CCP using stock phrases he had learned during the 1960s. He employed these phrases strategically to get projects approved and carried out successfully. This left me and others puzzled over whether such expressions of admiration were, as someone put it, from his "heart" or from his "mouth"—that is, whether they were deeply felt and meant or a necessity in the context of social or political pressure. Such narratives are interwoven and juxtaposed with several *amchis*' "oppositional practices of time," drawing on the concept first coined and developed by Eric Mueggler in the context of postreform social organization and ritual in a Lolop'o village (2001: 7).

Amchis construct and connect past and present by means of inherited books, instruments, and other aspects of their Medical Houses, including skills, knowledge, and authority that were often wholly or partially lost in the most extreme upheavals of the reforms. Memory practices are also evident in doctors' bodily techniques broadly conceived as the core of *amchi*'s medical work, namely "looking at illness" (including feeling the pulse) and making medicines. These skills span years, sometimes decades, of accumulated experience and continued "enskilment" (Ingold 2000, 2011) and thus form a direct connection among the past, present, and future work of *amchi*.

Through such memory practices, whether repetition of slogans from the Mao era, feeling pride and longing in respect to aspects of the time before occupation, as expressed in "oppositional practices of time," or ongoing attempts at revival and continuity, this work reveals discrepant temporalities and alternative accounts of events and lives that the party state cannot allow to be expressed, let alone included in official histories. These memory practices also show up the silences in state discourses on Tibetan medical development since 1951: the disappearance and destruction of doctors' and Tibetan medical institutes' material and immaterial belongings, the demolition of Medical Houses and the Lhasa Chakpori in 1959, the devastation of many private and monastic medical libraries, and not least the physical death and deprivation inflicted on physicians in the wake of the reforms.

AGENCY, THE CHINESE STATE, AND DYNAMIC MEDICAL TRADITIONS

An important question is the extent to which the state or individual practitioners have been responsible for the survival or transformation of this medical system during the most intense phase of reform, namely the Cultural Revolution and the period that followed. It is a question that has been addressed with regard to Chinese medicine's trajectory.

Based on CCP policy documents, historian Kim Taylor (2005) studied Chinese medicine's role in the Communist Revolution between 1945 and 1963. She suggests that Chinese medicine, or what subsequently became Traditional Chinese Medicine (TCM), was not as much a continuation of the past as a deliberate distillation of ancient concepts according to the dictates of the twentieth century and the PRC state. Mao's famous 1958 statement that "Chinese medicine and pharmaceuticals are a national treasure house" came from the period studied in Taylor's work. She traces official CCP policies designed to transform the unruly diversity of Chinese medical lore into simplistic sets of knowledge and practice. These could then be put to use in their reduced and practical form for the newly mobilized masses, especially in rural areas, as well as for promoting Communism. In the process, medicine was cleansed of scholarly interpretations and theories, links to religious and spiritual practices, and the lineage authority from bygone days. This model would later be globalized and readily applied to diverse cultural and social circumstances (for example, for East Africa, see Hsu 2008), while still being perceived as an "ancient" knowledge system.

In this picture of the heavy CCP involvement in the transformation of Chinese medicine and the making of TCM, one can see the "invention of tradition" at work, in which cultural and political practices of supposedly ancient origins are invented to lend legitimacy to current holders of power (Hobsbawm and Ranger 1983).

Volker Scheid, an anthropologist and practitioner of Chinese medicine, shows in a study of practitioners of the Menghe current of medicine in southeastern China (2007) how the CCP's construction of TCM was neither unitary nor entirely successful. Instead of eliminating lineage affiliations and sophisticated scholarship and practice, the CCP project opened up an alternative sphere for Chinese medicine. Here much (medical) power remained in the hands of doctors who had the lineage affiliations, associated medical techniques, and social networks. This might be read as an argument against the top-down, all-encompassing "invention" of TCM.

Such studies reveal a complex picture of state and individual practitioners' agency in the transformation of Chinese medicine during the high socialist period and the reform era after Mao's death in 1976. But for

Tibetan medicine, the current literature provides a less complex picture. There are highly politicized accounts and Lhasa-focused anthropological work, but work on Tibetan medicine during the Cultural Revolution is especially thin, represented in often short and contradictory notes. While Craig Janes holds that by 1973 Tibetan medicine as an institution had disappeared (1995: 20), Heather Stoddard notes that "medicine was the one domain of Tibetan traditional learning which was not completely interrupted by the Cultural Revolution" (1994: 141). Some of the more marginal *amchis* were able to negotiate rather than be wholly subjugated to radical state-led reforms. The CCP's creation of TCM and the spread of secularized Chinese medical techniques during the Cultural Revolution enabled Tibetan medicine to, in some cases, adopt revolutionary terminology and enable its practitioners to continue their work to a greater extent than other professions in Tibetan society. The core need for basic health care, especially in remote places with few alternatives other than reliance on the *amchis*, may also have contributed to the leniency.

This book also adds considerably to our current understanding of the actors involved in Tibetan medicine's revitalization and reemergence. Janes and Hilliard defined the Tibetan medical revival of the 1980s as a "restoration of the institutions of Tibetan medicine—the hospitals, clinics, and medicine factories—to their former integral position in Tibetan society" (2008: 35). They state that this accompanied a "'re-integrating' of Tibetan medicine into the public health and primary medical services." But when I expand the scope of inquiry to practitioners outside the institutions of Tibetan medicine, I find that the newly formed institutions of Tibetan medicine referred to by Janes and Hilliard were, in fact, only to a limited extent similar to institutions of Tibetan medicine found in the 1940s and 1950s, especially Medical Houses and monastic practices. The revitalization of Tibetan medicine, then, is far more than a top-down, state-led process pertaining to mainly government institutions; rather it is characterized by multiple agendas and actors with diverse projects.

GENDER

The intersection of gender with the political economy of Tibetan medicine in the 1950s and 1960s and through subsequent reforms is little understood. Only a handful of women working as doctors, such as Khandro

Yangga and Lobsang Dolma Khankhar, are known from academic works (Trinlé 2000; Tashi Tsering 2005), and they practiced at central medical or Buddhist institutions in Lhasa or later Dharamsala. Focusing on the Medical House enables a better analysis of the social and economic situation of *amchi* and gender in Tsang in relation to wider political economy, revealing the circumstances in which women and men inherited medical knowledge, how they fared, and how that differed according to gender, region, and economy. Through this case study, the effect of Communist social, economic, and political reforms can be appreciated in more depth.

THE RESEARCH

Officially approved, long-term anthropological fieldwork in rural areas of the TAR has so far been the privilege of few foreign researchers. Most have either had to make do with much shorter but repeated research visits or pursue longer stays through work in different capacities, often combining research with a role as student, English teacher, tourist, or business or NGO consultant.

"Officially Official"

My first fieldwork in rural Tsang took place in the summer of 2003. For this I had gained an official invitation and research visa from the Tibetan Academy of Social Sciences (TASS) in Lhasa, thanks to a research collaboration between that institution and the Austrian Academy of Sciences in Vienna, where I was affiliated. Together with a Tibetan co-researcher from TASS, I stayed for six weeks in Ngamring County (Ngamring Xian), both in the administrative center of Ngamring (also home to the largest monastery in the area, belonging to the Gelugpa school of Tibetan Buddhism) and in several townships (*xiang*) and villages in the southern, agricultural parts of the county. While there, I recorded twenty-one formal interviews, conducted in Tibetan, with healing specialists: sixteen *amchi*, two oracles, one tantric priest or *ngakpa* (who specialized in astrology and healing with mantras), and two biomedical doctors, as well as conversations with hospital and health bureau administrators at different levels. The interviews covered the practitioners' training, medical work, connections between Sowa Rigpa and Buddhism, the place of Tibetan medicine in governmental health care, the recently introduced NCMS insurance scheme, *amchis*' lineage affiliations, and the history of Sowa Rigpa in the area. I also conducted several interviews with elderly monks and others, focusing specifically on local history, and with patients concerning their financing and experience of government health care.[12] Owing to the official approval granted by TASS, as well as a letter from the local county administration (which explicitly allowed us to ask questions on "Tibetan culture, religion and medicine"), I also gained access—albeit limited—to statistics on medical treatments in the government facilities housed in the local Health Bureau. In addition, I was given unpublished and private documents, including handwritten histories of the People's Hospital and the Tibetan Medical Hospital in Ngamring. At the monasteries I obtained several local histories, some compiled by elders in the monastic community. Due to the relatively short period of time and visits to several sites, I felt more like an observer than a participant. That said, my official status as researcher and especially the approval of local officials gave me confidence to ask questions more openly, as well as to freely record interviews and generally feel secure in my role.

"Officially Unofficial"

My research experience during the second and longer fieldwork period, from September 2006 to August 2007, was rather different. My status then resembled that of an "officially unofficial" researcher and Tibetan language student, aptly described by Henrion-Dourcy (2013). Like her, I wanted to carry out long-term fieldwork in rural areas in Tsang and in the autumn of 2005 and spring 2006 had made several attempts to gain official permission through two Lhasa-based research institutions. But the necessary official invitations never materialized. The only other option known to me was to become a Tibetan language student at Tibet University, then see how far I could venture once enrolled.

The great advantage of being at Tibet University was clearly that I could improve my language skills and at the same time seek out knowledgeable doctors and scholars in Lhasa. Moreover, I could familiarize myself with official representations but also see what I could discover for myself of the recent history of Tibetan medical education, clinical practice, research, and pharmaceutical production. I studied works by the Mentsikhang's Jampa Trinlé (also discussing them with him), visited the various and growing Tibetan medicine museums in the city, and read Tibetan medical research papers and college textbooks. I often visited friends and acquaintances at the Mentsikhang, the TAR Tibetan Pharmaceutical Factory, and the Tibetan Medical College. The chance also arose to conduct biographical interviews in Lhasa as well as gain increasing familiarity with the classical Tibetan medical works that *amchi* frequently referred to.

I began to travel to Tsang on weekends, visiting established contacts and friends, and then extended my stays to the long holidays. This meant that my research in Tsang was scattered over the school term (October to early December, and March to June) but more sustained in the long holidays in between, bringing the total time spent in Shigatse and rural areas of Tsang to just over three months (see figure I.3). Given the usual restrictions and the need for travel permits for some places (specifically, the infamous Alien Travel Permit), this was a considerable achievement. Among earlier foreign researchers in rural Tsang, only Goldstein and Beall (1990) had been given permission for a twelve-month stay in Pala (northern Ngamring County), Fjeld (2006) for five months in an agricultural village in Panam, and Childs, Henrion-Dourcy (2017), and Diemberger (2007, 2010) for shorter repeated periods. Social science research undertaken by Tibetan researchers in the region is also scarce (e.g., Ben Jiao 2001). As a result, Tsang is a very understudied area of the TAR.

What traditionally had been referred to as Tsang was administered during the fieldwork as Shigatse Prefecture and divided into seventeen counties. The area is roughly equivalent in size to Washington state or Cambodia. Taking into account the region's enormous size and the constraints on research access, it is hardly surprising that Tsang is understudied, especially when it comes to contemporary life and recent historical developments.

In my application and upon arrival at Tibet University, I had informed its Foreign Affairs Department that I was conducting research on Tibetan medicine. This was never questioned further. It thus gave me the status of an "officially unofficial" researcher, in anthropologist Isabelle Henrion-Dourcy's terms, but, like her, I felt that it was "an ethically distressing choice" (2013: 208). Much less confident in my role than I had been during my 2003 stay, I was extremely vigilant and careful not to cause informants or translators trouble with the authorities. I spent considerable energy figuring out where the boundaries lay between safe and unsafe, and what this implied in terms of adjusting my conduct, my questions, and the

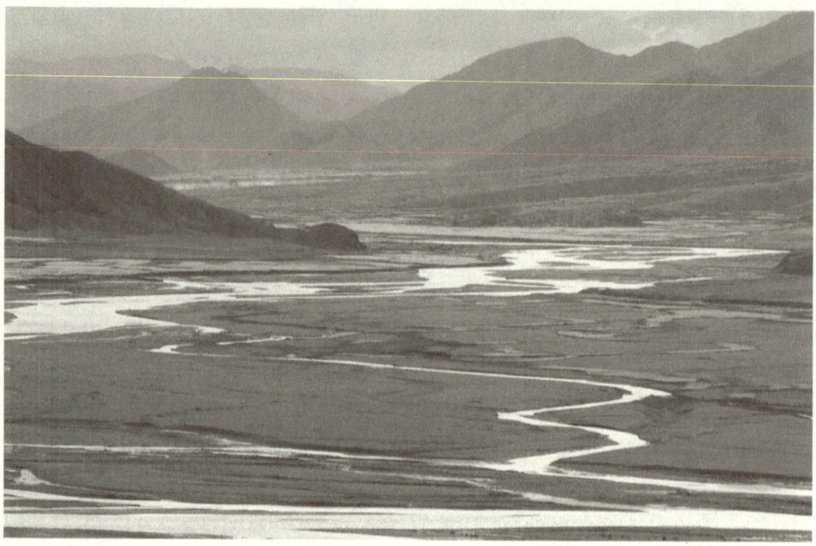

FIGURE I.3. Cultivated land in the summer in Ngamring, 2007. Photo by Meinrad Hofer.

visibility of my research as distinguished from my study of Tibetan language and medicine.

This was especially problematic when I was not with Yonten Tsering, one of my main interlocutors, who was originally from Ngamring, then resident in Shigatse, and of whose family I became a member. He always managed to smooth relations with officials and other Tibetans by following the party line, at least "from the mouth." His personal confidence and professional acumen, and the respect he commanded compensated at least in part for the great uncertainty I experienced. I felt to some extent protected by him. This perhaps explains why, despite his enervating praises of the CCP, Tibetans involved in medical and social projects seem particularly comfortable around him and seemingly empowered. This elderly doctor attributed to me the roles of medical student (*amchi loma*), researcher (*zhimjuk pa*), *amchi* (although I had at that point no medical training in this or any other medical tradition), family member (*acha*), and sponsor (*jindak*), depending on the context. When we were with his patients, he typically introduced me as a student from Tibet University in Lhasa, which carried high prestige, especially in rural areas. Or he introduced me as his medical student. In his family, I was called Acha—and or its honorific, Acha-la—which is used widely in Tsang for female relatives as well as acquaintances and close friends, in contrast to the Lhasa Tibetan dialect (where it means "older sister" or, with a different pronunciation, "wife"). I earned the title *sponsor* as a result of my fundraising efforts for some of Yonten Tsering's medical tours to the countryside and the reestablishment of a Tibetan medical clinic in the *amchi*'s childhood home.

Although I had explained to him that my work was that of an anthropologist, it was impractical for him to explain this to patients and officials, who would not know what the term meant. He preferred to describe me as a "student," *amchi*, or "medical student," which may allude to the difficult position of researchers in Tibet, and the PRC more broadly (M. Hansen 2006), perhaps colored by previous state-enforced research. Local officials are primarily concerned by potentially sensitive or political topics that will get them into trouble with superiors, and these are usually related to the political status of Tibet and the Dalai and Panchen Lamas. Such politically sensitive topics are, however, not clearly defined or openly articulated; rather they have to be figured out and one's behaviors constantly adjusted. This is part and parcel of what geographer Emily Yeh has called a "politics of fear" orchestrated by the Chinese state to control its citizens and researchers (2006: 97).

I also developed a close relationship with Ngawang Dorjé, whose whole family befriended me. They allowed me to participate in numerous ordinary aspects of family life in Lhasa and to independently hear accounts by several family members: his two children (one a biomedical health worker, the other a Tibetan medical pharmacist); Ngawang Dorjé's sister Ani Payang, who had been a nun and had undertaken some Tibetan medical training in her youth; his elder brother, who also lived in the household and had an excellent memory; as well as Professor Wangdu, who was a close friend and a scholar and professor at the Tibetan Medical College. Time spent with Ngawang Dorjé and Yonten Tsering allowed me to study and discuss some printed medical and historical sources with them. An additional benefit was that they were from the same area and generation and had known each other for a long time. Thus I gained different perspectives on comparable situations and locations. The close rapport I developed with these two individuals and their social network allowed me to carry out repeated interviews and have many informal conversations.

Most of my weekends were spent in Shigatse Town and surrounding villages, while during the university holidays my research extended into five other distant counties in Shigatse Prefecture. The choice of place, timing, and length of visit was, with the exception of a three-week stay in Ngamring County, neither strategic nor planned; it came about because I was invited to accompany Yonten Tsering and a few medical students on trips to provide health care in rural areas. Delighted to accept, I spent several days in the counties of Rinpung, Sakya, and Thongmön, where we visited townships and villages for a half or full day, in some cases remaining overnight. Yonten Tsering provided Tibetan medical treatments, assisted by the students, some of whom had taken medical lessons with him and were eager for hands-on experience. I knew these trips would provide ample opportunity to learn from him and participate in Tibetan medical practice. I went on similar trips organized by just the doctor, to Lhatse County and Ngamring.

In the doctors' homes and in rural areas I witnessed over one thousand consultations, of which I discussed just under two hundred, along with follow-up meetings, with Yonten Tsering. I also filmed many of the medical encounters and some of the interviews. I talked as much as I could with patients but managed to carry out a systematic review of the illness experiences of only thirty patients, including informal conversations with their family members.

These various roles, and extended exposure to and engagement with the two *amchi*, their families, and social networks, as well as a return visit to several of the *amchi* I had met in 2003 and meetings with new ones (not least through the Swiss Red Cross), allowed me to generate new texts, including field notes, transcriptions of many hours of interviews and videos, and practical notes on medicine. The many issues that arose during this anthropological participant observation, in particular with regard to some of the oral history interviews, are discussed throughout the book but especially in chapter 3.

APPLIED ANTHROPOLOGY AND PERSPECTIVES FROM BEIJING

During the second period of fieldwork, I was fortunate to obtain substantial data through a short-term consultancy role for the Swiss Red Cross (SRC), which at the time was the main international NGO (out of just a handful) operating in Tsang. On their behalf I carried out two Evaluations and Needs Assessments of two cohorts of graduates from the SRC-funded Pelshung Tibetan Medicine School (Hofer 2007a, 2007b). The results of these the SRC were used in deciding how to administer the last round of support for these graduates before the NGO withdrew from this sort of intervention. For the consultancy, I carried out fifty-one semistructured interviews of sixty to ninety minutes and two focus-group discussions during a training course at the Swiss Red Cross headquarters in Shigatse (the first in December 2006 and the second in March 2007). In addition, I visited six graduates in their home villages or the townships where they worked. This assignment helped me build a good rapport with the Pelshung-trained doctors of the Tashilhunpo Medical Clinic. Apart from forming the basis of my two reports—hence qualifying as "engaged" or "applied" medical anthropology (Lamphere 2003, 2004)—the substantial data generated during these encounters was crucial in advancing my understanding of the non-state-led revitalization of private medical training in Tsang and the work of the Tashilhunpo Medical Clinic. This practical engagement, rather than limiting my work, enhanced it. It gave me pleasure to see some of my research activities directly benefit these two groups of graduates, while I discovered many aspects that would otherwise have passed me by, for example the wider implications of the Pelshung *amchi* lacking official medical licenses and their anxieties about it. I would agree with the Tibetologist David Germano that "engaged and participatory research is not just more ethical but the knowledge it produces gets better, more diverse, more extensive and more useful. And it enables [those who have often been termed] 'others' . . . giving [our Tibetan] colleagues the tools and the space for self-representation."[13]

In addition to the fieldwork in Tibet and work for SRC, I conducted two short research stays in Beijing, mainly to study centralist representation, regulations, and state sponsorship of what was typically referred to there as "China's Tibetan medicine" or "minority medicine" (C. *minzu minjian yiyao/yixue*). Particularly useful was a meeting with representatives of the National Minority Medicine Association and a visit to their library, since they published periodic reviews of PRC-wide legislation on "minority medicine." I also visited the Beijing Nationalities Hospital, better known as the Beijing Tibetan Medicine Hospital. It has more recently been renamed again, this time as the Beijing Tibetan and Ethnic Medicine Hospital (Hofer 2011b), in line with recent shifts in the redefinition and translation into English of *minzu*, from "minority nationality" to "ethnic group" (cf. Bulag 2010a).

MEDICINE AS AN EXCEPTION?

Despite intense surveillance and the care I needed to take during my research, the topic of Tibetan medicine made me, generally speaking, less suspect to officials in Foreign Affairs, at Tibet University, at the county level, and in village administrations. Tibetan medicine was by then fully supported, recognized by all sides as an important aspect of health care and, of late, commerce. Moreover, my Tibetan friends and interviewees generally considered it to be an apolitical topic.

Given common anthropological practice, my various roles and positions during the research, and the still pervasive and intense political sensitivity, the personal names of research participants and interlocutors have been anonymized. Exceptions are those who wanted to be named in person, publicly well-known figures and published authors, and some interlocutors who have now passed away. The precise names of locations have also in some cases been amended.

CHAPTER 1

THE TIBETAN MEDICAL HOUSE

> A corporate body holding an estate made up of both material and immaterial wealth, which perpetuates itself through the transmission of its name, its goods, and its titles down a real or imaginary line, considered legitimate as long as this continuity can express itself in the language of kinship or of affinity and, most often, of both.
>
> —Claude Lévi-Strauss, *The Way of the Masks*

THE transmission of medical knowledge among lay *amchi* has been conceived of as a flow of medical knowledge and practices passed on from fathers to sons, this continuity over time being known as "medical lineages," or *mengyü* in Tibetan vernacular language and practice (Craig 2012; Hofer 2012; Schrempf 2007). My findings, however, lend themselves to broader anthropological analysis through the concept of the house, first coined and defined by the social anthropologist Claude Lévi-Strauss (1982) and then significantly developed and critically applied to ethnography of Southeast Asian societies (Carsten and Hugh-Jones 1995). Drawing on the reception of these debates in the study of Tibetan kinship and especially in social anthropologist Heidi Fjeld's (2006) study of the house as an important form of kinship organization in Tsang, this chapter broadens and fine-tunes existing scholarship on the transmission of Tibetan medical knowledge. Findings on residence and marriage patterns of *amchi*, the symbolic and cosmological significance of their physical houses and how *amchis'* socioeconomic position and medical authority were established and maintained within the broader social organization of central Tibetan society of the time likewise inform this inquiry. The concept of the Medical House is useful for tracing knowledge transmission as well as the practice of medicine outside of large, central medical institutions in the 1940s and 1950s. Particular medical practitioners were deeply affected when their houses were wholly or partially dismantled during the early Communist reforms.

Lévi-Strauss's two characteristics of the house as a form of social organization are particularly pertinent to the transmission of medical knowledge and the establishment of authority in terms of Medical Houses in Tsang. One is a relatively flexible endorsement of social forms other than descent in selecting heirs to medical knowledge and skill within named and unnamed Medical Houses. This is despite the use of the rhetoric of patrilineage. Similar to the noble houses in Europe, houses among the Kwakiutl discussed by Lévi-Strauss, or the *ie* in Japan discussed by Chie Nakane (1970), Medical Houses have been remarkably enduring social units. The continuity of Medical Houses will be explored through discussion of two "male" Medical Houses, the Mentrong and the Térap in Ngamring, and one "female" Medical House in Sakya, the Nyékhang, followed by discussion of Medical Houses as moral persons.

REVISITING THE HOUSE

Yonten Tsering and I had known each other for several years, and during the winter of 2006–7 in particular, we spent many days and weeks together. In the early summer of 2007 we drove from Shigatse to Gye, his home village, nestled on the side of a fertile valley in lower Ngamring. The wind gently moved the browning tips of still largely green barley fields as we went bumping along dirt roads in a rented jeep. We had begun to plan the reestablishment of a Tibetan medical clinic in his birthplace, a rural farming village of about six hundred residents. It was his dear wish that it should be located in the Térap House that had belonged to the previous two generations of doctors in his family (figures 1.1 and 1.2). As usual, in the trunk of the car were his two aluminum chests filled with about one hundred Tibetan medicines to treat people on the way. The driver had put on music, and the backseat was crowded with Yonten Tsering's students and supporters, myself included.

After several stopovers, we were in Gye by the next morning, in the house of Gyatso, an old acquaintance from previous fieldwork with whom

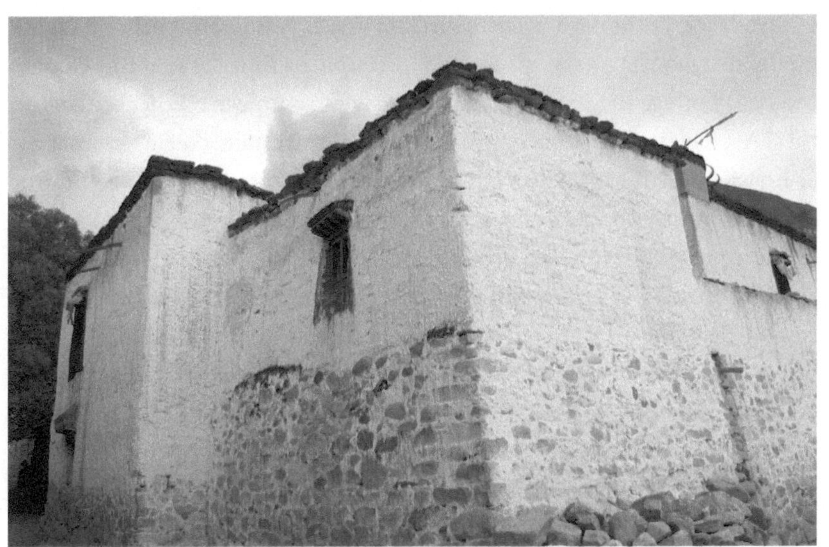

FIGURE 1.1. The Térap, 2007. Photo by Meinrad Hofer.

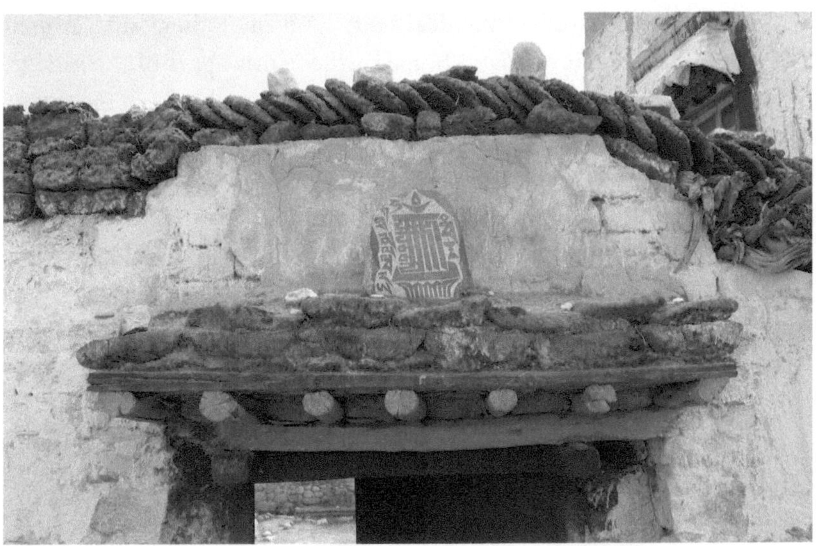

FIGURE 1.2. Entrance to the Térap, 2007. Photo by Meinrad Hofer.

I stayed. He is the father of Tashi Tsering, a young student of Tibetan medicine who was partway through a *durapa*, or BA course at the Tibetan Medical College in Lhasa, the most prestigious modern medical college in the TAR. Gyatso, a tax collector, was crucial to Yonten Tsering's endeavor as he was the official owner of the Térap House that had belonged to the doctor's family. Gyatso's parents had moved there in 1960, when landless farmers benefited from the first Democratic Reforms (Mangtso Chögyur), especially the land reforms implemented in the area. The doctor's family, by contrast, lost all rights to the house, its estate, and almost all personal belongings; they were relocated to a one-room shelter where they made do on less than the bare minimum over the following five years. With Yonten Tsering taking the lead, and Gyatso and his family present, we talked through the plans for the day: inspect Yonten Tsering's former home with a carpenter, meet the village leader to get his approval for the project, and in the afternoon study and pick medical plants in the vicinity of the village to see whether the clinic could rely to some extent on local materia medica.

"This is where I studied medical texts with my father," said Yonten Tsering as we entered his natal home in the central part of the village, peeping into a room where a thin shaft of light reached through the cracks of small wooden shutters. We opened them to let in light and air. The room was now used for storage, the walls blackened, but beyond several bags of clutter we began to make out a mural on one of the walls. It featured an *amchi* feeling the pulse of a patient (figure 1.3), someone grinding medicines, and another letting blood from a patient's leg: "My father had this made—it is very dear to me. I am happy to see it! This is nothing fake—it is real. It is part of our history and my memory," the doctor exclaimed as I quietly marveled over this almost forgotten treasure, only some time later pondering his use of the terms *history* and *memory* (*logyü* and *trenpa*). I then learned where the hearth had been—the center of sociality of the house, where medicines were made and his father once saw patients. Always practically inclined, Yonten Tsering continued, "However, it would be better to establish the new treatment rooms across the house, in the new northern court, as there is more light and warmth from the sun, also in the afternoons. This yard only gets the morning and midday sun," displaying his intimate knowledge of the sun's passage here, seemingly unbroken by the fifty-year hiatus.

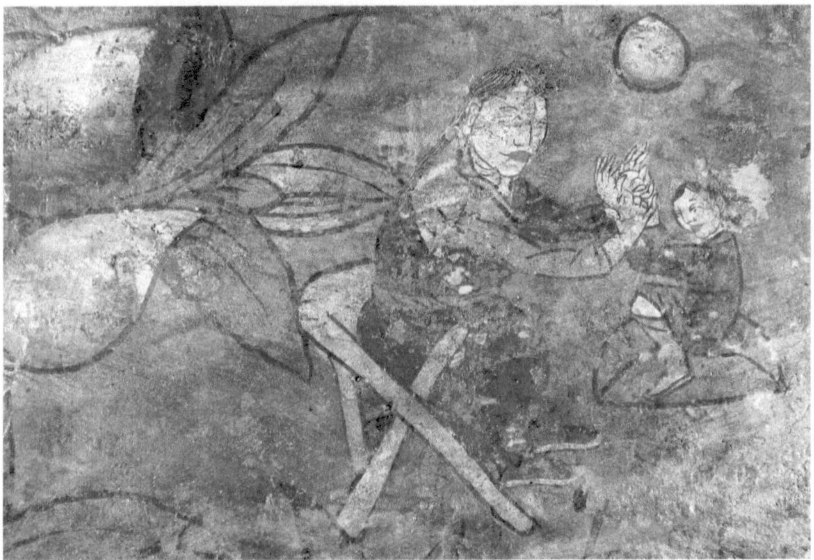

FIGURE 1.3. Detail of the Térap's medical mural, 2007. Photo by Meinrad Hofer.

MEDICAL LINEAGES: PAST AND PRESENT

Mengyü have so far been understood as major pathways for transmitting and reproducing Sowa Rigpa knowledge and skills in Tibet, and to lend authority, legitimacy, and status to medical practitioners.[1] Similar ideas and patterns of transmission are found in Chinese medicine, Ayurveda, and Yunani Tibb (the Arabic healing traditions of South Asia), as well as in Buddhist and Hindu religious domains.[2]

Tibetan medical lineages are sometimes recorded in Tibetan textual and oral accounts. Accounts of who was granted the authority to study a medical text or practice a particular technique from a given teacher fill thousands of pages in Tibetan medical histories and biographies of noted, usually elite, practitioners.[3]

The prominence of medical lineages as sources for and constituents of authoritative knowledge was established in the early days of the Tibetan medical system, in the twelfth-century *Four Treatises*. Here we read that "a medical doctor without a lineage [*rikgyü*] resembles a fox seizing the throne of the king and will not be honored at all" (Men-Tsee-Khang 2008: 298). This phrase uses the Tibetan term *rikgyü*, which is usually translated as "lineage" or "descent" and emphasizes proper lineage credentials. The

རིགས་རྒྱུད་མེད་པའི་སྨན་པ་
ཝ་ཡི་རྒྱལ་ས་བཟུང་བ་

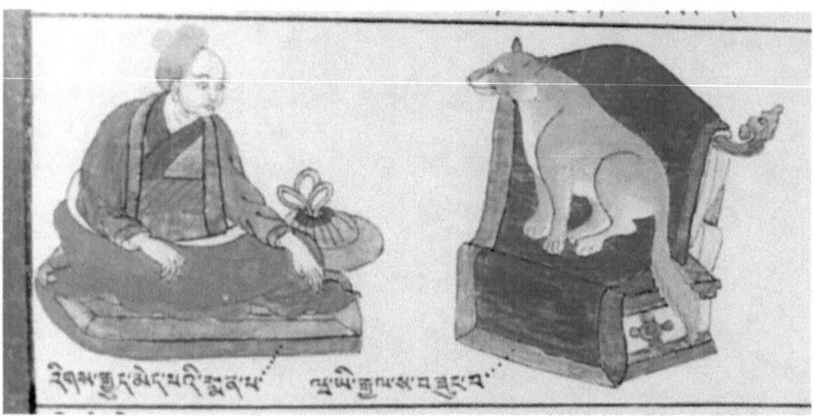

FIGURE 1.4. Detail from Tibetan Medical Thanka 37 on the Conduct of Physicians, Ulan Ude Set: "A medical doctor without a lineage is like a fox seizing the throne of the king." Courtesy of Serindia Publications.

phrase, or at least the sentiment, is repeated endlessly in medical works. We also find a visual representation of the fox on the king's throne in the famous Lhasa medical paintings (Parfionovich, Dorje, and Meyer 1992; figure 1.4). Such ideas on legitimacy and authority resemble wider Tibetan Buddhist and cultural ideals of who can become a scholar practitioner and how to be respected and successful in any of the ten Tibetan sciences, including Mahayana Buddhism (Barth 1990; Schaeffer 2003).

At the late seventeenth-century foundation of the Chakpori Medical College and other Buddhist medical institutions across eastern Tibet and Mongolia, the concept of *mengyü* continued to play a role. And *mengyü* is still important, even in secularized Tibetan medical institutions today, where classroom teaching, university exams, and degrees prevail.

In the historical and anthropological literature on Tibetan medicine, we find discussion of mainly two types of medical lineages. One, the prominent pathway within the family and along ties of kinship, is the so-called bone lineage or *dunggyü*. This refers to the ideal of transmitting medical knowledge along *dung*, an honorific term for *rü*, or what is translated into English as "bones" or "patrilineage." The other type is the teaching lineage (*lobgyü*) or master-discipleship discussed in the next chapter. Here a student sought out a physician or medico-Buddhist master, whose teaching and practices often connected closely with medico-spiritual rituals, for instance those of the Yuthog Heart Essence. Empowerments (*wang*), oral transmissions of medical texts (*lung*), the transmission of "secret oral" knowledge (*menngak*) to selected disciples, and oral didactic instruction (*tri*) were practiced in both kinds of lineages. The ritualized presence of *wang* and *lung* was more common in teaching lineages, where teachers and students were not usually related through kin. Instead relationships had to be forged through rituals and other social practices that demonstrated respect for teachers and teaching, and in return legitimacy for the student. Both pathways of transmission featured in my conversations with and observations of *amchi* in Tsang, the first prevalent among lay and the second among mainly ordained Buddhist and Bon practitioners.

Yet to merely analyze empirical findings on the transmission of medical knowledge among lay *amchi* in terms of bone lineages (*dunggyü*) and associated medical lineages (*mengyü*) is to leave out of those who do not fit local conceptions of "bones" as constitutive elements of medical lineages. In practice, many Tibetans in Tsang have gained medical knowledge and authority, even when they did not inherit the bones or pass on the bones of their fathers (i.e., belong to a particular patrilineage). Instead, they were accepted on the basis of being members or residents in a medical household (*mengyi kyimtsang*), through marriage (what social anthropologists refer to as affiliation), or through birth or adoption into the household (or filiation).

Scholarship on kinship and social organization in Tibetan societies has long documented the coexistence of ideas of descent (bones and lineage), affiliation, and residency in determining and creating social differences and groups in Tibetan societies.[4] In her analysis of social organization and domestic groups in rural Tsang, Fjeld (2006) applies and develops Lévi-Strauss's anthropological house concept to reconcile the tensions in analyzing descent, affiliation, and residency. This analytical category of the sociosymbolic house is particularly relevant to understanding the transmission of medical knowledge in Tsang and the social position and rank of lay Tibetan medical practitioners there.

BONES AND FLESH: GENDERED IDEOLOGIES OF DESCENT

Tibetan understandings of a bone lineage are grounded in theories of procreation and accounts of corporeal formation and constitution, in which the two substances of *rü* (bones, of which *dung* is the honorific form) and *sha* (flesh) are fundamental (Levine 1981; Fjeld 2006: 155–61). In the medical literature, as well as in lay concepts, *rü* is thought to be transferred via the white reproductive substance (*khuwa*) of the father to the bones of a conceived child, while *sha* (or what is called *trak*, or "blood," in medical texts and by Levine's informants among the Nyinba in Nepal) is transferred via the red reproductive substance of the mother (*khuwa* or *trak*) to constitute the flesh (Fjeld and Hofer 2010/11: 181–83). Of these, the bones form the "matrix of the body"—that is, they constitute the foundation for the person's physical and mental abilities—while the flesh has only limited implications for the constitution of personhood (Fjeld 2006: 158). While the bone lineage (*rügyü*, hon. *dunggyü*) is a direct and continuous line, the flesh lineage (*shagyü*) continues for no more than two generations. This is because the woman's red reproductive substances result indirectly from her father's bones (white substance) rather than directly from her mother's flesh (red substance), and therefore from her patriline rather than her matriline (Fjeld 2006: 159; Fjeld and Hofer 2010/11: 181–83).

Common practice, either the source or the result of this ideology, has been to pass on medical (and other kinds of occupational) knowledge to a male heir. Tibetans explain this in terms of kinship ideology, in particular ideas of patrilineal descent such those as just outlined. In the words of one of my *amchi* informants from Ngamring, "The circulation of 'flesh' and 'blood' [*sha khrag 'khor rgyug*] means they always change. Over time they become lighter and weaker [*sla ba*]. The bones [*rus*] on the other hand are harder [*mkhregs po*]. This is the reason bone lineages [*gdung rgyud*] remain strong and do not disappear easily." Another explained in a similar vein: "The color of the bone is white, and whatever happens, it will stay white; the color won't change. The color of blood, on the other hand, becomes lighter and lighter, and in the end it disappears."

This ideology of the transmission of medical knowledge from father to son is, however, not reflected in practice. Fjeld and I found that women born into medical households and in-marrying *magpa*s (called-in son-in-laws), or adopted children, also inherited medical knowledge and passed it on to both male and female heirs (Fjeld and Hofer 2010/11: 181–83). The house concept from anthropology therefore provides an apt framework to reconcile the widespread coexistence of a rhetoric about the ideal of patrilineal descent in the transmission of medical knowledge, and indeed practice, with other situations not conforming to this ideal, especially when we looked at cases in which women inherited and transmitted medical knowledge in Medical Houses.

In line with these developments in the study of Tibetan kinship, the house concept offers new ways to analyze the transmission of Tibetan medical knowledge as well as the socioeconomic status and authority of practitioners in Tsang. Many of Fjeld's findings regarding the social, symbolic, and economic aspects of houses in Panam in rural Tsang resonate with my findings on medical households in Ngamring, with the difference that none of the houses described below were to my knowledge polyandrous in the 1940s and 1950s (one however becoming so in the 1990s). At times these have even been referred to as Mentrong, literally "Medical Houses" (*sman grong*), while at other times they are called "medical households" (*mengyi kyimtshang*) or simply carry the name of a regular named House (Fjeld 2006: 126)—that is, without any explicit reference to *men* (medicine) but practicing and transmitting medicine across generations.

MEDICAL HOUSES IN TSANG

Despite the widespread verbal and practical insistence on the ideal of patrilineal descent for those who carry on medical lineages, medical knowledge has often been passed on to members of a family or a household who were not part of the bone lineage, such as *magpa*s, adopted children, and women, the latter especially (but not exclusively) when there were no sons (Fjeld and Hofer 2010/11; Hofer 2015). These persons were subsequently seen as perfectly legitimate heirs to family medical traditions, by virtue of membership and filiation in Medical Houses.

In the following example of a Medical House, remarkable continuity was facilitated by mechanisms other than transmission along the bone lineage, which was considered to have been "cut."

The Lhünding Mentrong

Situated in Lhünding Village at the foot of a hill topped by its local monastery is a named House widely known simply as the Mentrong, or "Medical House."[5] A seventy-year-old man, Rinchen Wangyal (affectionately and honorifically also called Rinchen-la or Mentrong Rinchen), explained the history of his Medical House to me in 2007:

> Our bone lineage comes from Jangpa Namgyel Drazang. He was born here at the Mentrong about six hundred years ago. His palace was later established up there [*points up the hill*], and at some point it was turned into a monastery. He was an extremely distinguished doctor, who during his lifetime helped so many beings in extraordinary ways. He was also a great lama. That's how it came about that people were saying that even eating the earth of the Mentrong would cure their coughs and colds. So famous and legendary was this place before its destruction! It is because of Jangpa Namgyel Drazang that we are called Mentrong. It means "the place where a doctor is born," and that remained our household name.

The life and medical legacy of Jangpa Namgyel Drazang have been recorded in several of his works and in medical histories.[6] His school, the Janglug (Jang School) was one of the dominant medical traditions in central Tibet (cf. Hofer 2012).

There is little doubt about the past medical achievement of the Mentrong. Medical works were written here, and its members tried and tested new techniques, some of which were subsequently propagated, such as the use of a uniquely shaped knife for bloodletting that is named after the Lhünding Mentrong.[7] Lhünding as a place for teaching medicine is mentioned by name in a history of the reign of the Fifth Dalai Lama and his regent, Sangyé Gyatso, for the year 1680 (Ahmad 1999: 328; Hofer 2012: 106). It is also prominently noted in the Fifth Dalai Lama's regent's orthodox medical history, *Khogbug.* Aiming to legitimate the medical and political authority of the Fifth Dalai Lama and his regent, this work claimed that the Janglug was united with another medical tradition of the time, the Zurlug, by Sangyé Gyatso. Yet according to local and family history, the medical tradition of the Lhünding-lug (a branch of the Janglug) continued well into the late nineteenth century at the Mentrong. It was during the time of his grandparents, Rinchen Wangyal said, that "the doctor's lineage was cut."[8]

As the preferred line of transmission, the brother of Rinchen-la's grandmother had received the medical lineage—that is, the texts, oral instructions on specific, sometimes secret practices (*menngak*), and practical teachings—from his father. He became a gifted doctor while still young—so much so that according to Rinchen-la's account, he aroused the jealousy of other doctors in the area and was allegedly given poisonous medicine and died. Although Rinchen-la's grandmother stayed in the house, married to an incoming *magpa* from an aristocratic family from Ruthog in western Tibet, she had not studied medicine. Due to the early death of her brother and their father, it was too late for this *magpa* to study in the direct teaching line of the Lhünding-lug tradition. After that no one could pass on the Lhünding medical tradition to either Rinchen-la's father or Rinchen-la's own generation. This is why he referred to the lineage as "cut."

Nevertheless with the material and immaterial wealth of the Mentrong painstakingly preserved, when Rinchen-la reached twelve, it was decided that the family medical tradition should be revived in the Mentrong. He was sent to nearby Phuntsoling Monastery to learn to read and write. After obtaining the *lung* and *wang* to the *Four Treatises*—permission to study the text—he studied and memorized three of its volumes while receiving practical instructions from a lay teacher named Jedrung Dzi (Rje drung 'Dzi), who taught medicine to two lay students at the monastery.

When Rinchen Wangyal returned to the Mentrong after several years of training, he was ready to read and further study medical texts. These included a large copy of the *Four Treatises* and the works of Jangpa Namgyel Drazang and their Lhünding-lug, still kept safely in the house. He began to make his own medicines from materia medica the family had preserved, combining this with newly collected herbs. He treated patients at home and made visits to patients in nearby villages. The Mentrong once again had a medical practitioner. Rinchen Wangyal thus combined the authority of the Mentrong—using its accumulated medical materials, texts, medicines, and instruments and its immaterial ritual power and efficacy—with the teachings and practical application learned from his teacher in Phuntsoling.

By virtue of the long-standing reputation of this Medical House and its medical lineage, Rinchen-la was known as the Mentrong *amchi*, or Mentrong Rinchen. This was despite "offending" two classic ideals of medical transmission: He was not born in direct patrilineal descent (that is, from the bones of his grandmother's father or her brother, the last *amchi* known in the patriline), as he was the son of the *magpa* from Ruthog. And he did not directly receive oral teachings of the Lhünding-lug (the Lhünding school). Yet he managed to reestablish the medical tradition in their Medical House and work as an *amchi*.

This shows how the indigenous concept of a named Medical House, when analyzed from an anthropological house perspective, allows us to account for continuity across generations, despite impasses in patrilineal descent. Members of Medical Houses, even decades later, on several occasions successfully sought out medical knowledge elsewhere and then continued work as a Medical House. This testifies to the importance Tibetans placed on maintaining the continuity of houses that were home to highly regarded professions, such as medicine. Due to subsequent political upheavals and reforms, Rinchen-la could not further develop as an *amchi* or recover the Lhünding-lug from the writings held at the Mentrong.

The Térap in Gye

In contrast to the Lhünding Mentrong's historically recorded and long-standing medical tradition, Yonten Tsering's medical lineage reaches back only four generations. Its members' names and work are remembered primarily within the family. His is a more straightforward, classic transmission of medical knowledge in the patriline, through the bones, from father to son. Yonten Tsering's grandfather established the Térap in Gye, moving it there from Napu, lower in the valley. Yonten Tsering's wife Yeshe Lhamo explained to me that Térap, the name of the house, was the short form of Tégu Rabpa, which her grandson spelled out for me as "*ste gu rabs pa*." As far as she was concerned, it meant "residence of good people." *Tégu rabpa* can also be translated as "place of generations" or "place of lineage," alluding perhaps to a desired continuity for this house.

At Térap, as far as Yonten Tsering remembered, there had been no shortage of male heirs, and in each generation they were trained at home, sometimes receiving additional scholarly and medical training elsewhere. He learned reading and writing at a nearby nunnery and then began to read and memorize the *Four Treatises* at home under the supervision of his father, studying every morning and then observing his father's work with patients. In 1954 Yonten Tsering enrolled at the newly founded Kikinaka Medical School of the Shigatse Labrang at Tashilhunpo Monastery, joining a class of fifty male students, half lay and half ordained. After four years of training, the class was discontinued as a result of political changes, and he returned home.

As he had been chosen as the one in the family to study medicine, he remained at home after marriage, while his siblings left to marry or join monastic institutions.[9] In 1956, during a school break, Yonten Tsering married Yeshe Lhamo, a woman from the named White House[10] in Targyü, by arrangement of their parents. Yonten Tsering's rank as a member of a *trelpa*, or taxpayer household, as well as the heir to a bone lineage of doctors—conveying high rank (*rik thopo*)—defined who was considered an appropriate marriage partner and thus future member of Térap.[11] Yeshe Lhamo's father served as a reserve soldier in the Tibetan army,[12] and her family was also from a *trelpa* household. The couple's socioeconomic status was similar, and during the land reform both families were labeled landlords and variously called *phyadag* or *phyado*. Yet there were several notable differences, chief among them that Yeshe Lhamo was and remains to this day illiterate, unable to even write her own name, and she is a few years older than Yonten Tsering.

I asked Yonten Tsering and his older sister, who had been ordained in Jonang as a nun, whether anyone considered passing the family medical lineage to her instead of one of her brothers. This prompted a great deal of laughter, followed by explanations that it had not been considered and would not have been right. Thus in their generation, Yonten Tsering was the sole recipient of his father's medical lineage, the lineage holder (*rikgyü dzinpa*).

Yonten Tsering's story follows the kinship ideal of patrilineal descent in the transmission of specialized, professional knowledge. Yet to this logic of patrilineality must also be added the differential perception of the mental capacities of men and women (Fjeld 2006: 159), in this case reflected in the reaction to my question. The preference of male heirs to medical lineages may also be related to the *polha*, the deity of the patrilateral kin group or bone lineage. Male heads of households worship the *polha* daily in the altar room, an activity Yonten Tsering carried out even after he moved out of the area in old age. Belonging to a bone lineage therefore not only embedded Yonten Tsering in particular social relations and professional expertise, but it entailed certain ritual obligations and the worship of deities related to the patrilateral kin group and the land (Blondeau and Steinkellner 1996).

As far as we know from current accounts, the transmission of medical knowledge over the past three generations at Térap neatly coincided with a patrilineally transmitted bone lineage. Marriage and educational choices ensured the continuity of both the social unit of the named house and the authority of the Medical House over time. In contrast to the Mentrong, the continuity of the bone lineage and the medical teaching associated with it had not been interrupted.

The Nyékhang

Both times I visited Sonam Drölma at her home in Tsarong District, Sakya County, she seemed surprised that a foreigner was interested in her story—and that I had made it to her house. In spring and summer the glacial melt carried away whatever had been rebuilt of the road in winter. The terraced fields and tiny hamlets, however, lay peacefully above the powerful pull of the river, as did the old footpath, which I followed along the upper part of the valley to reach her house. In 1941, Sonam Drölma was born into the Nyékhang, literally, "house dear and near [to oneself]." The Nyékhang was in a village at the base of the mountain, below the local Pusum Monastery of the Sakya order. Her grandfather and her parents lived in the household; she was the only child, and soon took great interest in her grandfather's medical work. At thirteen she began to study medicine:

> My grandfather was a layman, although with close connections to our Pusum Gonpa. He taught me to memorize the *peja*, mainly the *Gyüshi* [the *Four Treatises*], explained how to recognize the plants, how to make medicines, to read the pulse, and to check the urine. He explained everything. I watched what he was doing. He taught me, and I helped out. It was not like today's school; it all took place in an informal way.
>
> Grandfather let me collect plants, grind them, and give the medicines to the patients. They came to my grandfather, and he went to their houses. He also bought medicinal ingredients from India, via businessmen, or else we would collect them from the area. He made every single medicine himself—between sixty and a hundred types. He had a big wooden trunk full of raw materials, but that was burned during the revolution together with many other things.

Sonam Drölma's studies and training in medicine lasted until she was in her late teens, about 1960, when family members, especially her grandfather, were targeted by the new regime during its first local campaigns. They had to stop practicing medicine entirely but were able to preserve medical texts and instruments.

Both Sonam Drölma and her nephew, a learned Sakya lama and Tibetan medical physician, described the family medical tradition as a *khyimgyü*, short for *khyimtsang gyü*, meaning literally "lineage of the household" or "home lineage." This term emphasizes the corporate estate of the Nyékhang, the *khyimtsang* or "household," as an important social and symbolic category. It contrasts "doctor's or medical lineage" (*amchi gyü* or *mengyü*), which emphasizes the person or the medical craft; "bones," which references the patrilineage; and the name of a medical tradition's founder, usually men. The local term "household lineage" fits well with the anthropological concept of the house, which is wider and captures the idea that medical knowledge and skill was inherited and transmitted by and to men and women, to those affiliated by descent as well as by affiliation (i.e., birth, adoption, or marriage) and that they resided together in a household. Sonam Drölma was one of only a few lay Tibetan women to have inherited a Medical House, similar to, for instance, Lobsang Dolma Khankhar from Kyirong in southern Tsang (Norbu Chöphel and Tashi Tsering 2008; Hofer 2015).

Such an inheritance was possible to these two women as the only child in a household with no sons. They were given a solid education and medical training, receiving encouragement from their families and teachers as the perceived stand-ins for sons (or, at times, male students). As Sonam Drölma's Medical House had an excellent reputation and several centuries' standing, it is remarkable that it was inherited by a woman.

It was common knowledge among doctors in the area, and explicitly stated by Sonam Drölma and her nephew, that the Nyékhang's *khyimgyü* went back to Tsarong Palden Gyaltsen (Tsha rong dpal ldan rgyal mtshan, b. 1535). Historical accounts tell us that he was a Buddhist monk from an aristocratic family who was drawn to study medicine after a childhood illness, and that his teacher was Gongmen Konchog Pandar of the Gongmen tradition.[13] Sangyé Gyatso's medical history discloses that the inheritors of Tsarong Palden Gyaltsen's lineage, namely Tsarong's son and his nephew, established their own medical school, Drangsong Düpai Ling, and that they acted as doctors to local rulers and wrote many literary medical works (Sangyé Gyatso 2010: 320, 326; Garrett 2014: 183, 185).

According to these accounts, Tsarong Palden Gyaltsen must have left the order at some point to start his own family and teach medicine to his son and nephew.[14] The biographical account of an early twentieth-century

Tibetan politician, whose estate was in Tsarong, mentions a "medical monastery" (Tsarong 2000: 86). This is described as located near the Tsarong estate, a "two-story temple dedicated to the Medicine Buddha" with the eight monks residing there "conducting prayers and taking care of the daily offerings." I could not find out more about how the current Nyékhang was related to the Drangsong Düpai Ling medical school or the medical monastery mentioned in the historical accounts.

In the 1940s and 1950s, based on Sonam Drölma's information, the only doctor in this area was her grandfather. Sonam Drölma inherited his Medical House, as well as its material and immaterial wealth, comprising medical knowledge, skills, and a text collection associated with it. Having received a medical training and been married by arrangement to an in-marrying *magpa*, she began to practice at home as an independent *amchi* shortly before the reforms radically changed the trajectory of the Nyékhang.

RELATIONS BETWEEN MEDICAL HOUSES

Despite the relative proximity of Gye and Lhünding (about a three-hour walk), there was in living memory no medical exchange between practitioners of the Mentrong and Térap. Rinchen Wangyal insisted that after his teacher in Phuntsoling died in 1958, "there were no more good *amchi*," except at Tashilhunpo. This implies that he could not study with *amchi* from Térap in Gye. It is unclear whether this was due to distance and his own responsibilities, or perhaps due to medical households keeping their knowledge to themselves. At that time there would have been several *amchi* in the area who in principle could also have acted as teachers. Instead, when medical knowledge was sought outside one's Medical House, it was almost always from a teacher who was also a Buddhist monk or nun.[15] If Rinchen Wangyal's account of the intentional poisoning of the doctor of the Lhünding Mentrong is to be believed, there may have been competition between Medical Houses.

Such a lack of exchange between Medical Houses as was seemingly the case in 1950s Ngamring contrasts starkly with what we know of pre-Communist social and medical networks of family practitioners of Chinese medicine.[16] Furthermore, in Ngamring and Tsang more broadly Medical Houses rarely had more than one member per generation who inherited medical knowledge; thus usually only two, one parent and one child, practiced medicine at any one time.

Despite the social authority and continuity provided by lay Tibetan Medical Houses, difficulties in continuing Medical Houses across generations sometimes meant seeking knowledge from medical practitioners in monasteries, such as Phuntsoling or Tashilhunpo. This likely discouraged competition or sharing of lineage and family-specific secret knowledge, or *menngak*. One could also obtain Buddhist teachings from monastics, a commonly accepted and highly regarded practice.

MEDICAL HOUSES AS "MORAL PERSONS"

The second important feature of the anthropological house concept in relation to Medical Houses in Tsang concerns their status as "moral persons" (Lévi-Strauss 1982: 171–87). This concept opens up new ways to understand several phenomena usually studied and analyzed separately, such as the architecture and everyday social and medical practices related to houses. It allows material and immaterial wealth—economic position (in essence access to land) as well as the physical nature and cosmology of Medical Houses—to be included in the analysis. Material and immaterial wealth included primarily medical text collections, medical equipment, materia medica, medical knowledge and practice, as well as specific medico-Buddhist rituals intended to support the medical efficacy of practitioners and medicines.

To become a lay *amchi* in Tsang in the 1940s and 1950s implied significant interactions with the immediate physical, symbolic, and social aspects of Medical Houses. These were made and reproduced, establishing members as medical practitioners of a certain ilk: a particular, usually high *rik* (or kind), and their medical work's authority and efficacy. My analysis of Medical Houses as moral persons is inspired by several anthropologists working in the region (especially Fjeld 2006) and beyond,[17] and it follows Hsu's suggestion that the house, like the body, is a prime agent of socialization (1998: 2).

Buildings with Authority

In summer 2003, during my first visit to the Mentrong in Lhünding, as I was seated with Rinchen Wangyal in the open courtyard on the first floor,

I asked him, "What do you remember of the old Mentrong?" "I remember our old house very well!" he replied with a broad smile, his arms around his granddaughter, who was snuggled in his lap. "In our old house there was the *menkhang*, a small room solely devoted to medicine and the medical scriptures, though we ourselves did not practice medicine anymore. That had stopped two generations before. Nobody taught or practiced medicine in my parents' generation when I was young, but all the different books of medicine were there. Some of them were also kept in the *chökhang*." When I returned to the Mentrong with Yonten Tsering in summer 2007, Rinchen-la's sister, also called Drölma and on a visit from her nearby home at the Nyingkhang, gave a similar account: "Every now and then, Rinchen Wangyal and I sneaked into the *menkhang* when we were small. All the different kinds of medicinal plants and ingredients were there—I loved the smell. There were beautiful medicine spoons as well. We played with them until we were told to stop. Medical bags with ready medicines were also kept, but at the time no one knew medicine any longer. Nobody used these things, but we kept them as blessings." The siblings were remembering their childhood in the early 1940s, well before Rinchen Wangyal was sent to learn how to make use of the medicines he had played with. Their upbringing in the largest house of the village, Rinchen-la's education, and Drölma's eventual marriage to a member of the Nyingkhang, an old and famous *ngakpa* household, all indicate the Mentrong's privileged position compared to other households in Lhünding.

As mentioned earlier, the Mentrong comprised both the medical and the royal bone lineage of Jangpa Namgyel Drazang, the lay Buddhist scholar and teacher of the late thirteenth and early fourteenth centuries. These long-standing affiliations meant that the Mentrong enjoyed numerous socioeconomic privileges, including large landholdings, as well as certain ritual obligations.

The Mentrong building was located on the east side of the village, and its structure reflected this high sociosymbolic standing. It exemplified the symbolic ideal of Tibetan homes in Tsang, with the three floors of the house as a microcosm reflecting the tripartite macrocosm inhabited by humans and other beings: the *lhayul* (land of gods), *miyul* (land of people), and *nyelwa* (underworld) (Fjeld 2006: 265–99).[18] Most Tsang houses today have only two floors, and many commoner or servants' houses, like unnamed houses prior to the 1950s, have just one story.

The architecture and medico-ritual activities of Medical Houses corresponded to their socioeconomic position in the villages, together constituting the practical medical authority of each Medical House. The Mentrong's exceptional role in ritual activities during the yearly *cham* dances in the 1940s and 1950s held at the house contributed to the house's high moral and symbolic standing in Lhünding. On the other hand, owing to its structural survival to this day, the architecture of Térap in Gye is visible in more detail. Its socioeconomic standing was that of a *trelpa*, or taxpayer household, but because of its membership in a particular social subcategory, it was largely relieved from paying tax.

When Rinchen-la described the Mentrong as he had experienced it and remembered it again in the summer of 2007, a proud smile appeared as he described in his very polite way the size of the house: "Actually there was no need for it to be that spacious, but the house was really quite large. Yes, perhaps, it was even *very* large! [*He laughs.*]" He went on to detail its structure: Animals occupied part of the first floor. The second floor housed the all-important kitchen, bedrooms for members of the household and children, several storerooms, and the *menkhang*. Many rooms on the second floor were unused most of the time, reserved for guests when the need arose. The *chökhang* was located on the third, top floor, along with adjacent rooms used by visiting Buddhist monks.

Unusually for secular architecture in Tsang villages, the Mentrong featured a open central courtyard on the ground floor around which the whole house was constructed. It thus more closely resembled the houses of aristocratic families or Buddhist lamas in Shigatse or Lhasa, for instance the Lingtsang or Shatra mansions in Lhasa (Alexander, forthcoming; Larsen and Sinding-Larsen 2001: 119–21), which included up to three floors constructed around a central courtyard. It is not entirely clear why this was the case at the Mentrong but could be explained by the longstanding annual festival held there.

While it was common for monasteries throughout the region to hold *cham* dances at the end of each Tibetan calendar year, in Lhünding, rather than this taking place at the monastery, it was held at the Mentrong. Rinchen Wangyal explained:

> Once every year, on the 28th of the eleventh month, we would go up to the monastery, and my father would invite the protector Yeshe Gonpo [Ye shes

> mgon po]. He would come down with us to our house. Beforehand from the Mentrong *tsampa*, we had prepared a special *torma*. It had to be made from our *tsampa*—not any *tsampa* would do. Not even the *tsampa* from the monastery! Then when the protector had arrived here, on the next day the monks came down and performed the *cham* on the 29th, for the whole day. The protector, for only once a year, would have the cloth covers over his eyes removed and looked over the dances. We would offer all the food and drink to the monks and make donations. The villagers all came to watch, and by the evening everyone had left again. On the 30th of the month we would invite and carry the protector back up to the monastery. The *torma*, however, was kept in our *chökhang* inside a special chest for the rest of the year. All this gave great blessings to our house and to everyone present.

As this account indicates, the Mentrong played a crucial role in ensuring the proper ritual to close the old year and ensure the support of the village protector, guaranteeing prosperity and fortune for the whole village for the coming year. Quite apart from the medical provisions this house could offer to villagers, it also played a prominent part in an important Buddhist ritual for the benefit of the whole community.

This unique relationship between the Mentrong and Lhünding Monastery as well as between the Mentrong and the village, together with their royal background (*rgyal thog*) and large landholdings, classified the Mentrong as a member of the two main "high ranks" (*rik thopo*) in Tibet's traditional lay socioeconomic hierarchy. These comprised various kinds of lay nobility or *kutra*, the lowest of which was the *gerpa* category, and the *trelpa*, or taxpayers.[19] The Mentrong was a *gerpa* household, which meant they had large landholdings for which they were, however, not required to pay taxes in the 1940s and 1950s. Hierarchically, they were lower than other Tibetan aristocracy, whose members served in the government and as administrators and tax collectors on behalf of the Tibetan government. *Gerpa* were, however, usually seen as higher than *trelpa* households, who effectively leased land from monasteries, aristocrats, or directly from the government, and in exchange paid them taxes (*trel*). Most of the Mentrong's ancestral lands were found in and around Lhünding, while the land that had been inherited from the royal family of Ruthog in Ngari at the turn of the twentieth century was spread out in other places. In total the Mentrong had attached to their estate about seven landless farming households whom Rinchen Wangyal referred to as *yokpo* and who worked their land in the vicinity of the Mentrong in exchange for part of the yield and some payment; fields farther away were rented out and administered remotely. The landless farmers dependent on the Mentrong would later be termed serfs in Marxist parlance and "liberated" at the beginning of the Democratic Reforms in 1959–60 (cf. Shakya 1999: 247–48).

Social Status and Material Wealth

In contrast to the Lhünding Mentrong, the Térap in Gye was a *trelpa* household. This house was thus not technically a landholding estate in the traditional Tibetan organization but was required to pay taxes to the primary owners of the land, in this case the Khangsar Shekar, from which they had long-term leases.[20] Being a comparatively small landholder, the Térap had three workers who plowed and tended to the fields in exchange for a share of the yield. The Térap differed from other *trelpa* households in Gye and the surrounding area, however, regarding tax payments. In local terms, they were considered a *chödzé* household,[21] which was on a par and usually mentioned together with those of the rank of *shabdrung* and *jedrung*.[22] *Shabdrung* referred to families of lay tantric lineages (*ngakpa*), *chödzé* to medical families, and *jedrung* to members of aristocratic families. These three kinds of professionally and socially ranked households all enjoyed individually agreed tax privileges, as they served the government in one way or another.[23] In general their tax obligations were lower than those of regular *trelpa* households, and the *shabdrung* household of Nyingkhang was entirely exempted. In exchange for such privileges, the families of *shabdrung*, *chödzé*, and *jedrung* status—a seemingly Tsang-specific terminology—were expected to fulfill ritual duties and to serve the community through the activities of lay tantric households, for instance by carrying out protection rituals and averting hailstorms, providing medical treatment, or working as administrators for the government. This economic status and the associated tax privileges provided a financially stable existence for Medical Houses. Although no government health care was available in Ngamring, these tax levies allowed lay medical practitioners to work as doctors, which by all accounts required significant financial outlays for education and the

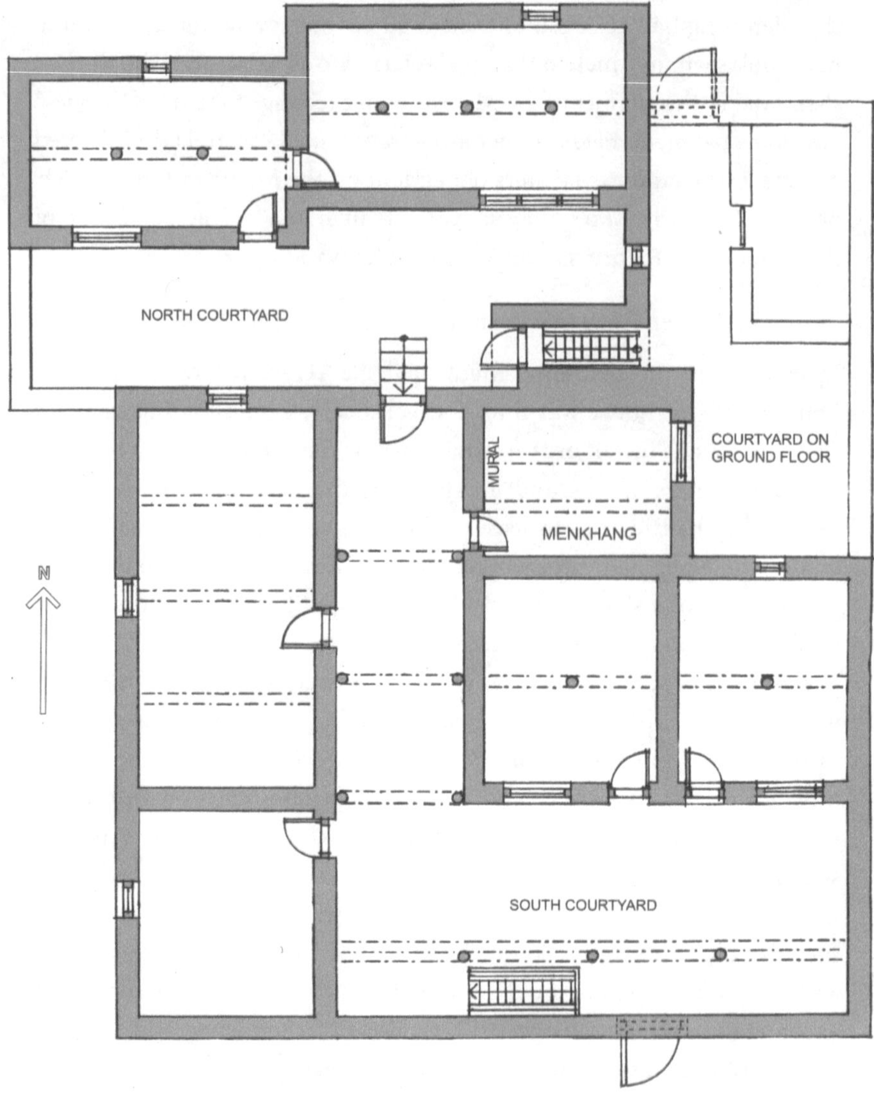

FIGURE 1.5. Plan of the second floor of the Térap. Drawing by Knud Larsen.

purchase of materia medica, as well as long hours spent in medicine production and consultations.

Though the Mentrong building was destroyed by the Red Guards during the Cultural Revolution, the Térap remains in Gye, its physical (in this case two-floor) structure intact and its medical tradition kept alive by Yonten Tsering. A key architectural feature of the Térap and the Mentrong was their *menkhang*, or medicine room, which set it apart from other named houses in the area. Yonten Tsering and his father spent many hours together in the *menkhang*, engrossed in medical studies, the preparation of medicines, Buddhist rituals, and visits with patients. The *menkhang* was positioned on the second floor, in the quietest part of the house, its northeastern side (figure 1.5). It featured the aforementioned mural depicting various aspects of medical work and a Chinese Buddhist deity of longevity surrounded by auspicious symbols in a landscape.

In terms of ritual purity, the *menkhang* was similar to the family's *chökhang*, which was located in the eastern part of the house. This is where most of the medical and religious texts as well as the *lha* (Buddhist deities) and thankas were kept. The *Four Treatises* states (in the chapter on the ethics of the physician) that "medicines should be regarded as precious jewels, nectar and sacrificial offerings [*mchod rdzas*]" (Men-Tsee-Khang 2008: 289). Medicines, instruments, and medical texts, as Buddhist works and ritual implements, had a status similar to that of Buddhist deities and were not to come in contact with impure practices (for instance, stepping over them). Similarly, they were to be kept out of impure locations (such as the ground floor) or highly "polluted" places or events and out of contact with certain groups of people, especially those of "impure *rik*" such as butchers and blacksmiths.[24]

The *menkhang*, rather than the *chökhang*, served as a place for Yonten Tsering's father to perform certain medico-Buddhist practices. One such practice was the Yuthog Nyingthig, or Yuthog Heart Essence, a Buddhist practice of great importance to Sowa Rigpa practitioners since the twelfth century CE (Garrett 2009). For the *torma* preparation in the context of this cycle of teachings, his father, Tsering Norbu, had drawn a fine visual guide (figure 1.6). Once the *torma* were made, they were placed in a special wooden chest for *torma* and kept in the *menkhang*. A thanka of Yuthogpa also hung there. In front of these Yonten Tsering's father practiced the Yuthog Nyingthig following a printed copy of the work from Lhasa's Chakpori Printing House, thereby empowering both practitioner and medicines.

Another important aspect of the material wealth of Medical Houses were their medical libraries. Text collections in the Medical Houses from before the 1950s survived the reforms almost intact in the Térap and Nyékhang, while all were lost from the Mentrong.

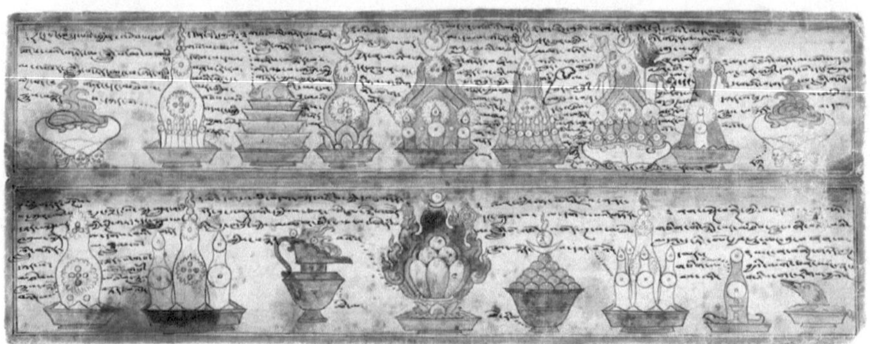

FIGURE 1.6. Instructions for *torma* offerings drawn by Yonten Tsering's father. Photo by Meinrad Hofer.

The surviving collections that I encountered during my fieldwork always included a *peja* of the *Four Treatises* and at least one work on medical compounding. In the collection of the Térap House were two editions of the *Four Treatises*, two commentaries on them, one large independent medical work with an extensive collection of recipes, two fragments of manuscripts, and one manuscript of a commentary on the *Third Treatise*'s chapter on pediatrics.[25] The collection of the female *amchi* Sonam Drölma had the most remarkable number and variety of medical and medico-religious materials. These ranged from illustrations to manuscripts and printed texts, and within the writings, from commentaries and original practical treatises (the so-called *nyamyik*, or "writings from experience") to recipe collections, medical notes, letters, and medical mantras.[26] Some of the titles clearly indicate a strong connection to the Gongmen medical tradition and to Tsarong Palden Gyaltsen's medical lineage, in which they were probably passed on. For instance, there is an undated manuscript of the influential medical work *A Hundred Verses Written from Experience* (*Nyams yig brgya rtsa*), by the teacher of Tsarong Palden Gyaltsen, Gongmen Konchog Pandar (1511–1577).[27] Tsarong Panden Gyaltsen himself was known for his expertise in treating *drumbu* and *drumné* (smallpox), on which he also wrote several works (Garrett 2014), some of them found among the surviving manuscripts and texts.

Two medical texts were saved from the collection of the Ruthog Amchi Tsewang, whose family practice is introduced in chapter 5. One of those was a unique *menjordeb* (see figure 5.2), a handwritten work on medical compounding that featured accumulated recipes and annotations in the hand of earlier members of this family medical tradition. These annotations suggest, for instance, how to substitute (*tsab*) medicinal ingredients of equivalent potency and effect for those that were not found locally.[28]

Since in the 1940s and 1950s medical texts were not commonly for sale or even printed in large numbers, these private medical text collections were simply the first port of call in the study and practical application of Sowa Rigpa. Because Sowa Rigpa was part of Buddhist learning, these texts gave equal blessings and prestige to Medical Houses compared with Buddhist scriptures, which were kept in the *menkhang* or the *chökhang*. Within Medical Houses, medical libraries were transmitted across generations. In some cases, even if the houses did not survive, these medical libraries were reinstated in the rebuilt homes of *amchi*.

— · —

Through ritual activities, socioeconomic position, and the physical houses, Medical Houses established and maintained their authority in a sociocultural nexus that resonates with Lévi-Strauss's conception of houses as "moral persons." Far from being inanimate physical structures, Medical Houses were made and maintained from within, through their symbolic order and associated rituals. These placed their members at the higher end of the traditional socioeconomic hierarchy in rural Tsang. Their inherited and actively maintained class status furthermore endowed them with responsibilities over specific village rituals or medico-spiritual practices, as well as medical work, which lies at the crossroad between material and immaterial wealth.[29]

THE MEDICAL WORK OF *AMCHI*

It was common practice at the Mentrong, Térap, and Nyékhang, my informants insisted, that *amchi*s treated all patients, rich or poor. This had been a contentious issue, as during the Communist reforms many doctors were accused of having exploited their patients. Yonten Tsering and Mentrong Rinchen-la said there were no set prices for consultations and treatment; those who could afford it made donations, and these usually made up for those unable to offer anything. "Those who were seriously sick and recovered usually gave most!" Rinchen-la commented with a smile when we spoke about this topic. Sonam Drölma said that her grandfather had never asked for medical fees, but patients gave a donation, however much they could afford. One difference from the medical practitioners in the monasteries discussed in the next chapter is that lay *amchi* generally treated anybody in the laity, as well as monks and nuns at monasteries without a doctor, which was apparently often the case. By contrast, monks and nuns treated mainly other clergy.

Seeing Patients

At Térap, patients were seen on the first floor, either in the kitchen or the open courtyard, the social center in Tsang houses. Occasionally concessions were made and special patients were treated in the *menkhang*, which was otherwise used as a study and pharmacy.

Although the *Four Treatises* promises that the treatment of patients leads to Buddhahood (Clark 1995: 233), and compassion and generosity benefit *amchis*' own Buddhist practice, allowing outsiders to enter the Medical House could threaten the household's ritual purity. Resulting impurities had to be countered by appropriate purifications and rituals to avoid *drib*, or pollution. *Drib* was regarded as reducing the auspiciousness and efficacy of medicines but also caused illnesses and misfortune more broadly. Whether *amchi* also went to other people's homes, and on what terms, differed from place to place and person to person, some saying they went to others' homes only when specifically called, while others went to other villages voluntarily. Presumably social class was an issue here. Be that as it may, informants related that due to the scattered population, it was often necessary to diagnose at a distance, either through urine, which a family member of the sick person brought to the *amchi*, or by "stone diagnosis." It is possible, however, that the grounds for such remote diagnoses related to the social background of patients.

Yonten Tsering was at first hesitant to explain stone diagnosis. He was worried about his credibility as a doctor today, as this was, in his words, "religion [*chö*] rather than medicine [*men*]," deflecting the thorny issue religion had become for *amchi* since the start of Communist reforms (cf. Adams 2001) by adding that "anyhow it cannot be compared to actually reading a patient's pulse." While discussing, with a monk at a remote Nyingma monastery, treatments that today fall outside strictly medical definitions—for example, the exorcism of a spirit through ritual, which was still recommended and practiced by monk and nun practitioners—Yonten Tsering became more willing to explain the technique of stone diagnosis:

> A sick person first needed to make a prayer and then walk seven steps toward the east, close his or her eyes, and then pick up a stone from the ground. It might be any color, size or shape. Then this needed to be wrapped in a piece of cloth and brought to the *amchi*, since they might live far away. According to the shape, size, and color of the stone, the *amchi* would make a diagnosis and prescribe a treatment. One would still ask after problems of the sick person. This technique is close to a divination [*mo*]; it belongs to the realm of *chö*.

He considered this to have provided accurate diagnosis in many cases but nevertheless judged it to be no longer relevant. Medicine (*men*) and religion (*chö*) had to be separated, since the socialist transformation, he averred, attempted to separate the centuries-long tradition of "combined religious and medical traditions."[30]

The core diagnostic technique used in Medical Houses was the classic *ta rek dri* approach of visual observation, palpation of the pulse, and questioning. Details are now hard to recover as practitioners have since passed away. However, judging from the subsequent generations' accounts as well as some of the medical works they studied, it was likely personal virtuosity that made practitioners rely more or less on certain aspects, as all diagnoses have vast internal differences and repertoires. Among the works Yonten Tsering's father had passed on to him, we find techniques not present in the classic *Four Treatises* work, such as ear vein diagnosis. This was used mainly in young children, where the pulse is difficult to determine at the wrist. This diagnosis is discussed in one of Yonten Tsering's manuscripts, a handwritten commentary on the gynecology and pediatrics chapters of the *Four Treatises*, influenced by Khyenrap Norbu's work on childcare and pediatrics.[31]

Apart from preparing medicines according to techniques and knowledge derived from classic and family-created works or specifically for patients, Yonten Tsering's father applied external therapies, such as moxibustion, cauterization, golden needle therapy, and bloodletting. He had learned these mainly through hands-on practice with his father, rather than from Lamenpa Kachen Norbu, a doctor and teacher at Tashilhunpo and the personal physician to the Ninth Panchen Lama. He passed these skills on to his son, when he had returned from his education at Tashilhunpo.

Making Medicines: A Culture of Recipes

Almost all medicine prescribed in Medical Houses was compounded on site using both local and foreign ingredients. Collection of local raw materials either by the *amchi* or by their landless laborers took a lot of time as it involved journeys of several days to several weeks to places where the desired plants grew and minerals were found. A few were easily accessible in the immediate surroundings of the *amchis*' residences or by exchange with people one knew. The same was true of animal ingredients, which were commonly used. These derived from domestic animals and hunted wildlife, including the musk deer (*ladzi*) for its gland and the Tibetan deer for its horn (*sharu*).

Foreign ingredients from warm climates in the south were essential to treat cold diseases. These account for many of the ingredients in many Tibetan medicines, and they were expensive as they came via trade or pilgrimage, mainly from India and Nepal. They included, for instance, the three dried fruits *arura*, *barura*, and *kyurura*, sandalwood (*tsendan*), the so-called six supreme medicines (*sangbo druk* or *sang druk*) of nutmeg, cloves, cardamom, saffron, cubeb, and bamboo pith, and animal parts such as rhinoceros horn (*seru*). The relative ease and cost of access to local versus foreign ingredients at the time appears to be the reverse of today's situation, which is related to the great expansion of the Tibetan medicine industry. As one *amchi* explained, "In the old society the *sang druk* were really valuable and precious medicines, because they came from far away, from India and so on. Those included *aru*, *baru*, *kyuru*, *dzati*, *sukmel*, *ka ko la*, etc. Today it is the other way around! The plants from inside Tibet have become the *sang druk*."

The principal place where medicines were prepared, ground, and mixed in Medical Houses was the *menkhang*. Raw and ready-made medicines were dried elsewhere, including on the roof and in covered parts of courtyards. Yonten Tsering still possessed and treasured several instruments in use at the time. He also kept an old three-layer wooden box to store raw materia medica and two large grinding stones in Gye. These bore the traces of several generations of doctors, a thick portion of the hard stone ground away through their efforts. Here medicines had been made according to classic formulas and the family's own pharmacological traditions, as recorded in some of their manuscripts and practically learned as a craft. The whole medicine-making process was replete with adjustments factoring in the availability of raw materials and possibly their substitution (*tsab*); perceived efficacy and quality of the raw materials as defined by their taste (*ro*); and importantly, the individual patient's condition.

Other medical items and instruments kept in the house were medical spoons, ideally made of silver, decorated with precious stones, and used for measuring the doses of powdered medicine, and a large medical bag made of snow leopard skin, filled with smaller leather bags. This bag was used primarily when visiting patients in their own homes, where ready-made medicines were relied upon and the *amchi* was unable to compound or adjust them en route.[32]

— · —

Named Medical Houses in rural Tsang were central social units and physical places for medical education and professional practice. State-sponsored health work (either Tibetan medical or biomedical) was mostly absent until well into the late 1960s and early 1970s. The fact that during the 1940s and 1950s private Medical Houses enjoyed tax benefits can be read as a form of Tibetan state support for their services. Medical Houses enjoyed economic wealth due to their *trelpa* and *gerpa* status, and this sustained the medical practice, as patients did not always pay for treatment. Although lay practitioners made up a relatively large percentage of Tibetan medical practitioners during the 1940 and 1950s, there has so far been little research on their work and history, which this chapter has gone some way to remedy. It describes and analyzes the transmission of knowledge, as well as the socioeconomic position and work of *amchi* in Ngamring and surrounding areas through the anthropological house concept. A combination of particular social relations, rank, professional knowledge, and ideas about moral purity worked to secure and maintain the authority and successful continuation of Medical Houses among lay practitioners over time. The Democratic Reforms and subsequent Communist reforms in Tsang from 1959–60 onward diminished, and in some cases permanently eroded, the hitherto long-standing medical and social authority of Medical Houses and their members.

Established Medical Houses were not the only places to learn, transmit, and practice Sowa Rigpa. New Medical Houses were formed, and medicine was practiced in other professional houses, for instance those of lay tantric priests. Importantly, medical teachings and practice were also present in monastic settings and among itinerant Buddhist teachers cum doctors.

CHAPTER 2

MEDICINE AND RELIGION IN THE POLITICS AND PUBLIC HEALTH OF THE TIBETAN STATE

> It was our old custom in Tibet that religion and politics were joined. People's efforts in getting better comprised medicine [*men*] and doing religion [*chö*].
>
> —Yonten Tsering, 2007

In addition to lay Tibetan physicians studying and working in Tsang Medical Houses, *amchi* also learned Sowa Rigpa through master-discipleships or teaching lineages and practiced as monks and nuns. Sowa Rigpa has long been considered one of the ten Buddhist sciences,[1] and many works in the tradition have been written by monk-scholars, whose lives and works are recorded in numerous biographies and medical histories (Garrett 2008, 2014; Schaeffer 2003). An estimated nine out of ten doctors depicted in the famous set of medical thankas from seventeenth-century Lhasa are monks. The others are male lay doctors (I have found no records of female doctors in these paintings). Despite the iconic image of monks studying and practicing medicine, monks and monasteries actually played a relatively minor role (compared to the Medical Houses) in providing Tibetan medical treatment in Ngamring during the 1940s and 1950s, especially to the laity. Although scholars have assumed female doctors to have been absent, new findings show that local nuns studied and practiced medicine and that their learning and work differed from those of monks and lay men and women doctors. Politics and religion were tightly connected in the Tibetan state administered by the Lhasa Ganden Phodrang government in the 1940s and 1950s. State health campaigns, such as one focused on child health, however, exerted limited influence on health care provision in Tsang.

RELIGION, MEDICINE, AND PUBLIC HEALTH IN THE GANDEN PHODRANG STATE

Modernity, Michel Foucault (1973, 1977, 1980, 1981) argued, requires new forms of governance that rely less on coercive mechanisms of control but more on new apparatuses, including hospitals, prisons, and schools, which produce new knowledge and truth about the body and its sexuality, movement, and so on. The role of hospitals and medicine for asserting and dispersing knowledge and power in modern and colonial nation-states in Asia has been acknowledged and theorized in this vein (e.g., Arnold 1993). Yet we know little about Tibetan modernisers' use of such new forms of control in building modern Tibet under the Thirteenth Dalai Lama and his government.

In the early twentieth century, concerns of the Dalai Lama and the Lhasa government over the health of its citizens began to be expressed in new ways. Their most visible expression was the 1916 founding of the Mentsikhang, the Institute of Medicine and Astrology in Lhasa. Its mission, in contrast to the monastic Chakpori College, was to train doctors from and for geographically and socially diverse constituencies, including doctors from the secular aristocracy and the Tibetan army. Other widely documented reforms and institution building of the time included the modernization of the Tibetan army, tax reforms, and installation of telecommunications. These are generally considered to have been at the height of their implementation and experimentation between 1913 and 1923, with many measures intimately linked to British involvement.[2]

An important reform of that era was the Lhasa Mentsikhang's child health campaign. This early twentieth-century initiative was intended for rural areas and mirrored similar initiatives in other rising nation-states in Asia in that period. Republican-era China and Japan promoted public health under the terms of *weishang* and *eisei* and established biomedical clinics, health stations, and dispensaries, and carried out public health and vaccination campaigns (Rogasky 2004; Furth and Leung 2010). The production of health statistics in the context of medical work rose to importance at these historical moments in other modernizing (and colonizing) nations. All this was absent, however, from Tibet's modernization project, despite or perhaps because of the British efforts in spreading Western medicine and carrying out vaccination campaigns in Tibet (McKay 2007). Indigenous efforts were less comprehensive, relied almost entirely on key Tibetan medical and Buddhist ideals, and remained largely limited to Lhasa and its surroundings.

Lay Tibetan *amchi* and Medical Houses enjoyed partial or entire tax exemption, while monastic doctors received provisions for their medical training and practice either from the monasteries or from lay donations. But with few exceptions doctors did not work directly for the centralized state, or for that matter organize themselves into nationwide or even regional governmental or private professional associations. Medicine has, however, been used at times to expand the power and knowledge of the Tibetan Buddhist state and its central government institutions. Both Buddhist and medical notions of self and self-control were crucial in the continued transition from pre-Buddhist to Buddhist notions of self and nation in Tibet (Adams 1992).

TIBETAN MEDICINE TO BUILD AND SERVE THE NATION

From 1916 to 1924 the Mentsikhang, upon the initiative of two Buddhist monk-physicians and supported by the Thirteenth Dalai Lama, spearheaded a lesser-known reform of the newly modernizing Tibetan government, the so-called child health care campaign.[3] Van Vleet has argued in her study of this campaign that, in stark contrast to such campaigns in surrounding regions of the period, it drew on indigenous modes of conceiving and promoting child health in Tibetans' newly forming ideas of governance and national prosperity (Van Vleet 2010/11).

This program began in 1916, when the Thirteenth Dalai Lama issued an edict to implement this postnatal health care program based on the medical manual *On Childcare: Treasure of the Heart Benefiting Beings* (*Byis pa nyer spyod 'gro phan nying nor*; Van Vleet 2010/11), commonly known as *Treasure of the Heart*. This text had been written the same year by the Dalai Lama's most senior personal physician, Jampa Tupwang (d. 1922), who from 1913 had served as Chikhyap Khenpo, the highest monk official and head of the monastic branch of the Tibetan government in Lhasa. The program aimed to distribute eight compounded medicines "to the family of every child newly born within the Lhasa Government's jurisdiction" (Van Vleet 2010/11: 354). Accompanying these was advice for rituals and childcare during the first year of life, and the directive that a natal horoscope be issued for each infant. These horoscopes were to be created by the Mentsikhang, under the directorship of Jampa Tupwang's student, Khyenrap Norbu (Van Vleet 2010/11: 354).

In the medical collections of *amchi* discussed so far, I did not come across copies of the *Treasure of the Heart* or hear any living memories of the campaign. The absence of sources makes it difficult to ascertain where and whom the child health campaign reached, especially in the outlying Tibetan areas and among those not in direct communication with the Lhasa government. Yet the related documents clearly show how the Thirteenth Dalai Lama, high-ranking politicians, and doctors conceived of Tibetan medicine during building of the Tibetan nation-state. They also indicate how these efforts reframed and reformulated certain areas of Sowa Rigpa's largely elite medical knowledge: with the help of short, mass-printed texts that were easy to distribute widely, medical and astrological knowledge could reach a far greater audience than had the classic, usually bulky medical literature.

Another text published in the context of the child health campaign was *Mirror of the Moon: Methods of Giving Birth Helpful for All* (*Byis pa btsa' thabs kun phan zla ba'i me long*) by Khyenrap Norbu and published in 1924 (figure 2.1). I found a printed copy and a fragmented handwritten copy in the collections of *amchi* from Tsang. Similar to *Treasure of the Heart*, this text relies on key concepts in Tibetan physiology and classical works, yet also summarizes them to make this knowledge understandable to a much wider readership. Especially notable is the author's address to pregnant women (Hofer 2011c). For the first time, the text acknowledges women as sources of knowledge for the book, pointing to "the wise women of Tibet who have given birth" as authoritative sources for ways to support women in childbirth (Hofer 2011c). It also mentions five unnamed medicines, referred to as "medicine number 1" and so on, suggesting that the text was given out with numbered ready-made medicines, akin to *Treasure of the Heart*. This indicates another substantial deviation from the common pattern, in which Tibetan medicines made by *amchi* were named rather than numbered. These childcare and childbirth medicines

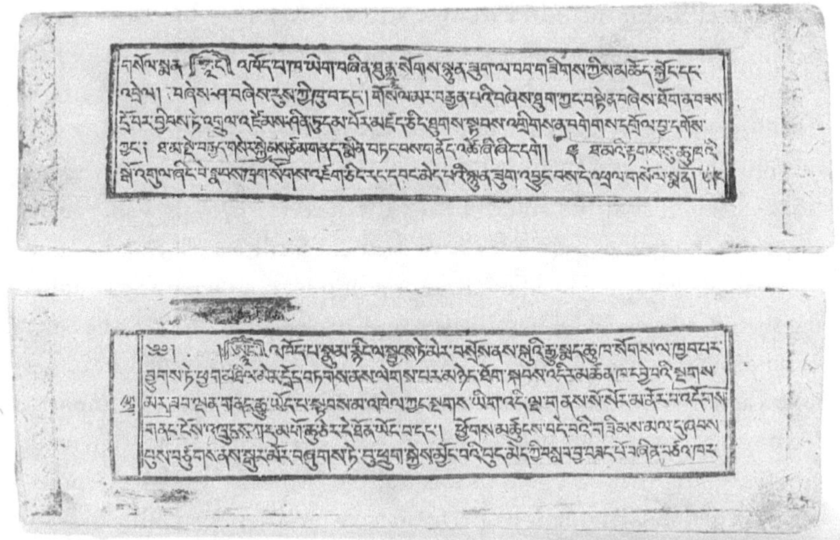

FIGURE 2.1. *Mirror of the Moon* text on how to assist women in childbirth, by Khyenrap Norbu. Private collection of the author.

must have been produced on a large scale, perhaps indicating the earliest known manufacture of Tibetan medicines.

Government support of the child health campaign, or possibly that related to the childbirth text, was ultimately insufficient (Van Vleet 2010/11). The campaign's contribution to forming new subjectivities among ordinary Tibetans and fostering their sense of belonging and citizenship in a modern "imagined community" remained limited.

Clearly the Tibetan government under the Thirteenth Dalai Lama made distinct attempts to promote health care and medical provisions in ways that legitimized new forms of modern Tibetan governance and reproduced indigenous medical ideas. These ideas were quite different from those of the British political mission, present in Tibet between 1904 and 1947, and its medical mission. The British approach was wholly dedicated to the promotion of modern biomedical clinics and dispensaries, staffed mainly by Indian Medical Services (IMS) doctors (McKay 2007). These Western medical clinics and their doctors, although well attended for certain conditions, were hampered by insufficient backing from the Tibetan government, and were thus unable to provide the full range of public health and medical care the British envisioned for Tibet (which were effectively implemented in India and China at the time). There were rare instances, however, when private efforts by Tibetan political and Buddhist hierarchs complemented the British medical endeavors.

Political scientist Charles Cassinelli and missionary Robert Ekvall (1969) recount that the ruler of Sakya was concerned, probably in the 1940s, by the inadequacy of Sakya's medical facilities. At first he sponsored a convention of local medical practitioners in the hope of improving their methods, but it had "little result" (324). Then, in 1941, the Sakya Tri'chen, Ngawang Thuthob Wangchuk (1900–1950), decided to undertake a smallpox vaccination campaign using vaccines privately imported from India. Some of his people were opposed to the use of "foreign medicine," arguing that vaccination was not the "Tibetan way." In response, the Tri'chen had divinations performed, which supported his plans to vaccinate the people of Sakya, and "officers and others with manual dexterity, including members of the royal family, were taught to perform the operation. They then vaccinated the entire population of Sa sKya [Sakya] proper, who were gathered by headmen and District Officers at convenient spots." The campaign, according to the authors, "met no serious resistance from the subjects, and it was a success" (Cassinelli and Ekvall 1969: 324).[4]

Although several leading Tibetan medical physicians, among them government politicians and the director of the Mentsikhang, were open to using vaccinations, the Tibetan government at that time never funded vaccination campaigns or biomedical facilities from its own budget. Financing of the biomedical facilities was left almost entirely to the British, and only a few private shops in the markets of Lhasa and Shigatse sold Western medicines (McKay 2007, 2011). Tibetans in most rural areas of Tsang, in villages like Gye and Lhünding, with the medical pluralism prevalent there in the 1940s and 1950s, were largely unaffected by the efforts of either Lhasa or the British missions to provide public health and child health care or Western medicines. To my knowledge there were no local vaccination campaigns like the one carried out in Sakya. The Mentsikhang's mission to increase lay or monk physicians in outlying areas led only to a minute increase in doctors serving peripheral areas. Until the early 1960s, when the People's Liberation Army and Chinese medical personnel began to be sent farther afield and local Tibetans started to be trained in Western medical methods and techniques, local lay and monastic doctors continued their work.

MONASTIC MEDICINE ON THE MARGINS

There is no evidence from my research in Ngamring that "every main monastery" had a doctor in the 1940s and 1950s (Clifford 1994) or that the Lhasa-initiated child health and childbirth campaign left any visible traces there. When a monastery did have a doctor, he provided medical treatment mainly to the monastery's resident monk population or trained monastic and sometimes lay doctors in medicine. Less commonly they also treated the laity, especially in the large establishments. The practicing nuns more or less followed this pattern.

Prior to the reforms, Ngamring Dzong was home to an estimated forty to sixty monastic institutions and communities representing all Buddhist denominations as well as the Bon religion. To my knowledge, and contrasting with the situation in Republican and early Communist China, there were no surveys of traditional medical practitioners prior to the reforms.[5] I talked to a number of elders in five districts in Ngamring as well as all the abbots of the more than fifty monasteries that had been (re)built by 2003, after their destruction in the 1960s.[6] The few establishments that had a resident medical practitioner prior to the 1960s were smaller monasteries and those of the Nyingma school. *Amchi*, whether lay or Buddhist, were generally few and far between, partly due to the scattered residences and small size of Tibetan villages.

The largest Gelugpa monastery in the area, Ngamring Chöde (home to four hundred monks), with an attached village of about thirty lay households (mainly serving the *dzong* administrators and the monastery), had no monks trained in medicine. This was despite its strong earlier ties to Jangpa Namgyel Drazang, his Jang medical tradition, and the royal sponsorship of Sowa Rigpa (Hofer 2012). When a monk fell ill, either religious observances and rituals were performed or, in certain cases, a lay *amchi* was called to diagnose and treat him. Only in the early 1950s did Ngamring Chöde receive an order from the Lhasa government recruiting monks from large Gelugpa monasteries for training at the Lhasa Mentsikhang. Lobsang Duden, the oldest monk of the monastery with personal experience of the time (he was treasurer of the monastery in the

1950s), remembered that two monks were recruited for studies in Lhasa. For eight years he sent payments to the capital for their expenditures. He also recalled paying *amchi*s when they were called to treat monks at the monastery. Another elderly man, who had served the *dzong* as a *yokpo* (servant) and lived in the lay hamlet in Ngamring, remembered never having consulted a professional doctor prior to the 1960s, relying entirely on home care and Buddhist prayers and offerings.

I found no evidence in Ngamring that "every monastery in Tibet had an *amchi*," or that in Tibet a "public health care system was in place" (Clifford 1994: 61). Yet Lobsang Duden and others summarized the availability of *amchi* in Ngamring as such: "Every *lungpa* [place] had its own *amchi*," referring to the presence of both lay and ordained Sowa Rigpa practitioners, including in Medical Houses and monasteries. Who were these *amchi* at monasteries and nunneries, how did they study, and whom did they treat?

Nyingma Practitioners as Doctors

Tutob Gyeltsen was the elderly abbot of the Nyingma monastery Chaug Gonpa in the far northern part of Mü Valley, which I visited twice. He had learned medicine from one of his Buddhist masters who was also a doctor, and complemented those instructions with extensive independent study. Alongside empowerments, transmissions, and practical instruction in Buddhist teachings, Pema Kelsang gave Tutop Gyeltsen the *wang* to study the *Four Treatises*, which he memorized over a ten-year period. He also studied several other medical texts and was initiated into medico-Buddhist practices, such as the Yuthog Heart Essence and others. In addition, he was instructed in the practical skills of pulse diagnosis, medicine preparation, and moxibustion, and given *menngak* relating to medical compounding techniques and empowerment of medicines (*mendrup*). Tutop was thus considered by his teacher to hold Pema Kelsang's medical teaching lineage and allowed to pass it on to his students. There were no formal examinations during his ten-year studies. The most important thing in becoming an accomplished *amchi* was to attain positive outcomes of treatment after substantial practical experience. Once this happened, Tutop stopped consulting his teacher and practiced independently, partly necessitated by his transfer to a different monastery.

Key to Tutop's acquisition of some of the medical and Buddhist practices was his access to medical works held in the various monasteries where he stayed at the time, as well as those kept by his teacher. Despite the widespread destruction and personal attacks on Tutop Gyeltsen during the Communist reforms, in the 1970s he managed to recover several medical texts that he had hidden at the beginning of the reforms. These included a block-printed copy of the *Four Treatises*, medical manuscripts, and a handwritten collection of recipes, on which he based many of his medical formulas without following them rigorously. He in turn instructed a student in these works and in the practices he had learned from his teacher.

Pharmaceuticals were, however, only one component of the way he treated patients. As a lama he also imparted religious blessings (*shabden*), did puja, and distributed sacred pills made during monastic and public rituals—referred to as *mani rilbu* and *tseri* (short for *tsering rilbu*, or "long-life pills"). Such pills were not made according to medical standards, but consisted mainly of *tsampa* and some herbs, their efficacy deriving from blessings and mantras said over them at the monastery during rituals of several days or weeks, including public long-life empowerment rituals and personal meditative practices of the monks. Blessed substances were later distributed to lay people and deemed to bring long life when taken as a general preventive against illness or worn as protection.

Tibetan medicines, in contrast, were compounded from a wide range of local and foreign ingredients, then given out sparingly and in small doses after consultations. Lay patients made offerings of food, money, and dried medical plants for treatments, and Tutop treated whoever needed it, whether or not they could pay. Monks did not usually offer much in return for medicines. Tutop's rationale of treatment identified about a fourth of all conditions to be treatable by *men* (medicine). During one of my visits to this monastery in 2007, Yonten Tsering explained how the *Four Treatises* set out a related etiology and this sort of rationale for treatment. This had been commonly followed before Communist reforms complicated the relation of what medicine or other kinds of approaches could treat:

> In the *Gyüshi* there is a differentiation of the existing 404 kinds of diseases into four groups. The first 101 are called *kundagi dönné*,[7] the second 101 *shenwang ngöngyiné*,[8] the third 101 *yongdrub tseginé*,[9] and the fourth 101 *lanang tralkyiné*.[10] For the first group of illnesses there will be no benefit from medical treatment; instead what is required are prayers or pujas to the Medicine Buddha and to perform religious activities. The reason is

> that these illnesses are caused by the *dön* or spirits.[11] So for these [illnesses] puja will be more effective. The diseases of the second group come from previous lives. So again for these, whatever medicine you take, there will be no benefit. However large and good the clinic you go to, or expert a doctor you see, there is no benefit. Again, here puja and religious activities will give the best benefit. However, for the third category, a puja will show no great benefit, but for the illnesses in this group, you need to take medicines, whatever kind: Tibetan or Chinese. So, let's say you have *chuser*; then you need to take medicine for this disease. For the diseases of the fourth type, even without medicine and *shabden* you will get better, all on your own. If you do take medicine the recovery may be easier, like when someone falls down he or she can stand up on his or her own, but it will be easier if someone helps them. This was our old custom in Tibet; religion and politics were joined. People's efforts in getting better comprised medicine [*men*] and doing religion [*chö*].

Tutop Gyeltsen was reluctant to talk much about how he continued to apply his treatments according to his judgment of the root of a patient's condition when I visited in 2003 and we didn't know each other well. However, four years later, I spoke with a younger monk at his monastery who recounted several examples:

> A few years ago, there was a girl who tried everything for her illness. She had fallen sick a long time ago, and all three doctors in the area were consulted. Then, at last she came to see Tutop-la [the abbot]. He checked her urine and said, "You have a *dön* in your body. First we need to kick out this *dön*. After that, the medicines will work." She had a problem with her intestines and always had diarrhea, and there had been no effect from medicines. She had received *tangmen* as well as Tibetan medicine, both Communist and Tibetan medicine from three different people.

"So she was cured?" I asked. "Yes, she was cured. First they needed to make an effigy, and then a brief puja was held to remove the *dön* into the effigy. We held the *peja* onto the *dön*, subdued it, did some prayers and meditation, and offered the *dön* to the *Yidam*. Then she took Tibetan medicine prescribed by our abbot and got better." The Buddhist training and context in which Tutop had been educated and still practiced provided him with the ability to advise and act upon a given diagnosis in a more flexible manner than most lay *amchi*. Into the 1940s and 1950s, lay *amchi* acknowledged the diverse origin of illnesses found in medical texts, and commonly recommended that patients seek out Buddhist lamas and practices for conditions they judged beyond their ability to influence through their own Sowa Rigpa treatments.

The authority of the Medicine Buddha for doctors and patients was universally accepted, whether in a monastic or lay environment. Doctors paid their respects to the Medicine Buddha as the teacher of the *Four Treatises*, and he was the object of prayers and practices for both doctors and patients. Patients mainly related to the Medicine Buddha through offerings and prayers, the story widely known that the Medicine Buddha had made a vow that he would forever heal sick people and those with physical deformities (Dorje 2014). Doctors tried to emulate the Medicine Buddha in their way of relating to patients. Such practices changed dramatically during the reforms, and many were reluctant to speak openly to me about the subject, even long after religious practice had regained state sanction in 1979. This was especially so in government hospitals.

The boundaries between various kinds of medicines or benefits (*penpa*) and what is today considered quintessential Sowa Rigpa treatment (i.e., pharmaceuticals) were much more fluid among monk-doctors before the start of the Communist campaigns. This extended also to broader ideas beyond the body-mind and one lifetime, through notions of karma and spirits needing to be placated and remedied through combined medical and Buddhist practices, as Tutop's work and formation show.

Because the monasteries where Tutop lived and trained prior to the reforms were small, he treated lay patients as well as fellow monks and occasionally nuns. There were many interactions between him and the lay population because of the monastery's role in rituals for lay people, and medical practice was quite naturally another way to interact with lay people from surrounding areas.

Bonpo Medical Practitioners

In 2007 I met and interviewed the eighty-four-year-old Amchi Rabgyal in northern Ngamring. His training shows that multiple authorities for medical knowledge and practice existed in Ngamring's monasteries, including sources such as the *Bumshi* (the Bonpo equivalent of the Buddhist *Four*

Treatises) and its commentaries by renowned Bonpo masters. Like Tutop's, Amchi Rabgyal's training and work showed little influence from the developments in medical training at the Chakpori and Mentsikhang in Lhasa, and they differed from mainstream medical practice that relied on the *Four Treatises.*

Rabgyal lived about three hundred kilometers northwest of Tsatsé township in Nyingo *xiang*, a sparsely inhabited region where even administrative townships of large districts housed populations of just one hundred people. Inhabitants relied mainly on pastoralism, herding yak and sheep, and on trade. The sacred Tarko of the North Mountains dominates this astoundingly beautiful area, with large turquoise lakes and snow-capped mountain ranges rising over six thousand meters. Tarko of the North is a powerful mountain deity and the most important patron of the spirit mediums of the area who invoke him (Bellezza 2005: 22; Diemberger 2005).

Born in 1923, Rabgyal became a monk when he was about fourteen years old. He joined one of the four Bonpo monasteries on the shore of Dangra Yumtso Lake.[12] His medical and religious teacher there was Patzul Rinpoche,[13] who taught him Sowa Rigpa for two years and had been a student of Khyungtrul Jigmé Namkhai Dorjé, a famous Bonpo lama, scholar, and doctor (Millard 2009, 2013; Kværne 1998). Patzul Rinpoche instructed Rabgyal and four others; some focused more on medicine and others predominantly on astrology. After Patzul Rinpoche left the monastery to help with the establishment of Jigmé Namkhai Dorjé's Gurgyam Monastery in Ngari, a lama and *amchi* from the Kham region took over responsibility for teaching Rabgyal and his fellow classmates in medicine and astrology. Khyungtrul still occasionally visited the monastery.

The main medical text used was the Bonpo work known as the *Bumshi.* Rabgyal memorized large parts of the *Bumshi* and received the empowerment and reading transmission, as well as practical instructions by Khyungtrul Jigmé Namkhai Dorjé during one of his visits. In 1942, at nineteen, Rabgyal completed his medical and religious studies and soon after left the monastery to become a wandering mendicant monk, going on pilgrimage and conducting prayers and rituals in exchange for food. He lived this life for about ten years before opting to leave the order. During that time he studied Khyungtrul's comprehensive four-volume commentary on the *Bumshi*, the *Khyungtrul Menpé* (*Khyung sprul sman dpe*), published in 1949, of which he obtained a copy. When we met, Rabgyal held copies of this text, as well as several medical manuscripts, many of them on compounding.

It is remarkable that Rabgyal could study the *Bumshi*, which he and his teachers considered as the precursor of the *Four Treatises*. Rabgyal's good fortune can be explained by his monastery and teacher being at the forefront of the revival of Bonpo medicine under Khyungtrul, giving him privileged access to the *Bumshi* and its commentary.[14] These Bonpo medical works were not widely available, even among *amchi* who were followers of Bon (Millard 2013). Many instead relied on the *Four Treatises* passed on in the Buddhist tradition, where this text is held to have been first taught by the Medicine Buddha and then promoted by Yuthog Yonten Gonpo. Bon followers, by contrast, consider the *Bumshi* to be the teaching of Shenrab Miwoche, the founder of their religion, and think it was later propagated by his student Tribu Trishi, making the *Bumshi* the precursor to the *Four Treatises*.

Rabgyal said there were well over a hundred different medicinal plants plus various minerals and wildlife that he had used in the preparation of medicines at the monastery. However, once he left he no longer had access to these because he lacked the funds. To make medicines in his repertoire, he needed to import ingredients from India and elsewhere, and this was very expensive. He remarked, "If you want to be an *amchi*, you need wealth. However much you may apply yourself in your studies and however much compassion you have, without finances you can't treat people."

None of the other *amchi* had been quite so explicit about the finances required for making medicine. Yet it was common for lay doctors to have a higher socioeconomic position and often to benefit from tax breaks. Monasteries received donations from the laity that could be used for medical raw ingredients. Through an unlikely coincidence of political and personal circumstances, Rabgyal eventually established his medical practice after the Communist reforms began.

— · —

Both Tutop and Rabgyal chose to study medicine out of personal interest. In both cases, kinship relations were not a prime consideration in the selection of students or teachers. They combined the study of medicine and Buddhism or Bon, and in line with the conventions of Buddhist and

Bonpo learning, their training emphasized the memorization of texts. Also in common with Buddhist learning, three elements were thought to complete a medical transmission: receiving the empowerment (*wang*) for a practice, listening to a teacher read a medical text (*lung*, often translated as "oral transmission"), and receiving instructions on how to do a practice described in the texts (*tri*).

After their training, the obligations of monk doctors were very different from those of lay *amchi*, whose work was influenced by social and financial concerns tied to the continuity and prosperity of Medical Houses. Tutop practiced medicine as part of his role as a Buddhist lama combining Buddhist and Sowa Rigpa healing, and using donations from his transactions with patients, he complemented locally available materia medica with traded foreign ingredients. Rabgyal, meanwhile, as a Bon mendicant monk and later a layman, was at first unable to practice as an independent *amchi* owing to lack of funds. The medical knowledge and skill gained prior to the 1960s by both of these *amchi* nonetheless weathered prolonged periods when they could not practice: for Rabgyal, when he was a mendicant monk and after leaving the order, and in Tutop's case, when as a monk and abbot he was labeled an exploiter of the poor during the Communist reforms.

BUDDHIST NUNS AS DOCTORS

I often discussed the topic of women's education in traditional and contemporary Tibet with one of my main interlocutors from Ngamring, the *amchi* Ngawang Dorjé. He was in an interesting position to do so. His sister had received a Buddhist and medical education as a nun in the 1950s, when this was by all accounts uncommon. His younger daughter was a biomedical health worker, and his son a Tibetan medical pharmacologist. Ngawang Dorjé's opinion was that before the 1960s the main way for women to gain a Tibetan medical education was by becoming a nun. Through this they could learn to read and write, and then seek out a teacher with medical knowledge while carrying on with their Buddhist practices. He held that if women inherited a family medical lineage, it would be weaker than one inherited by men and more easily lost. There are accounts in the literature of nuns practicing medicine, but very few.

Among the list of twelve Tibetan women doctors of the first half of the twentieth century that the exiled Tibetan scholar Tashi Tsering has compiled, two were definitely nuns: Taykhang Jetsunma Jampel Chodron (c. 1882–c. 1959), who bears the title Jetsunma (Venerable), and Do Dasel Wangmo, whom I personally interviewed. In addition, Khandro Yangga, who eventually became an expert in Tibetan medical cataract surgery, started out as a nun but then married and had children. Biographies of these three nun doctors and their teachers reveal that two were from Kham and one from central Tibet. They were born into wealthy families with a wide political or Buddhist network and all had accomplished doctors as close family members: Taykhang Jetsunma Jampel Chodron was the niece of Taykhang Jampa Tupwang (d. 1922; Tashi Tsering 2005), the Thirteenth Dalai Lama's personal physician and author of the *Treasure of the Heart*; Do Dasel Wangmo's mother was an accomplished physician in the medical lineage of the famous eastern Tibetan physician Mipham (Tupten Chödar 2008; Michalsen 2012);[15] and Khandro Yangga's grandfather was a doctor (Trinlé 2000; Tashi Tsering 2005). The two latter women had no brothers (like Sonam Drölma of the Nyékhang), and as such were likely to have been given better access to medical knowledge and received more encouragement than women in households with sons (Hofer 2015). All in all, these three women belonged to an exceptionally fortunate religious and political elite. They had kinship relations with medical practitioners, in most cases men, and these nuns thus gained medical teachings from Buddhist teachers in addition to medical training within the family. We cannot assume that other women who aspired to become doctors, or even received a medical education, were as likely to succeed under the usually less favorable conditions they found themselves in. At this point we cannot be sure whether Tibetan women doctors prior to the 1960s started more often as nuns or as lay women.

In Ngamring, I found out about three nuns who studied and practiced medicine prior to the reforms. What do their histories and social background add to our understanding and the seeming scarcity of nuns working as Tibetan medical doctors?

Ani Payang and Ani Ngawang

Ani Payang was a woman in her late sixties who at the time of my research lived in Lhasa, where I met up with her several times. Her two elder brothers also contributed their recollections in their Lhasa home.

Ani Payang was born into the Nyingkhang in Ngamring, into a family with a long-standing *ngakpa* tradition. Her father was a Nyingma practitioner in the *nyag thong* lineage, serving the Fourteenth Dalai Lama by carrying out major purification rituals once a year and smaller ones at other times. This family was well connected with an elite circle of Nyingma practitioners. For example, Ani Payang and her brothers and their father had been to an audience with the Fourteenth Dalai Lama upon his visit to Shigatse Dzong. Through her father's Buddhist networks, a lama from Kham named Kyemen Rinpoche[16] came to stay at the Nyingkhang in the 1940s. He gave Nyingma Buddhist teachings to her father and other local disciples. While there, the Rinpoche suggested that Ani Payang ordain as a novice nun and learn medicine from him. This was well received by all sides; her older brother recalled, "Kyemen Rinpoche said that although my sister was young she possessed good knowledge [*shérap*]. He thought she was intelligent [*changpo*] and that it would be good to teach her to become an *amchi*." Ani Payang added:

> I wanted to become an *amchi*. I thought that I would be able to cope with being in remote places, even if the Rinpoche took me all the way to Kham. That's what I thought. But in fact what happened was that although I liked studying, I couldn't manage. Because I was so young, I dearly missed my family and my brothers. I was soon given the nickname "Ten Thousand Tears" as I couldn't stop crying. Later my father got permission from the Rinpoche to take me back home.

The group of six nuns and two monks that Ani Payang had joined lived as disciples of the itinerant expert doctor Kyemen Rinpoche. Out of this group, Ani Ngawang gradually became Kyemen Rinpoche's main disciple. Little is known about Ani Ngawang's background. Ani Payang held that she served the Rinpoche over a long period and received many of his teachings, as well as gaining hands-on practice when he treated the patients who came to see him almost every day (except when he was on retreat). Ani Payang, by contrast, did not get far in her medical training, as she left for home after having taken the first steps in the study and memorization of the *Four Treatises*.

Contrary to assertions in medical texts that women are not allowed to attend or participate in certain phases of mercury processing (Dawa Ridak

2003: 420; Gerke, in preparation), Ani Payang and her two brothers were sure that Ani Ngawang had access to them. Among these was the making of *tsotel*, the production of mercury sulfide powder, an important ingredient in the *rinchen rilbu*, or precious pills, that Kyemen Rinpoche made. Ani Payang recalled:

> One time I remember they had made *tsotel*. I then received one *rinchen rilbu* made under the guidance of the Rinpoche. It was Rinchen Tsotru Dachel. I had heard that one of the precious pills was worth 100 *dotsé*.[17] Not many people could afford this, but the *kutra* [aristocrats] could. They could offer this kind of money to the Rinpoche, but common people received them without paying anything. These *rinchen rilbu* were so precious! After you ate them, your face would become chubby [*sha rgyags pa*] and a healthy radiance appeared [*mthangs chen po*]. These precious pills were very rare at the time. When I got mine, I gave it to my mother. Today, you can't find precious pills like that! Actually, the same with the Rinpoche's regular medicine—he didn't give much, sometimes just for two days, only a little bit, but it worked so well. This lama was really very different [*ma gcig pa*] and knowledgeable; it was a great blessing to stay with him.

As we can see from these accounts, Ani Payang and Ani Ngawang's teacher of Buddhism and medicine certainly did not think that women were unsuitable to become doctors or that they lacked the mental capacities for it. He had called Ani Payang "intelligent" (*changpo*), and he passed on the bulk of his medical knowledge mainly to nuns. Significantly, Ani Ngawang later taught medicine, including the making of *tsotel*, to both nuns and monks, who continue to practice and purify mercury according to the oral instructions of Khyemen Rinpoche and Ani Ngawang at Chiu Gonpa Tekcholing Nunnery in Nyémo today (figure 2.2).[18]

As in the case of Tutop and Rabgyal, there were no stated medical fees for consultations or medicines given by Kyemen Rinpoche and Ani Ngawang. They instead received donations and offerings from the laity, which in a Buddhist framework were understood to increase merit and ensure good karma, especially when given to a monk or nun.[19] Receiving medicines in this setting can be understood as another form of religious transaction between monks and nuns and the laity. Patients probably did not

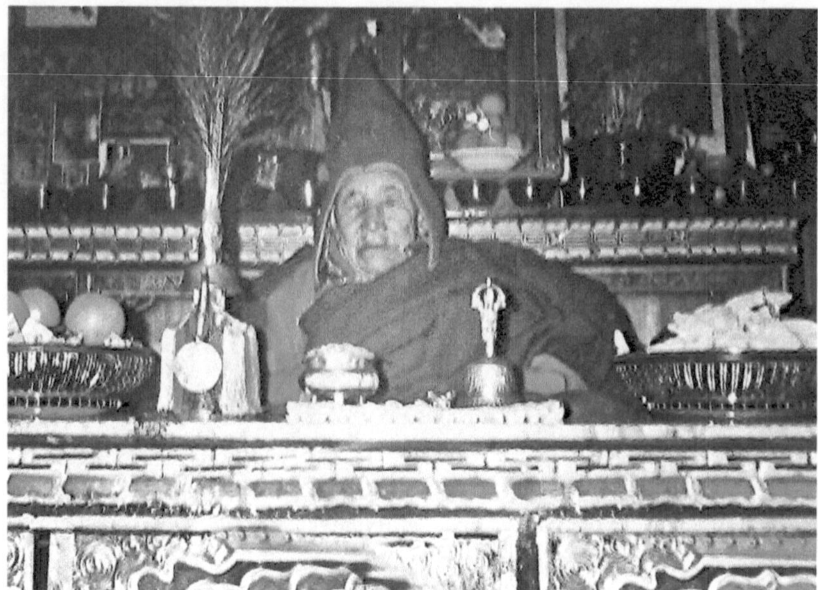

FIGURE 2.2. Ani Ngawang in old age at her nunnery in Nyémo. Source: Ani Payang.

think of medical treatment provided by monks or nuns as significantly different from other recompense they received in return for their offerings, such as blessings, blessed substances, and ritual services. That even people who could not afford to give large donations still received the extremely valuable *rinchen rilbu* is remarkable but also fits into the Buddhist framework, since some of the underlying principles of these pills are also common in Tibetan Buddhism. Understanding medical treatment as a part of Tibetan Buddhist interactions between monks and nuns and the laity, at least in the context of this Nyingma lama and his disciples, lends support to Geoffrey Samuel's (2012: 165) interpretation of Tibetan Buddhism as a "practical religion," with its main goal being the protection of communities and the good health and prosperity of its members.

Ani Pema Lhamo

At Pangyul Monastery in Ngamring, Ani Pema Lhamo (c. 1922–2005), a nun from Dewachen Nunnery, studied Sowa Rigpa with the abbot, Söpa-La. Dewachen Nunnery, with twenty nuns, was located a little farther up the valley from Pangyul Monastery, but it did not have its own practicing doctor or medical scholar. Both establishments practiced the Gelugpa school of Tibetan Buddhism.

Ani Pema Lhamo's training continued over many years and was not formalized, consisting mainly of memorization practices of the *Four Treatises* followed by practical experience through helping and asking questions. She had many opportunities to observe clinical work while serving the abbot of Pangyul over a long period. She was the abbot's niece, which perhaps explains their closeness. Ani Pema Lhamo was remembered by many lay people as well as her students in the valley of Pangyul Monastery. By all accounts, she was the abbot's only medical student and the only heir to his medical lineage. Upon his death, she received his medical texts, medicinal ingredients, and medicine-making equipment, such as grinding stones. Today these are held at the old site of Pangyul Monastery, the only material testimony to the medical activities at Pangyul and Dewachen in the 1940s and 1950s.

Among the works in the text collection are a number of practice-oriented treatises but no entire print or manuscript copy of the *Four Treatises*. A possible reason for its absence might be that the printed *Gyüshi* texts were bulky and more difficult to move or hide and had therefore been destroyed. Or perhaps the other texts were rarer and she went to greater lengths to hide them. In any case, the collection includes only one handwritten copy of a commentary on the third volume of the *Four Treatises*, a clinical handbook entirely dedicated to the etiology and pathology of named diseases and their diagnosis and treatment.

Most texts in the collection treated the compounding of medicines and included lists of recipes written by hand, with occasional annotations indicating adjustments. One four-page manuscript, for example, discusses the compounding of *khyung-nga*, or Garuda 5. The Tibetan name refers to the Garuda, the mythological bird widely venerated in Indic-influenced cultures in Asia. The manuscript features four charts listing the five raw ingredients for this drug: *aru*, *ruta*, *shudag*, *menchen*, and "*gli*" (short for *ladzi*). Each is allocated a function, as the "meat," "bones," "muscles," "heart," and "blood" of the medicine, a symbolic reference to the five components of the Garuda bird, who offered his body and power as medicine. This is an interesting document, as each list uses a slightly different order of ingredients and indicates a different quantity depending on availability (figure 2.3). If all ingredients from the first list are available, the medicine

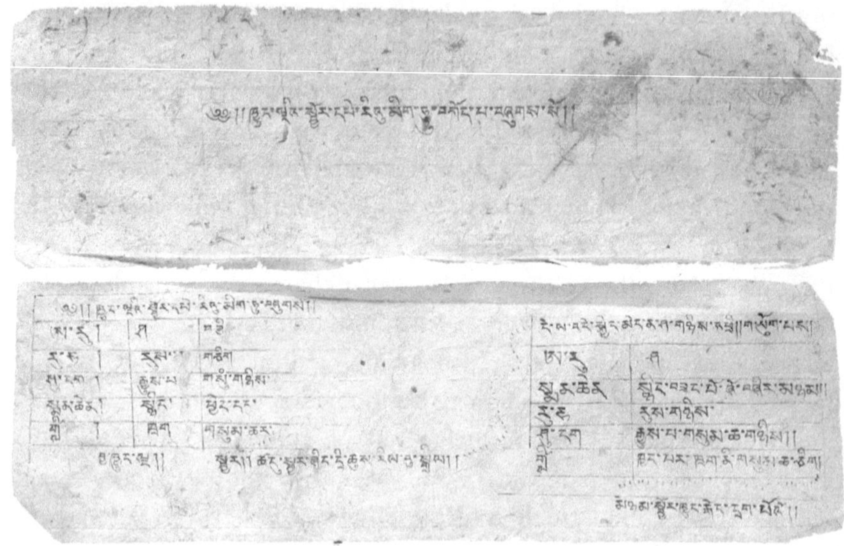

FIGURE 2.3. The section of a medicine compounding manuscript describing preparation of the Garuda bird medicine, *khyung-nga*. Photo by Meinrad Hofer.

would contain four units (*zho*) of *aru*, one of *ruta*, thirty-two of *shudag*, one-half of *menchen*, and one-third of "*gli*," or musk. In this compound *aru* is the only imported ingredient. As this ingredient must have been sometimes unavailable, one list shows the amounts of the other ingredients adjusted to compensate. None of the local ingredients was ever absent in any of the four charts, which is noteworthy especially with regard to musk, which is present only in tiny amounts in *khyung-nga* made today. Here it makes up one-third of the ingredients and hence is the "blood" of the compound. This underlines the perception of many *amchi* that while foreign ingredients were precious in the old days, the precious items are now the local ones, including musk.

Other medicines Lobsang, currently a monk at Pangyul, learned to make from Ani Pema Lhamo were *zhijé byed 6*, *tigta 8*, and *trültang*, which are all relatively basic medicines with few ingredients. These medicines are today regarded as classical formulas, mainly because they are mentioned in the third volume of the *Gyüshi*, and perhaps also because they are found in the pharmacological works of Khyenrap Norbu, which are still popular among many *amchi*. Ani Pema Lhamo's collection included one of Khyenrap Norbu's texts on medical compounding, the only printed manuscript.[20] It featured eighty-four medical compounds and has likely contributed to the current perception of many of these drugs as classical formulas. Here a work produced at the central medical institutes in Lhasa found its way into medical collections in peripheral Tibetan areas and added to the local "culture of recipes." Whatever the origin and materiality of the texts, the production of medicines was characterized by great fluidity in almost every regard: names, amounts, and ratios of ingredients in suggested preparations could all be adjusted to changing social, environmental, economic, and clinical circumstances.

Because Ani Pema Lhamo came from an aristocratic family and was the head nun of Dewachen Nunnery, she endured great hardship during the successive Communist reforms, as she refused to leave the order. Just before the large-scale destruction of religious objects and texts began, she entrusted the treasured medical texts to two junior monks, one of whom I met and interviewed. He recounted how he had hidden four bags of books and thankas, burying them in an old house behind some junk. He returned the texts to Ani Pema Lhamo when she began to reestablish Dewachen Nunnery in the early 1980s, and then began studying medicine with her. The monk recalled that her knowledge of local plants helped them through the years when all went hungry due to the failure of the communes and local production teams. They were regularly excluded from communes and production teams after refusing to publicly confess their "wrongs," including the exploitation of poor people. Both monks had learned how to compound a few simple drugs from local medicinal plants, enough to care for common illnesses among the monastic community. They could not, however, import any ingredients to make medicines.

Notable in Ani Pema Lhamo's story is her teacher's choice to transmit his medical knowledge and medical collection exclusively to a woman when he had many potential male heirs to his lineage. Lobsang explained that it was because she was a relative and he believed she was intelligent, worthy to be taught Sowa Rigpa.

Despite widespread Tibetan preconceptions regarding the lower mental capacities of women, Ani Pema Lhamo was remembered fondly by many of the *amchi* I met from the area and lay people in the valley, especially for treating patients from all social backgrounds. Yonten Tsering confirmed that she treated many patients but pointed out that "she was not a very scholarly [*khépa*] *amchi*." He characterized her teacher, however, as "very scholarly." These comments are interesting because I heard several times that woman *amchi* were sometimes described as "not scholarly," while this criticism was never leveled against male *amchi* (Hofer 2015).

— · —

Together, the life stories and work of Ani Ngawang, Ani Payang, and Ani Pema Lhamo show that male Buddhist teachers passed on medical knowledge to female disciples and nuns in Tsang. Moreover, in two cases they chose women as principal heirs to their medical lineages, even when male monks and disciples could have received that privilege. Why was this the case? Without fuller knowledge of these teachers and their students, we can only estimate that either they were exceptional men and women, or that, at least in Ani Pema Lhamo's case, the kinship relation with her teacher made the difference. This would apply to the three better-known women *amchi* who studied medicine as nuns, but not Ani Payang or Ani Ngawang.[21]

The nuns discussed so far were not ordinary nuns. Ani Payang, like the three women discussed in the literature, hailed from a well-situated family with an extensive Buddhist and social network and financial means. None of the female Tibetan medical doctors known to us so far was from a low-ranked family. It seems likely that the elite social status of those female Tibetan medical doctors whose records have reached us today eclipsed gender as a defining category in terms of women's perceived (lower) mental ability and ideas related to women inheriting medical lineages and knowledge.

These cases from Tsang confirm Ngawang Dorjé's opinion that being a nun gave a woman potential access to medical knowledge and perhaps made it easier to succeed as a doctor. Ordination opened the road to literacy, teachers, and texts, and it freed women from looking after households, husbands, and children. They could devote more attention to their training, practice, and the labor-intensive work of collecting and making medicines. Still, the nuns from Ngamring who worked as doctors were sometimes not perceived as the equals of male doctors and were considered by some to be "not very scholarly."

Our knowledge of the number of Tibetan women doctors and the details of their lives is still very limited. This is partly due to their absence from the textual record, difficulties in personal access, and the fact that many are elderly or deceased. Yet even in recent times, when women have come to constitute the majority of Tibetan medical students and a substantial proportion of practitioners, very little is known about what has changed in the way they live and work and how they think about many aspects of their medical tradition. With few notable exceptions (e.g., Craig 2012), the expanding anthropology of Tibetan medicine has missed highlighting gendered constructions of Tibetan medical theory and practice. To rebalance this situation, we need to address the expectations and beliefs that Tibetan people have projected onto men and women, and what this has meant for the medical domain.

Some traditional limitations for women in accessing education and medical training were denounced by Communist reformers eager to promote gender equality of a Maoist hue. Communist newspapers in 1963 claimed that "it was almost impossible for a woman to learn Tibetan medicine in the old society" (Union Research Institute 1968: 592). This was part of a campaign to promote the work of the female doctor Khandro Yangga at the Lhasa Mentsikhang (Adams and Dovchin 2001). Her recognized specialty was eye surgery. However, when women's and children's health came onto the Communist health care agenda, she was removed from the Department of Eye Medicine at the Mentsikhang and made head of a newly founded Department for Women and Children's Health (Hofer 2011a: 112–13), in accordance with another set of gendered expectations.[22]

Small Gelugpa and Nyingma monasteries and Buddhist teachers in peripheral areas in Tsang sometimes treated lay patients as part of their Buddhist practice and transmitted medicine to the next generation. These smaller establishments and independent teachers were more willing to teach adept female Buddhist and medical disciples, as compared to the large Gelugpa medical institutes run by the Tibetan government or Tashilhunpo Monastery in Shigatse. These did not, with the exception of Khandro Yangga, include female students in their official training programs.

EXPANDING BUDDHIST MEDICAL AUTHORITY IN TSANG

During the coexistence of Communist and Tibetan government structures in Lhasa, the Mentsikhang began to promote a socialist outlook and looked to increase patient numbers in line with the Communist mission to provide "medicine to the masses" (cf. Janes 1995). At the same time, the Panchen Lama's Tashilhunpo Monastery in Shigatse chose to expand Buddhist authority in the training of medical doctors.

Tashilhunpo was the largest monastery in Tsang and the fourth largest in Central Tibet, housing over three thousand monks. It was the primary landholder in Tsang and maintained close ties to all Gelugpa monasteries there, appointing abbots and offering higher degrees of monastic learning.[23] Despite recurrent tensions between the Dalai Lama and the Panchen Lama—not least a tax dispute that led to the exile of the Ninth Panchen Lama from 1923–24 to his death in 1937 and initially the exile of his successor as well—Tashilhunpo Labrang and Monastery retained great political and religious influence in Tsang into the 1940s and 1950s. Tashilhunpo exerted a thus far unrecognized but important influence in Tsang by training lay and monastic students in Sowa Rigpa. This monastery thus imparted Buddhist and medical authority to male doctors from the region, and it was attended by several *amchi* from Ngamring whom I interviewed.

The Tenth Panchen Lama and Kikinaka Medical School

Efforts to mobilize indigenous means to improve health care in the region had been negligible under the Panchen Lamas, though they promoted medical scholarship and a few doctors at Tashilhunpo took on students and treated patients.[24] This changed under the Tenth Panchen Lama, Lobsang Trinlé Lhundrub Choekyi Gyeltsen (1938–1989). In 1952 his advisers had secured the Panchen Lama's political influence in the region with the help of the Chinese Communist Party (CCP) and settled the tax dispute with the Fourteenth Dalai Lama (Goldstein 2007). In April 1952 the Panchen Lama, age fourteen, traveled to Tashilhunpo Monastery for the first time for formal Buddhist training. While holding important offices in the new CCP political organizations in Beijing, he became known for some unexpected undertakings. Tibetan historian Jamyang Norbu writes that the Panchen Lama "realized that the antiquated system of administrative and ceremonial functions, which was still in place in Tashilhunpo at that time, was inadequate for the challenges of the modern world. Thus, in 1956, he opened Chensel Labdra to three hundred students from his estates. The school featured a revolutionary curriculum; it included Tibetan,

Hindi, and Chinese language, photography, driving, horseback riding, and shooting" (Norbu 1997: xxv). In addition, the Panchen Lama formalized a medical school at Tashilhunpo in 1954, locating it in a small park called Kikinaka,[25] southeast of the main monastic premises, naming it Kikinaka Medical School.[26] The exact intentions of the Panchen Lama and his advisers remain unknown, but, given his position, he and his advisers must have been aware of contemporary controversies over the role of Chinese medicine in health care provision in the PRC.

Policies in the early years of the PRC, between 1949 and 1954, included efforts to improve Chinese medical practitioners through Western medical training, the unification of Western and Chinese medicine, and a campaign known as Western Medical Practitioners Study Chinese Medicine (Taylor 2005). Although Mao was initially not a supporter of Chinese medicine, in 1953–54 he accused the Ministry of Health several times of neglecting the role of Chinese medicine in forming a "new medicine" that could be used widely and efficiently throughout the PRC (Taylor 2005; Scheid 2002; Fang 2012). It might be no coincidence, therefore, that in 1954 the Panchen Lama established a new Tibetan medical school.

However, Kikinaka had no classes in Western medicine nor were any attempts made to change the Tibetan medical curriculum to reflect Mao's efforts to form a single medicine (based on the principles of dialectical materialism) rather than two separate medicines. At this time there were no statements from either central or regional authorities regarding the fate of Tibetan medicine in the Communist health campaigns for central Tibet. Given the Panchen Lama's role in the Gelugpa hierarchy, his initiative to establish Kikinaka was likely an appropriate move: Sowa Rigpa was considered one of the ten Buddhist sciences, the Chakpori Medical College is a Gelugpa monastery, and there were Menpa Trazangs, or medical colleges, attached to several major Gelugpa monasteries in eastern Tibet and Mongolia (Bolsokhoyeva 2007; Van Vleet 2014; Sabernig 2007, 2014). The eastern Tibetan monastic medical colleges, such as Kumbum and Labrang, were also likely known to the Panchen Lama. It is not known to what extent he might also have mirrored the early twentieth-century mission of the Mentsikhang in Lhasa: to expand outreach of government-sponsored medicine beyond the monastic elites to include lay students from the aristocracy, the army, and non-Gelugpa clergy.

Kikinaka Medical School: Curriculum and Reforms

The first class of students at Kikinaka was made up of fifty students, half of them monks, the other half lay students from medical families (Trinlé 2000: 558; Hofer 2012). This was a much larger group than those studying in conventional master-discipleships or Medical Houses. The forms and content of studies differed little, however, featuring memorization of the *Four Treatises*, study of some of its commentaries, hands-on learning of diagnostic techniques under the supervision of a master, medicine collection trips, and collective compounding, as well as some practical application of external therapies. Students were divided into groups, with each assigned three main teachers who had served as personal physicians to various Panchen Lamas.[27] Apart from common prayers to the Medicine Buddha each morning, the commonly received *wang* and *lung* to medical works, and the making of medicines, group activities were few, with all hands-on clinical instructions taking place in the residences of the teachers, who supervised and corrected students while seeing patients.

The only significant departure from training in both Medical Houses and teaching lineages for those who finished the entire course of study and memorized the whole of the *Four Treatises* was an official final exam in the presence of the Tenth Panchen Lama. At their graduation ceremony, successful candidates received a *bumrampa* degree, which was awarded to eight monks out of the fifty students. All were Gelugpa monks, who were expected to memorize more of the *Four Treatises* and work harder on the scholarly side of the training.

In the medical training program and medical practice at Tashilhunpo, Kikinaka made few concessions to modern ideas of how to organize teaching and medical work. The Mentsikhang in Lhasa, in contrast, enthusiastically implemented such adaptations in the 1950s (Janes 1995: 15–16). Under Khyenrap Norbu and his main student and Communist Party member, Jampa Trinlé, the Mentsikhang for the first time established a publicly accessible clinic rather than focusing only on medical training. Mentsikhang doctors were sent to rural areas around Lhasa to treat patients, and increasing patient numbers became a high political priority, as the institution was very aware that it would require the approval of the new rulers to dodge the "anti-feudal bullet" (Janes 1995; cf. Trinlé 2004, 2006). These efforts eventually paid off, and the Lhasa Mentsikhang was one of the few Tibetan government institutions to continue into the new regime of post-1959 reforms and Communist governance. Kikinaka's failure to adopt a similar approach probably contributed to its demise after the reforms began in earnest.

Most important, though, was the Panchen Lama's fall from grace with the CCP in the early 1960s, which ended his efforts in the medical domain, at least until the 1980s. In 1958 the school began discharging its students,[28] as Yonten Tsering recalled: "Our government was about to be reformed and restructured is what we were told, so my father came to take me back home. That's when they said that high-class children should go to school in China for education, but my father loved me so dearly and was afraid of me going to China. I really wanted to go . . . but he wouldn't let me. Instead, we went home and then took the opportunity to go on pilgrimage to India." Although the school reopened briefly in the early 1960s, in 1962 it closed entirely and its head teachers were imprisoned on charges of being "reactionaries" and "carriers of gods and spirits."

The fact that Kikinaka Medical School was set up solely for the study of Sowa Rigpa and no Tibetans from Tsang were trained in Western medicine during the first eight years of Communist rule reflects a unique juxtaposition of circumstances, differing substantially from other areas on the fringes of the PRC. The only Western medical establishment in Tsang at that time was the People's Liberation Army (PLA) hospital in Shigatse. It began to offer basic training only in the early 1960s, with the aim of sending health workers along with Communist work teams to remote parts of Tsang. There are no extant early written accounts of the work and local reception of PLA medical teams in Tsang. Their work is mentioned only in a few propaganda publications (e.g., Epstein 1983: 386–400; Strong 1959; China Tibet Information Centre 2005), where they are hailed as crucial agents in "winning over the masses" in rural areas. Doctors are discussed as carriers of revolutionary messages and work in the writings of Gayong, a Tibetan cadre from Rebgong, Zeku Township, Qinghai (translated into English and analyzed in Weiner 2012: 199–209).

The Outreach of Kikinaka Medical School in Tsang

Despite the relatively brief existence of Kikinaka Medical School, it trained dozens of *amchi* in Tsang and provided them with uniquely privileged training at Tashilhunpo, the most powerful Gelugpa institution in Tsang.

It increased the medical and Buddhist authority and credentials of doctors from both Medical Houses and monasteries, but not for nuns or lay women. Immediate results in Ngamring were that lay *amchi* like Yonten Tsering added to their family-based medical training, furthering expertise and practices, and that the local monastery of Samdrub Ganden now had Ngawang Dorjé as both a monk and a doctor. He obtained the *bumrampa* degree but had to leave the order when the Democratic Reforms began and attacks on the clergy increased.

During the integration of Tibetan medicine into official government health care institutions in rural areas in the 1970s and 1980s, both of these Tibetan doctors, as well as seventeen other graduates from Kikinaka whom I interviewed, would rise to the highest positions in the local governmental health bureaucracy system. These included the head of Shigatse Prefecture Health Bureau, the director of the Shigatse Mentsikhang (est. 1982), and directors of several local county People's Hospitals. Many of them played important roles in the revitalization of Tibetan medicine in government, private, and Buddhist educational initiatives, as well as in the institutionalization and expansion of Communist health care at county and township levels in Tsang.

In line with the efforts of the Lhasa Tibetan government and the Thirteenth Dalai Lama to support Tibetan medical practitioners and health care, the Panchen Lama's initiative in the 1950s fitted well with Tibetan rulers' efforts in the medical domain. This served not only to improve the health of the population but also to demonstrate benevolence toward their subjects, as is clear in the writing of the Thirteenth Dalai Lama, in the context of the child health care campaigns and others, which continued to link medicine with Buddhist tropes and institutions.

— · —

Tibetan medical practitioners in Tsang did not constitute a homogenous group with a single professional organization or body controlling their medical education and work. *Amchi* in most cases came from higher social classes, with lay *amchi* having access to land and gaining religious merit from their profession. Furthermore, whether lay or ordained, *amchi*s' status was enhanced by the identification of Sowa Rigpa as one part of the tenfold system of Buddhist learning and its propagation by the Medicine Buddha.

Members of some Medical Houses and some monks and nuns sought training from Buddhist masters. Within selected Buddhist and Bon institutions there existed medical lineages and practitioners, but only Kikinaka Medical School represented to some extent a shift from the traditionally limited transmissions to a small number of students prevalent in Tsang toward substantially expanding the number of doctors.

Although the Tibetan government in Lhasa attempted to improve health care beyond the capital through campaigns (especially the child health campaign), from what I can ascertain its activities reached only selected and probably elite members of society, namely administrators. Activities to improve health care on the margins were more piecemeal and ultimately were cut short either by the Tibetan government, in the case of the child health campaigns, or by political changes such as those that prompted the closure of Kikinaka. The Tashilhunpo Labrang and Sakya local political units in Tsang supported biomedicine only with regard to the smallpox vaccination campaigns. The British played an important role in the twentieth-century eradication of the disease in the area, through their medical clinics and activities in and around Gyantse, their rapport with the Tashilhunpo administration, and Sakya's direct import of drugs from India.

The measures taken by the Tibetan government in Lhasa and its prime medical institute, the Mentsikhang, to increase access to health care in the early twentieth century remained limited into the 1950s. To maintain that a public health system was in place in central Tibet in the 1950s, or even before the early 1970s, is an overstatement.[29] Through the de facto tax exemption for members of the threefold social substrata of *shabdrung*, *chödzé*, and *jedrung*, the Tibetan government indirectly supported medical practice among lay *amchi*. Over several generations members of these medical households created new, distinct medical traditions through their practice and engagement with teachers and texts. The forms of transmission may well have shared many basic tenets with those in Lhasa, but there were manifold local expressions. This was fostered through a variety of medical treatments, the compounding of drugs embedded in local "cultures of recipes," and prevalent diagnostic techniques passed on within Medical Houses and through oral instruction, hands-on learning, and direct instruction. It was largely due to local rather than national networks that there existed a situation where, in the words of one of my interviewees, "every *lungpa* had its own *amchi*."

Changes for *amchi* across the sociocultural spectrum, including Medical Houses, monasteries, and nunneries, began to gain momentum in Tsang in 1959–60 and increased during the subsequent socialist transformation and accompanying reforms to the rural Tibetan socioeconomic fabric. The shift in political circumstances drastically altered how Tibetans considered their own past. In the medical domain this required, for example, faithful repetition of an official discourse that held there had been no affordable medical care in "old Tibet," that it had been the sole preserve of the elites. This early experience of a new history regime continued to shape memories and stories among *amchi* I encountered, as well as contemporary biographical and autobiographical writing.

CHAPTER 3

NARRATIVE, TIME, AND REFORM

> Tibetan medicine is a medical science that comes from Tibetan people's experience of struggling with various diseases. It is an important achievement in the national medical treasure house. It should be improved. It needs to serve politics, people, and production.
>
> —Heizu Yang, chairman of Lhasa City Commission, 1961

> When the Democratic Reforms started, I could not continue to practice as an *amchi*. I was accused of being a representative of the exploiters' class.
>
> —Mentrong Rinchen, former *amchi* from Ngamring, 2003

ELDERLY Tibetan doctors in Tsang who experienced the first radical sociopolitical and economic Democratic Reforms beginning in 1959 were subjected to waves of destruction. The demise of *amchis*' medical authority was due mainly to their intrinsic ties with what the newly arrived CCP considered Tibetan "feudal elites," whose influence was to be undermined on the "road to socialism." Some Tibetan medical practitioners were able, however, to create spaces for their work within the new regime and continued against the odds. One doctor even started to practice at that time despite his previous high rank. Interwoven throughout accounts of this period are critical reflections on how successive regimes of state-enforced modes of remembering and narrating Tibet's past have shaped and are still influencing conflicting meanings and temporalities in their narratives. Whether such narratives can now be expressed or must remain silent today is a pertinent question (McGranahan 2010)—as is

TABLE 3.1. Timeline of key events and CCP reforms in Central Tibet, 1951–1976

1951–59	Gradualist approach to implementing reforms in (central) Tibet; United Front work to win over Tibetan elites
1956	Preparatory Committee for the Autonomous Region of Tibet (PCART) established to create an administrative system parallel to the Tibetan government but along Communist lines
1959 (MARCH)	Escape of the Dalai Lama; Lhasa Uprising
1959–62	Democratic Reforms (including land reform)
1965	Tibet Military Region renamed Tibet Autonomous Region (TAR)
1963–66	Socialist Education Movement (SEM)
1966–76	End of redistributed land ownership, start of rural production brigades and communes; the Great Proletarian Cultural Revolution

the question of the extent to which the *amchis*' narratives express "oppositional practices of time" (Mueggler 2001: 7).

While the political history of the early reforms beginning in the 1950s and especially in 1959 in central Tibet has been addressed in a number of scholarly works (see table 3.1),[1] the developments in Tibetan medical practice and the field of health care more broadly have received little attention. Written accounts have focused almost exclusively on central government institutions and tend to be polarized.

Craig Janes (1995: 16–19) refers to the period of 1959 to 1966 as a time of "cautious growth" for Tibetan medicine; despite the demise of the Tibetan government and the successive implementation of reforms, the Lhasa Mentsikhang survived as one of the few Tibetan government institutions in the new regime, even expanding its services. Several officially published, if brief, CCP-endorsed accounts of this period also exist. Foremost among these are the historical and (auto)biographical accounts written in the Tibetan language by Jampa Trinlé (2000, 2004, 2006), a longtime director of the Lhasa Mentsikhang, as well as biographies in Chinese of two noted Lhasa-based *amchi* (Yinba 2008; Su Qiong 2008). Extant English-language accounts published through Xinhua's news outlets (e.g., China Tibet Information Centre 2005) and its Foreign Languages Press (e.g.,

Zhen and Cai 2005) mainly bolster the legitimacy of the new regime. They report on its "success" in "winning over the masses" through free distribution of medicines and health care services, specifically referring to the role of traditional medicine in this endeavor, stating, for example, that after the 1951 liberation "conditions changed a lot. Radical changes occurred in Tibetan medicine, whose goal became to serve the vast masses. The old medical institutions underwent thorough change. As an integral part of Chinese medical treasures, Tibetan medicine was well inherited and developed" (Zhen and Cai 2005: 33–34). It is not clear from their account what kinds of changes they refer to or whether these changes took place immediately following 1951 or later. It is sure, however, that their account provides a stark contrast to book-length modern autobiographies of Tibetan medical doctors who later went into exile and became the personal physicians of the Fourteenth Dalai Lama. Foremost among them are those of Tenzin Chödrak (2000) and Lobsang Wangyal (2007),[2] who offer harrowing accounts of their experience of the reforms, their prolonged prison sentences, and their eventual appointment as prison doctors. Several short historical accounts written by exiled Tibetan physicians on the Mentsikhang and its post-1959 fate also exist.[3]

Because these works share an almost exclusive focus on the doctors involved with the Lhasa Mentsikhang and the Dharamsala Men-Tsee-Khang in exile, we lack an understanding of actors outside of these central institutions. During the initial phases of my research, I aimed to address the absent voice of marginal actors through the use of oral history interviews, thus offering an account of Tibetan medical practice inspired by subaltern studies (cf. P. Hansen 2003). It became increasingly apparent that Tibetan doctors, whether classified as landlords, peasants, or serfs, far from being silenced, in fact had been forced to speak up as part and parcel of their socialist transformation; they had often experienced a socialist form of oral history through China's "oral history regime" (Bulag 2010b: 97). My recording of rural *amchi*s' life histories and testimonials no longer seemed the sole preserve of a Western social scientist, as I was led to confront my interlocutors' earlier experiences as well as the wider social and political circumstances that influence the recording and making of oral history.

Enforced narratives and variously publicized memories of the past, especially during the first twenty years of socialist reforms in Tibet, as elsewhere in China, have been an important tool in legitimizing the CCP and building socialism. The CCP termed these practices the "speaking of bitterness," or in Chinese, *suku* (Anagnost 1994; Bulag 2010b). Despite the radically changed circumstances and decades having passed since these earliest CCP-driven forms of remembering, traces of "speaking bitterness" are still part of political discourse in Tibet to this day, even when this has long been abandoned in most of the PRC (Makley 2005). *Suku*-style metaphors were present in some of my informants' ways of talking about the pre-reform and early reform period. One elderly doctor, for example, used these as means to educate young students, and it served him as a means carry out his own projects successfully without obstacles from the authorities. This doctor was able to work as an *amchi* throughout the reforms and played an important role in preserving and revitalizing Tibetan medicine during the 1970s. The mastery he had gained in employing the statist remembering of the "old society" combined with near-constant praises for later political regimes enabled this remarkable continuity.

NARRATING BITTERNESS

"Recalling of past [suffering] and thinking over [the source of] present [happiness]" (C. *yiku sitian*, Tib. *sngar dran deng bsdur*) involved narrations of personal life history staged in public. These were often highly corporeal performances, including crying over abuse and "serfs" physically attacking their former "lords." The core narrative had to be structured around the crucial dividing line of 1949, the year demarcating the "old society" from the "new"—the former associated with bitterness, suffering, and sadness, the latter with happiness, sweetness, and liberation.

Throughout the 1950s, Mao considered central Tibet a special case that was not ready for socialist reforms (Shakya 1999: 244–45; Goldstein 2007, 2013). In the spirit of the United Front (a political organ made up of mainly "minority" [*minzu*] leaders in the CCP) and through specific policies targeting minority nationalities, reforms had been delayed for central Tibet in an attempt to win over Tibetan elites. They were then expected to lead the broader Tibetan masses, according to the seventeen-point agreement of 1951, toward "demanding socialist reforms." Yet after the Lhasa Uprising and the 1959 escape of the Dalai Lama along with most members of the Tibetan government, this gradualist approach to bringing reform to central Tibet, which had been disputed within the CCP, changed radically (Shakya 1999: 247). The CCP instead appealed directly to the Tibetan masses to raise their class consciousness and find new ways to legitimate CCP rule. A prime means, as observed by Anagnost, was "speaking bitterness," which for the first time brought ordinary Tibetans in direct contact with the PRC's demands.

Once reforms had been nominally "asked for" by the Panchen Lama and Ngapö Ngawang Jigmé, the heads of the Preparatory Committee for the Autonomous Region of Tibet (PCART), a two-stage implementation of the Democratic Reforms began. These comprised for instance the Three Antis and Two Reductions and the land reforms (Shakya 1999: 246–62). Political mass meetings and "speaking bitterness" sessions choreographed by Communist cadres became an important political tool, following the template set in early Chinese Communist meetings and the practices from the period of the foundation of the PRC in the late 1940s (Bulag 2010b: 98–100). This inflicted an entirely new political culture on ordinary Tibetans in towns, villages, and pastoralist camps. In many cases Tibetans had to learn to cast the "old society" as a time of backwardness and feudal exploitation and to conceive of people as "reactionaries," "exploiters," and "landlords," and as such as representatives and remnants of the old society (Shakya 1999). These people were then verbally attacked in public and asked to confess their wrongs. In towns and some villages, graphic displays of the "Wrath of the Serfs" were meant to raise class consciousness among Tibetans (Harris 1999).

Anthropologist Charlene Makley (2005), writing on the 1958 reforms in Labrang in eastern Tibet, explains that Tibetans' first encounters with "speaking bitterness" were not during small discussions and work team sessions but in the dramatic public meetings and struggle sessions.[4] There "Tibetans were required to produce and listen to testimonials of their participation in the Communist-led revolution, that is, life-stories attesting to their consciousness of past class-based oppression in the 'Old Society' and their present 'liberation' in the 'New Society'" (47). Public "speaking bitterness," under the duress of the reforms in central Tibet, became a marker of the most vicious public encounters, culminating in public "struggle sessions" (*thamzing*), a hallmark of the Socialist Education Movement (SEM, 1963–66), and further intensified during the Cultural Revolution (1966–76).

The accusations against those who held on to the "old society" were increasingly regular, sometimes daily, features of life in Tibetan towns and villages, as reported by my interlocutors. Not limited to spoken narratives, they were also published (Dhondub Chödon 1978) and featured heavily in official written documents, newspapers, and books. These included direct quotes from interviews with "former serfs" and use of their first-person life stories and accounts to prove their "bitterness" in the "old society" and happiness in the new one. Topics ranged from industrialization and land rights to women's rights (Hsi and Kao 1977; Strong 1959; Epstein 1983), and they often included references to Tibetan medicine and health care in pre- and post-"liberation" Tibet.[5]

In *Tibet Leaps Forward*, Hsi Changhao and Kao Yuanmei report an interview with "Comrade Drolkar," whom they describe as "a medical worker and deputy-director of the health bureau of the autonomous region" who had been born into a "serf family" and only after liberation was given access to medical study in the "interior" (1977: 97). They found the interview she gave them "very informative." "Under the reactionary feudal serfdom in old Tibet," said Drolkar, "the million serfs enjoyed no freedom whatsoever, not to speak of medical care. Reactionary lamas and witch doctors, capitalizing on the people's superstitious ideas, sold quack 'pills' made of clay or incense ash to the sick. Their greedy practices brought great harm to the toiling masses" (97). The authors then report on a smallpox epidemic in Tibet, when a man called Jampa, his brother, and many others were cast outside their village by reactionary local government troops, leaving the diseased to perish under the eyes of the local manorial lord, who did not allow Jampa to enter the village even after he survived the epidemic (98). Instead, Jampa had to "wander here and there, turning home only after liberation." In contrasting the "feudal reactionaries'" neglect of the extraordinary sufferings experienced by Tibetans, the writers assert: "Chairman Mao and the Central Committee of the Chinese Communist Party were gravely concerned about the health of the hundreds of thousands of liberated serfs in Tibet." They then praise the work carried out in the health and medical domain, from a medical corps "marching alongside the PLA army into Tibet in 1951" to the "thousands of health workers and barefoot doctors giving medical aid to fellow commune members" by the mid-1970s, thus unfavorably comparing the earlier situation with "modern medical treatment" that now reliably reached remote parts of Tibet. There are numerous such examples, in many cases supported by photographs of the work of medical teams among Tibetans.[6]

Such "speaking bitterness" testimonials continue today. In 2009, March 28 was officially declared a public holiday to "commemorate" the "complete emancipation of a million Tibetan serfs" and its fifty-year anniversary for the first time officially "celebrated" in Lhasa. On this occasion, a special issue of *China's Tibet* was published with the title "Pacification and the Democratic Reforms of TAR" (Zhang 2009). Along "speaking bitterness" lines and with numerous "eyewitness accounts," it retold the great changes and improvements brought to Tibetans by the Democratic Reforms. These are contrasted with the backwardness and crudeness of the "old society." Addressing the medical sphere, an article by Sochong relied on interviews with a Tibetan named Ngawang Dorjé, who is quoted at length. Many features of Sochong's account are similar to those first published in the 1970s (such as those in *Tibet Leaps Forward* and prominently in Epstein 1983): it focuses on shortcomings of medical care in the old society, which is identified as incredibly "primitive," with people relying on sending their urine to be diagnosed by faraway doctors and unable to check whether medicines were effective (Sochong 2009: 25).

At times the conversations of individual Tibetans closely mirror these official accounts. How, then, did the people I worked with negotiate and translate China's pervasive "socialist oral history regime" in their own retelling and remembrance? For my informants the socialist oral history regime had been experienced early on, either through speaking bitterness during the reforms or through the ongoing propagation of first-person written life histories during the post-Maoist era.

OPPOSITIONAL PRACTICES OF TIME AND REFORM

These officially sanctioned forms of narration were far from the only or even the dominant ways of conceiving the past among *amchi* and their families with whom I spoke and spent time. Most rarely structured their stories around the widespread themes of "liberation," "old society" and "new society," or the various state campaigns and reforms. In numerous conversations and interviews they instead offered stories we may interpret as what Mueggler has termed "oppositional practices of time" (2001: 7).

Anthropologist Eric Mueggler developed this concept in his extraordinary ethnography *The Age of Wild Ghosts*, which describes the suffering of a Yunnan Lolop'o community as a result of Maoist policies, in particular the destruction of their ancestral system of Tsi'ci headmanship during the Great Leap Forward. In Mueggler's analysis the stories, songs, dances, and ritual chants the Lolop'o shared with him are understood as an overarching narrative in which the relation of the Lolop'o to the state, from personified external other in the 1940s to internal abstract other in the 1990s, becomes complete. "Time" and "oppositional practices of time" powerfully demonstrate individuals' and communities' relation to the state and their own dream of community. Similarly, profoundly different interpretations and narratives as well as the contrasting fates are apparent in accounts of Medical Houses and their members' experience of socialist reforms. Although in pre-1959 times the members of the Mentrong and Térap Medical Houses were socioeconomically quite similarly positioned, as the reforms began they experienced vastly different consequences. These relate in significant ways to how they engaged and negotiated the state and its discourses during and after the reforms. While the Mentrong's narrative in many ways mirrors the retelling of experiences of reform that have been widely published in exile, the Térap of Yonten Tsering remains largely committed to the state-orchestrated historical account, including its core division between "old" and "new" society.

The Mentrong

This is how Rinchen Mentrong remembered the start of the reforms when we first met in 2003, talking in his courtyard in the presence of his then-young granddaughter as well as my coresearcher from the Tibetan Academy of Social Sciences:

> When the Democratic Reforms started in 1959 I could no longer continue to practice as an *amchi*. Everything changed, but the destruction, like of the medicines and books etc., did not start immediately. In the beginning I had to stop practicing, as I was accused of being a "representative of the exploiters' class" [*mangdag*]. So I gave the medicines away. I gave them to a doctor and lama from Nyémo, who stayed in Lhünding at the time. He was here to build a new monastery and also practiced as an *amchi*. However, after a year

> or so he got political reeducation and later on was executed by the Chinese. He had been a good *amchi*. . . . Then in this area there were no good *amchi* anymore and there was no possibility to study with anybody. That place called Phuntsoling had good doctors before, and in Tashilhunpo Monastery there were some too, but I couldn't go there, and my teacher in Phuntsoling had died. Being labeled a representative of the exploiters' class was a serious accusation, so then I did farmwork and later on went to do business.

The medicines referred to were the ones his family had kept in the *menkhang* of their large Mentrong, but patients and local villagers considered even the material components of the house to have medical properties: "They sometimes scraped off some of the earth of the outside walls and ate that, considering it medicine!" Rinchen told us, laughing. We continued our conversations when I visited again in 2007, little changing in the way he presented, often proudly, the Lhünding Mentrong's social position and ritual functions in the village before the Democratic Reforms and the events that followed their commencement.

Rather than using the socialist tropes of "old society" and "new society" to structure his narratives, Rinchen-la simply used the word *ngönma* (before, earlier)[7] to refer to practices just prior to the start of the reforms, and *ngönma ngönma* when relating the situation of his family and Tibetan medical history in a longer perspective, or *logyü* (literally the "tidings of the years" but now the general Tibetan term for "history"). For example, when asked how medical work was remunerated before the reforms, he recalled seeing up to fifteen patients a day: "*Ngönma*, there was no system of set prices for consultations and medicine; people gave a donation if they could afford it, and if they couldn't they were treated anyway."

Already in 1958, Communist cadres had visited Lhünding and begun to investigate local people's situation. The Mentrong was labeled a *mangdag*, literally "owner of many," referring to families who had owned land and employed *yokpo*. In the indigenous social categories, these families belonged to the *kutra* or *gerpa* groups. The label *mangdag* was at first merely nominal and without effect in terms of access to land. This changed with a campaign that freed *yokpo* families from their obligations toward their estate (part of the Two Reductions). They then no longer "belonged" to the estate of the Mentrong. Despite Rinchen Wangyal and his family's high status as *gerpa*, they were not accused of being counterrevolutionaries, a fate that befell members of the nearby Nyingkhang to tragic effect.

The first substantial change to the life of Rinchen-la and his family came with the start of the second part of the Democratic Reforms, the land reform of early 1960. All of the Mentrong's land was taken away from the family and redistributed, along with the land belonging to the monastery and one *trelpa* household, among twenty Lhünding households who were defined by Communist cadres as poor (*nang ulopon ga*). The Mentrong's stored grain and many of their belongings were similarly reassigned. The process was managed by an outside Communist cadre who worked closely with the members of five local families who had "become Communists," said Rinchen. Having lost their land, the Mentrong were given back a small piece, which Rinchen then worked (instead of practicing as an *amchi*) so that the household could survive. Because the family did not immediately lose the right to live in their house (unlike Yonten Tsering), they remained at the Mentrong until the start of the Cultural Revolution. Others from the village, mainly the former *yokpo* who worked on the Mentrong's estate in return for part-yield part-payment, also moved into their house. The Mentrong household members had to make do with two rooms. The tradition of holding the *cham* dance at the end of the old Tibetan year at the Mentrong was discontinued in 1960.

Rinchen Wangyal had to attend regular public meetings in which his class status was problematized and his former "exploitations" dramatized. Over the year such attacks increased. He was harshly struggled against on several occasions in the village and the nearby new administrative center for the valley, Targyü *xiang*. Attacks intensified during the Cultural Revolution, as Rinchen-la explained:

> Before the Cultural Revolution there was much talk already about "destroying the old." We had to destroy our religious statues, books, thankas, and other objects, or give them to others to destroy. In that first phase, from among the twenty poor households [*tempa*], five of them had joined the Communists [*tang*] and were most active in agitating against us. Of course they were encouraged by the Chinese. Members of these five poor households were the first to agitate in the village, and they insisted that we hand over our *chökhang*'s silver and copper bowls as well as others things that were there.

> At that time we were able to preserve a few things and some of the books. But then when the Cultural Revolution began, the *mimang* [populace] came so suddenly and quickly to our house, and they were so enraged, they destroyed everything. Now there is nothing left. We couldn't do anything—they came so suddenly! Whatever they could find they would take. There was no way to do or say anything. If I'd say something I would be immediately locked up. So we could only allow them to take whatever they wanted. I wasn't endowed with any rights.
>
> We had the *Gyüshi*, collected works of Jangpa Namgyel Drazang and many *Menngag* works, a short version of the *Kangyur* and statues. Most works in the *chökhang* were medical books. But they destroyed everything, tore them apart and left them there at first. Then they came back and threw it all into the river and the fire. Everything was destroyed and nothing left.
>
> The monastery and the Mentrong house itself were destroyed by the members of all of those twenty poor households during the Cultural Revolution. First those five households attacked the *chökhang* and the inside of the monastery. When that wasn't enough, they destroyed the buildings too.

Rinchen offered this narrative during a recorded interview in the summer of 2007. Rinchen-la, his granddaughter, a friend of mine helping with translation, and I were on the roof of the Mentrong building, which had been rebuilt at a different location. During the interview, the elderly man pointed to various places in the village as he explained to us what had happened. His account contained no trace of "speaking bitterness" narratives referencing the unjustness of the "old society." On the contrary, Rinchen spoke with pride about his family's history in Tibetan society and explained lucidly what happened when the reforms began. In his opinion relations among different families in the village had been harmonious but the "Chinese" had managed to capitalize on local poor people's willingness to support them for personal gain. When asked how he felt about the people in the village who had inflicted so much pain on him, he responded, "Actually, they didn't only destroy the monastery and my home. Moreover they severely struggled against me, very hard [*'thabs rtsod*]. They dragged me to Tarkyü and also out here in the village. Even so, now I don't feel any hatred. I think that was my karma. From the inside of my heart I don't feel hatred toward them."

Although Rinchen was quite willing to speak with me and we had several conversations, both recorded and informal, he never specified the accusations that had been made during the public struggle sessions. His memory of the various reforms and campaigns he had been exposed to were vague, and the Cultural Revolution seemed to seamlessly follow the Democratic Reforms. Makley encountered a similar situation during her research in Labrang. She calls the absence of actual descriptions of "struggle sessions" or "speaking bitterness" accusations the "loudest silences" within "oppositional testimonies" (Makley 2005: 63). Similarly, Rinchen never explicitly reiterated Marxist ideology. Given the massive quantities of Marxist ideology and media (in Chinese and in Tibetan translation) to which Tibetans had been exposed, Makley interprets this as narrators' repudiation of the validity or relevance of state ideology in structuring their memories. The farthest Rinchen went in using reform-specific language was the Tibetan term *drelrimgyi taptsö* (class struggle).[8] He used this expression like a loan word from an alien language, even laughing when he introduced it into our conversations, seemingly implying that this period had been an incredibly ignorant time.

The Ngakpa Nyingkhang

In many ways Rinchen's narratives resemble the kinds of experiences narrated in the biographies by Tibetan aristocrats from Tsang that were later published in exile (e.g., Carnahan and Rinpoche 1995). And they are also comparable, in their "oppositional practices of time" and (to some extent) ridicule of Communist propaganda, to accounts from members of the Nyingkhang, to which the Mentrong is related through marriage. Here a sense of absurdity pervaded the kinds of labels and punishments the oldest brother and father of the Nyingkhang had to endure. I heard their narratives initially from Ngawang Dorjé, the doctor from Ngamring who had since our first meeting moved to Lhasa. I often came to their house after enrolling at Tibet University, and I became friends with various members of his family, several of whom had grown up in the Nyingkhang. I interviewed those with firsthand experience of the reforms in Ngamring in the 1960s several times, including the doctor Ngawang Dorjé, his older brother Wangdu, and their younger sister Ani Payang, who had joined Khyemen Rinpoche as a nun to become an *amchi*. Many encounters quickly turned into lively conversations involving them all, or sometimes just Ngawang Dorjé and Wangdu, since they lived in the same house. These conversations featured events that affected other named houses and the members of the so-called *shabdrung*, *chödzé*, and *jedrung* social groups in Ngamring, which had been given tax exemptions or levies by their primary landholders.

One afternoon in their Lhasa home, Ngawang Dorjé's oldest brother, Wangdu, explained what happened in 1959, when the reforms came to their valley and he and his father were sent to jail:

> They said that I was a member of a "secret youth organization,"[9] that I was in an organization called "Above Eighteen up to Sixty,"[10] and last I was accused of being an "owner of history's exploited serfs."[11] Since they couldn't use the youth organization label for my father, he was named a "reactionary" [*lokchöpa*] and also the "owner of history's exploited serfs." We had no idea about the meaning of these labels! We just listened, but we never actually did any of the things they accused us of. In fact, we had never even heard about these various organizations' names that they claimed we were a part of! [*He laughs.*] My father was sentenced to twenty years in prison but only stayed for two, three years and came home sick, then they sent him back. He went back and forth for several years before he passed away. Since he was already old, he used to laugh and say, "How kind the Chinese are, giving me twenty more years in this human life!" My father was very strong headed—he was a fervent religious practitioner, and many times he had stood up for the common people. He was often against the old leaders who were taking too much tax, arguing with them to protect those who were poor. In the 1950s he even made a case against two local *ponpo* [leaders] and took it all the way to the court in Shigatse as they were taking more than Drepung asked them to. Even so, we were sent to prison early on—in 1959 and 1960. Then in 1969 many people went to jail.

Wangdu, after shorter periods in a local prison, was himself sent to a labor camp in Kongpo between 1969 and 1974.

> There I continued to be called a "reactionary" and "history's oppressor and exploiter of serfs." Others were also still wearing the "history hat,"[12] short for the "history's oppressor and exploiter's hat." Those they said

> had killed people were given the "evil people's" hat.[13] Everyone was given different hats at the time. In Kongpo we had to work very hard, and that also depended on our "hats." Whatever work we were asked to do, that's what we had to do. Our work was mainly cutting down trees and also producing various things.

Instead of "happiness" and "liberation," the beginning of the reforms tore apart the family, and its members were exposed to prolonged prison sentences and several years in labor camps. These initial sentences were based on the (incorrect) accusation that the family had actively supported the March 1959 uprising in Lhasa. The sentences were initially unrelated to the family's newly defined Communist "class status," which was that of the *ngazab* or *ngadag*, an "owner of many." Compounded by this *ngakpa* family's traditional role in carrying out protective rituals for the Dalai Lamas, the punishments intensified and were prolonged.

Members of the Nyingkhang House practiced a range of nonstatist remembering at their home in Lhasa. The older brother, Wangdu, who had never worked for the government, was most outspoken. His sister, Ani Payang, often burst into tears when remembering the incredible kindness and compassion of Khyemen Rinpoche and her father, and their fates. Ngawang Dorjé, although slightly more reserved and retired from a government job, was also willing to share his family's experiences. When either brother talked about the time before the reforms, it was with pride in their long-standing *ngakpa* tradition and the services they had rendered to various lamas as well as local villagers, such as averting hailstorms and producing protective pills. Yet they also balanced these with recollections of their father's strong social conscience: how he had stood up to two local Tibetan leaders working as administrators and tax collectors on behalf of the Drepung Monastery, who exacted extra taxes from local landholders for personal profit. Because of their father's elevated position and reputation, he was able to defend the landholders. He even took one case to court at the Tashilhunpo Labrang in the mid-1950s. Nevertheless, the family was accused of having "exploited" poor people, and on these grounds lost their land, home, and belongings. Ngawang Dorjé eventually became a government worker in the 1970s, alongside his lifelong colleague Yonten Tsering.

Like most Tibetans, Rinchen and his family, as well as Ngawang Dorjé, Wangdu, and Ani Payang, had learned to switch aspects of their narratives or simply remain silent. Depending on who was present, they learned to say, or not, what they judged necessary to keep out of trouble and maintain good relations with those wielding power in the state system (work superiors and their children's teachers or employers, for example). This ability to switch must also have affected what I was and wasn't told, depending on whom I was with. Yet in general I believe I gained a high level of trust from this family, who saw me as loyal (coming to visit over a long period of time), interested in religion and local (medical) history, which they rated highly, and connected to the outside world and knowledgeable about Tibetans in exile.

STATE-TIME AND SPEAKING BITTERNESS

Although in the pre-reform period Yonten Tsering of Térap enjoyed a high social position similar to Ngawang Dorjé and to some extent the members of the Mentrong, he put forth near-constant praise for the government and the Communists, and he remembered the past quite differently. He narrated many of his memories of early reforms in a "state-timed" manner, making ample use of the Communist themes of "old" and "new society" and even using the key Communist road metaphor.

On our first morning in Gye in the summer of 2007, Yonten Tsering told me at Gyatso's house,

> You should remember that in Gye before the Democratic Reforms, there were four "high-class" families [*torim thopo*]. One was my own, one my elder brother's, one my elder sister's family, and one the previous owners of the house we are in this morning. The other people who lived in this village were very poor. They worked on the fields of these four wealthy families; we did not do much of the hard work ourselves! I would say about half of our wealth wasn't really ours; it should have belonged to the commoners [*miser*]. When the Democratic Reforms began, everything was taken away from these four families, and it was distributed among the commoners. We exchanged houses: the high-class people had to live in the houses of the poor people, and the poor people were sharing

> among them the houses of the wealthy. This was a great movement. I love the Communists for what they did!

We were on our way to visit the Térap Medical House, which was to be revived and would once again provide medical care. Although I was no longer surprised to hear the government being lauded by this elderly *amchi*, listening to his eulogies about the reforms next to people who had experienced them as intrusive and violent made me deeply uncomfortable. In homes and monasteries, others had already related to me, with varying degrees of caution, the heavy personal toll the early reforms had taken on their lives and those of other local residents. People who had owned or administered land and estates, as well as monks and nuns at local monasteries and nunneries, were particularly affected as "landlords," "exploiters," or worst, "counterrevolutionaries." From 1959 onward they were increasingly singled out from the masses, now renamed *mangtso* (the people). This replaced the earlier term *miser* (commoners), a denomination of the pre-Communist system.[14] The *mangtso* mainly comprised the previously poor groups in the villages.

From the expressions of the driver and my research assistant, Pema, I knew I was not alone in my discomfort, but Yonten Tsering continued unabated: "The Communists helped the *mangtso* a lot. Now everyone here can lead a happy life! Before, this village was under the manor of the Khangsar Shekar, which belonged to the Shigatse Labrang and the Ninth Panchen Lama, Chökyi Nyima. They had to pay tax to them. Although they behaved/acted much better than the Drepung Monastery, who was taking so much tax from the people, they still took a lot."

It was in Gye Village, in fact, that Yonten Tsering had first been forced, or volunteered, to espouse such speech practices, so that, fifty years later, he could tell me proudly and always in a relieved manner: "We were never touched!"

Even when I was alone with him, he narrated positively the enforced labeling exercises and their consequences: "The government policy was good at the time and they established different classes; we became *ngazab*. People were surprised that even though we were from that background we didn't have problems. My father was so wise. He said, "All these material belongings, they don't help us, we give away everything." It often struck me how Yonten Tsering appeared to focus unremittingly on the bright side of the difficulties he and his wife endured when they were first relocated to a tiny one-room shelter, working a small piece of land. He recalled:

> We ourselves lost almost everything. At first I also lost my treasured medicines, all the texts. Then later, when the mutual aid groups [*rogré*] were started, the work group leader came to me and said: "You must work as a doctor." Then the Communists gave back one horse, and I gained access to the medicines and texts. They were moved to a small room in my old house. They were saying that I should work for the health of the *mangtso* in the village and for the farmers and pastoralists of the entire area. Even though I was labeled a *ngazab*, they said my behavior was good. The communalization had not yet started, so the work team leader said that while you are away from the production team, we will send someone else to fill in for you. So from 1958 until now I continued to be a doctor. I never stopped. For the first fifteen years I worked alone, going here and there. At the beginning I had a very good stock of medicine. Compared to others in Shigatse, I wasn't rich, but there in Mü Valley I was certainly of "big family,"[15] so I had lots of good medicines, also from India. At the time of the Democratic Reforms, I got back the stock of medicines, with them saying, "Actually it is yours." So then I treated people and never took any payments.

The group listening to Yonten Tsering comprised a government employee, Gyatso; his college student son; my driver and my research assistant (both from Lhasa); a couple of students from Shigatse; and my brother, who was visiting from abroad. Having seemingly held back, one of them eventually responded, "You speak of so many improvements under the Communists. Some are certainly there, but overall, not that much has changed for the better. The situation today is almost the same as in the 'old society.' For those who work for the government things have improved, but for others life is very hard. Also, today mostly the previously high-class families have become government workers once again, not those who were previously poor." Someone else chimed in, "Also, why should so much destruction have been necessary to bring these alleged improvements?" Without missing a beat, Yonten Tsering countered with a common slogan from Maoist times, internalized and repeated alongside many others when he worked as a Communist cadre:

> The road is full of pebbles, but in the end there is a bright future for everyone! I will give you a clever and satisfying answer. There was no destruction in 1959. All the monasteries were intact, but land and wealth were redistributed and that was good. The destruction of the monasteries was because of a big mistake, namely the Cultural Revolution. The Gang of Four made this big mistake, starting in 1966. It lasted for about nine years, and afterward everybody apologized for this mistake. People whose relatives died were given money, the monasteries were reestablished, and old things that were taken away in the Cultural Revolution were given back.

There was no satisfaction visible on the faces of the driver or my research assistant, who smiled gently nevertheless, knowing the man well enough from our time spent together. Yonten Tsering's statements and responses were the closest I had heard any Tibetan come to mirroring and repeating the party line concerning both the unjustness of the "old" "feudal" society, as retold in countless "speaking bitterness" sessions, and the Cultural Revolution, which otherwise offered a rare chance for Tibetans (and Chinese) to express their actual experiences. His praise of the various reforms was surely related to the requirements of being a party member, a suspicion I confirmed later in my research.

The group's challenges to Yonten Tsering's statements were, by extension, challenges to the state and its widely imposed narrative. His response suggests they had crossed the limits of what could be spoken without fear of repercussion and entered the realm of what we have called "oppositional practices of time." This was transgressional even within the confines of a private home where members had been profoundly exposed to exile historical narratives, and thus clearly had engaged with such discourses. As if to mend the situation and avoid potential conflict among those gathered, Yonten Tsering ended the discussion, saying, "Everything we have discussed just now was said in jest," adding that such conversations were not the purpose of our trip and "we had better do some work."

Essentially the *amchi* was suggesting that what we had talked about should not be taken seriously, at least not those parts that challenged the teleological narration of how everything has gotten better on "the road to socialism," with its many promised advancements and ever-increasing improvement to the lives of people in the PRC. Instead, the group was supposed to have been "only joking." Except that they really were not. They had willingly expressed disagreement with Yonten Tsering's profound adoption of state rhetoric, even if they revered him deeply for his exemplary and selfless efforts in providing medical care to local villagers.

Based on other explanations and conversations, as well as the memories of Yonten Tsering and his wife, Yeshe Lhamo, the fate of Térap House can be reconstructed: The *amchi*, Yeshe Lhamo, and Yonten Tsering's parents had to leave everything behind, the four of them moving into accommodation previously occupied by a local *miser* family: a one-story stone building with one room, without a window or wooden pillar, and with a low entrance and a mud floor. They were allowed to take from their former home a mattress and blanket each, a kettle, teacups, and a small amount of *tsampa*. Four *miser* families, including the one previously living in the small shelter, were given deeds to the doctor's land and his family home, ensuring an embodied, literal reversal of the local social order. The doctor family's belongings and livestock were split between them, with Yonten Tsering "given" only a tiny piece of land, which he and his wife henceforth planted and tended. The distribution of goods, land, and property was executed in public fashion, so that it could be witnessed and create new revolutionary subjectivities and introduce Tibetans to the Communist class consciousness.

After some time, Yonten Tsering and his father, Tsewang Norbu, were allowed to practice as *amchi* again, but his father was by then old and unable to help much. The family's medical and Buddhist texts, thankas, medicine, and medicine-making equipment, once allocated to spaces on the first floor of their original Medical House, mainly the *menkhang* and *chökhang*, were moved to its ground floor. This area had previously been used for animals and was perceived as an "impure" part in the house. Now, however, not only was the doctor's family living in a ground-floor accommodation (the previous *miser* one-room house), but their medicines and religious objects were also no longer respected in traditional ways, when they would have been placed upstairs, and in the *menkhang* and *chökhang*.

Yonten Tsering used this ground-floor room of his old Medical House to make medicines and see patients, as it had been declared a public clinic. At the same time, he conducted medical rounds, soon combining his work of "carrying the medical bag" with a job as a Communist cadre, for which he cut his hair and joined the party.

In many ways the subsequent medical practice of the increasingly reformed Yonten Tsering became simplified. He had been asked to use "only simple remedies" in treatment and to make reference neither to Tibetan medical theories nor to spiritual treatments, which were judged feudal, of the old society, and inextricably linked to religion. It was clear that the stone diagnosis and *torma* offerings his father used to perform, and which he had also learned, were no longer to be part of medical work and were considered reactionary and superstitious.

The remedies were also simplified, the Térap's rich stock of medical raw materials diminishing rapidly from what Yonten Tsering and his father had preserved, including the ingredients brought back from their 1958 pilgrimage to India. Yonten Tsering collected locally available herbs and some minerals, but given his busy workload "for the revolution," there was little spare time for this. Foreign ingredients in Tibetan medicine were no longer available or not affordable, so whatever he made was largely derived from local flora and fauna. He, his father, and his wife did the collecting and compounding outside of working hours. By the time the communes started and the Red Guards began their violent attacks, there were only three types of medicines that the young *amchi* could prescribe to patients, apart from external therapies.

By all accounts, neither Yonten Tsering nor his immediate family was personally exposed to physically violent struggle sessions. He insisted that his father died a natural death, when his life force had been consumed and not because of violent attacks or prison sentences, as had been experienced by others. He did once add that his father had not taken his own life, a telling comment on the dire situation at the time and others' responses to it. Being a party member, working as a Communist cadre, and providing medical care under great personal hardship most likely gave Yonten Tsering the status and capital of a "reformed man."

As he described life and social divisions in the "old society," Yonten Tsering repeated many of the common tropes of speaking bitterness narratives, confessing the wrongs of the old system of which he was a part and taking the side of those who had been "exploited." Yet he also remained full of praise and admiration for his father and many teachers who were intricately linked to the pre-1959 sociocultural fabric of life.

Over time I learned that praising the government to this extent was not just a long-standing habit from his work as a cadre and government employee. It also showed a good deal of insight into current Tibetan realpolitik—how one can get along and do good from within the system—even if many Tibetans would be uncomfortable working within such narratives and discourses of the state. This was evident from the reactions of some of the people present during our conversations in Gye. Yonten Tsering was, however, able to straddle these diverse expectations and stances, thereby getting on with his social projects and practicing medicine with a deeply engrained Buddhist-cum-socialist medical ethic that will be discussed in detail in chapter 6.

Yonten Tsering's practices are partially mirrored by other Tibetan cadres of that generation, heads of monasteries and village elders from central Tibet. Diemberger (2010) discusses their crucial role in the widespread reconstruction of Tibet's cultural heritage in the 1980s and 1990s, showing how they profoundly shaped contemporary Tibet precisely because of their ability to deal with the complexities of political and moral demands across the divides of Mao- and Deng-era Tibet. She argues that they are best accounted for through analysis of Tibetans' life narratives (124).

In public, I witnessed Yonten Tsering's masterful performance of "speaking bitterness" style narratives throughout my fieldwork and with many different groups of people, including family, students, patients, monks and nuns, health bureau officials, and party comrades. It was so pronounced that at times my acquaintances and I remarked on how uncomfortable we were with them, even if Yonten Tsering continued to enjoy the utmost respect for his medical work and professional achievements, as well as his charisma. It was certainly no coincidence that the *amchi* was frequently asked for help with paperwork, such as that required for the government registration of other people's clinics. People knew he would say and do the right things, know whom to contact, and get papers stamped and approved so that they could proceed without obstacles. Perhaps Yonten Tsering's caution, not only in his own speech but also what he allowed others to say in his company, paid off after all? A scene I witnessed between Rinchen Wangyal and Yonten Tsering particularly illuminates how he found his own balance with regard to state discourses and requirements. When a conversation between the two turned to the very political topic of the Dalai Lama and exile, Yonten Tsering got up, saying he was tired, and left the room. Rinchen Wangyal looked at me apologetically and with a soft smile remarked, "I do not know a more careful person than Yonten Tsering." Yonten Tsering thus avoided discussing the Dalai Lama and exile, but also showed that he would not criticize the Dalai Lama either, which might have been expected given his position and status.

That even Rinchen had to be "careful," however, was and remains a fact of living in contemporary Tibet, no matter how remote one might be (Yeh 2013; Henrion-Dourcy 2013). Being "careful" has everything to do with the near-constant presence of the state and its demands on Tibetan citizens to adopt a correct position vis-à-vis Tibetan "politics," and by extension "correct" practices of "state-time" and "speaking bitterness" in narrating the past, even into the new millennium. Moreover, it is an indication of a wider "politics of fear" (Yeh 2006).

THE STATE AT HOME: PRACTICING VIGILANCE AND DIPLOMACY

In summer 2007, on my third day as a guest at the Mentrong, I was in the open courtyard area sitting at a low table with Rinchen, his sister Tsering Kyi, Rinchen's granddaughter, my research assistant, and a man in his forties whom I did not know and assumed was a visiting relative. Rinchen-la's daughter-in-law moved back and forth between the kitchen and our table, offering tea and biscuits. It was midafternoon and the courtyard was especially calm, the house having heaved with patients all morning and over the two previous days, as the Mentrong had offered up their home as a clinic for the duration of Yonten Tsering's stay (figure 3.1). He had just left for Lhünding Monastery, to give consultations to a visiting elderly rinpoche and the monks there, his two medicine trunks borne up the steep hill by student helpers.

I continued to be puzzled, at times upset, by Yonten Tsering's persistent praise for, perhaps identification with, government authorities. That morning, he had volunteered it generously. Two elderly patients had sought his treatment, and when they had been diagnosed and given medicine, repeated their *kadinche* (thank you) so many times it seemed they would never leave. Perhaps searching for a response that would help them leave, the *amchi* said, "There is no need to be grateful to me; these medicines were given by the great kindness of the Communist government. *They*

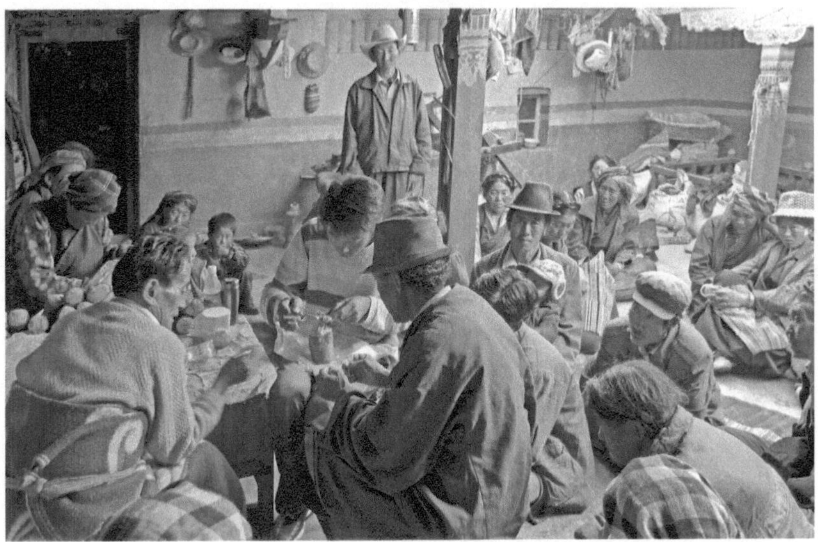

FIGURE 3.1. Yonten Tsering seeing patients at the Mentrong, 2007. Photo by Meinrad Hofer.

deserve your gratitude." It worked: the patients acknowledged his words and left, medicines in hand, thinking they had been provided by the government. In fact, the medicines had been purchased with private donations from the *amchi* and two sponsors that I had helped bring in.

I recounted this episode and my amazement over it to the Mentrong household members, asking what they made of such effusive statements by Yonten Tsering. After a short pause, Tsering Kyi responded, "I think he is right," looking in an unusually penetrating way at me. The middle-aged man I supposed was a visiting relative added that he thought perhaps Yonten Tsering said these things only "from his mouth" and not "from his heart." Rinchen nodded and, letting some time pass, added, "Yes, that's possible." It was an awkward moment, although at the time I did not pick up that something was amiss. I asked some questions arising from an earlier interview with Rinchen, related to the extent and composition of the Mentrong's land and how they had administered it before it was taken away. Rinchen willingly explained, but instead of the proud manner I had witnessed before, he recounted the Mentrong's socioeconomic situation matter-of-factly, acknowledging that, yes, they had indeed owned disproportional amounts of land compared to others in the village. It was then, for the only time in all our conversations, that he used the term "old society." All of their land had been taken away during the reforms, and the family accused of having exploited the people who had worked it. There were no proud smiles or further details.

Following another prolonged silence, I asked why they thought Yonten Tsering might not have had the same problems as the Mentrong. Rinchen and his sister seemed at first lost for words, then speculated that perhaps it was simply because he was not from a *gerpa* or *kutra* family, certainly not a family as influential as the Mentrong (due to its family connection with the king of Ruthog). The discussion then turned to other matters, and I was also happy to leave it at that.

Once the conversation was over, Tsering Kyi asked me to join her in a different room. Glancing repeatedly at the door as she spoke, she explained that when she had said she agreed with Yonten Tsering it was only because the man present was the village teacher of her niece and a loyal party member, adding, "He doesn't speak much in favor of the Communists, but he is convinced of them in his heart." She wanted to make clear to me her disapproval of Yonten Tsering's exclamations, even if they had helped him and his family stay out of trouble. I apologized profusely, feeling terribly guilty for having instigated a situation where my hosts, in their own home, were pushed to alter their communication because I had not understood that the presence of the village teacher meant they had to be "careful" with what they said.

It nevertheless brought to the fore the widespread ability of, and necessity for, Tibetans to engage in narrations of their past and present in accordance with their judgment of the audience, in particular the presence of the state. Robert Barnett describes precisely this phenomenon in the context of oral history research in post-Soviet Central Asia and postsocialist China: "The oral-history interview is not a two-way process between a dispassionate outsider and an Other with rich experience. Whether an interview is conducted alone, in a group or mediated by relatives . . . , it is never between two parties: it is always at least a three-way process in which the state is sitting visibly or invisibly at the table, sometimes encouraging, sometimes threatening, sometimes enticing, sometimes intervening" (2010: 85).

With the village teacher at the table, the state was highly visible and present to the Mentrong family but invisible to me as the outside researcher. They knew we were in a three-way conversation, the state altering and interfering in narratives demanded of Rinchen and his family, as it had done in early socialist life. Once again, it had required them to relate their past along the party line and acknowledge the CCP state's dividing power between the "old" and the "new" and how that juncture needed to be interpreted.

Whether perceived by Yonten Tsering as a challenge during some of our conversations, visiting in the form of the village teacher, or seen in a visiting government-employed *lechepa* (worker), the state was not only an incredibly powerful force in people's lived experience of past reforms but also remained profoundly present when this past was narrated during my fieldwork.

ABSENT NARRATIVES

Apart from the spectrum of memory practices so far discussed, we also have to acknowledge situations and people where the chance of remembering and retelling has not arisen or been realized. In discussion of the gendered nature of narrative possibilities, the anthropologist Carole McGranahan (2010: 768) writes that the possession of one's own life story is not a given, that what people narrate is not just a question of *how* but also of *if*. This encapsulates in many ways my experiences and observations in recording and documenting the life stories of female Tibetan doctors and other women.

Very few Tibetan men and women voluntarily pointed me to female doctors who could share their life stories with me. Except for Lama Tenzin Phuntsok referring me to his aunt, the female doctor Sonam Drölma, I stumbled across them or followed other leads. Once I started to speak with female doctors, I discovered that they talked about the lives of male family members or teachers in preference to their own, even when they were accomplished practitioners in their own right. This made it difficult to understand in depth their experience and memories of the reforms, or to make any meaningful comparison with male doctors. For example, when I finally met with Sonam Drölma many years after her nephew's suggestion, we could meet only twice, due to the remoteness of her residence and my failure to obtain the right permit for the area. Another challenge was the combination of self-deprecation and a greater ease in talking about male teachers or family members, who were considered more "knowledgeable" in medicine (cf. Hofer 2015).

How Sonam Drölma experienced the early reforms was hence difficult to grasp, but she shared some observations. I noted that, like members of the Mentrong and Nyingkhang, she did not use the names of various reforms (except for the Democratic Reforms and the Cultural Revolution) or provide details of what they implied for her personally. She also did not use the terms "old" and "new society." Instead she remembered day-to-day details of the enormous changes in cultural practices at that time:

> We were asked to be like the Chinese. So my grandfather was not allowed to be an *amchi* any longer. They burned the medicine kit, and we were accused of exploiting "poor people." Eventually my grandfather said, "Now we have to stop; we can't practice any longer." We were also not allowed to practice religion. When my grandfather died at age eighty, sometime in the 1960s, we secretly lit butter lamps inside a chest, so they could not be seen.
>
> Actually my grandfather had never charged medical fees, but they said that he was taking money and exploiting his patients. Actually he had never asked for medical fees; the patients gave a donation, however much they could afford. They said he had to stop taking from the poor, etcetera, and he went to prison many times.

Because of these upheavals, for a long time Sonam Drölma was not allowed to practice, and she felt that her "skills went down."

What are we to make of these difficulties in documenting women's life stories? To be clear, their almost completely absent narratives, either in writing or in oral history interviews, do not imply that Tibetan women have in any way been less exposed to the state oral history regime or that women and issues of gender were irrelevant to the Communist cause in Tibet. Both are topics we need to learn much more about. Rather, they show gendered possibilities or obstructions.

— · —

During the implementation of Democratic Reforms in villages in Ngamring, the continuity of Tibetan medical authority and of most *amchis*' work was significantly compromised. This was not due to directives or campaigns specific to Tibetan medicine at that time and place, but rather to the socioeconomic foundations on which its practitioners had depended in terms of training, household economy, class, and moral authority. These bases further crumbled with each successive CCP campaign and reform aimed at eroding the traditional structures of Tibetan society and the individuals who upheld them. Yonten Tsering and a few others were able to continue their Tibetan medical work, either because of their pre-1959 social status, their political choices, or their rhetorical abilities. Most of the *amchi* discussed in the previous two chapters sooner or later stopped practicing, some forever and some until policy changes after the Cultural Revolution reopened possibilities for working in Tibetan medicine.

One route to remaining in the healing profession was for *amchi* to train in Chinese-style biomedicine, as health care in rural areas was clearly rising on the Communists' agenda from 1960 on. Villages and newly formed township administrative headquarters in Ngamring, even in the midst of the devastations of the Cultural Revolution, were constructing a health care system for members of rural production brigades and communes—the hallmark social organization that brought to an abrupt end the redistributed land and property. These converted the entire farming population to a largely military-style organization of their daily lives.

The differential relations to the state illustrated in the narratives of members of the Mentrong and Térap to some extent explain their different fates with regard to their physical existence, how their members fared in an increasingly violent class struggle, the continuity or discontinuity of their medical authority, and the possibility of recovery.

CHAPTER 4

THE MEDICO-CULTURAL REVOLUTION

> Like everything else in Tibetan culture and education, so also Tibetan medical theory and all precious cultural objects were destroyed. With a lack of Tibetan medical students, almost all hope for Tibetan medicine was lost. It was like a verdant tree drying out.
>
> —Jampa Trinlé, *Gso rig lo rgyus*

> Tibetan medicine and pharmaceuticals are a part of the motherland's medical treasure house.
>
> —*Barefoot Doctor's New Tibetan Medical Compounding Manual*

It was not until the height of what is generally known now as the Cultural Revolution (1966–76) that basic Communist health care arrived in rural Tibetan villages, delivered by the "barefoot doctors" (C. *chijiao yisheng*), locally known as *amchi kangjenma* or *menpa kangjenma*.[1] Although this radically different story of how Communist health care spread beyond Lhasa and other administrative centers after 1969 is largely undocumented, examination of the role of Chinese and Tibetan medicine in this endeavor in rural Tsang illuminates the state of Tibetan medical knowledge at that time and permits comparison with rural and urban China proper.[2]

Stark shifts occurred in official policy and attitudes toward rural Tibetan medical doctors and Tibetan medicine practice, as is evident in accounts of *amchi* from Ngamring and textbooks available to them. One was the revolutionary Chinese medical work *Chinese Herbal Medicines Common in Tibet* (Tib. *Bod ljong rgyun spyo krung dbyi'i sman rigs*; C. *Xizang changyong zhong caoyao*, 1971–73), and the Tibetan medicine–specific

TABLE 4.1. Key dates and texts relating to the medico-cultural revolution in Central Tibet

AUGUST 1966	The Great Proletarian Cultural Revolution begins in Lhasa
SEPTEMBER 1968	The *People's Daily* national newspaper reports favorably on the work of the barefoot doctors and the Cooperative Medical Scheme as "newly emerging things" in two "model communes" in Shanghai Municipality and Hubei
1968/9	The barefoot doctor movement takes root across the country
1969	First publication of the *Barefoot Doctor's Manual* (*Chijiao yisheng shouce*) in Shanghai
1972	First Chinese and Tibetan bilingual edition of the *Barefoot Doctor's Manual*
1973	The *Sino-Tibetan Herbal* is published in Tibetan and Chinese editions
1974	A separate section for Tibetan medicine is established at the People's Hospital in Ngamring, fully formalized with two government-appointed Tibetan *amchi*
1975	"Tibetan medicine and pharmaceuticals" are included in the "motherland's medical treasure house"
1975	Publication of the Tibetan medicine–specific *Barefoot Doctor's New Tibetan Medical Compounding Manual* (the *Tibetan Medical Manual*)

Barefoot Doctor's New Tibetan Medical Compounding Manual (*Sman pa rkang rjen ma'i bod sman sbyor sde gsar bsgrigs*, 1975). Both complemented a bilingual edition of the famous *Barefoot Doctor's Manual* (Tib. "*Rkang rjen sman pa'i" slob deb*, C. *Chijiao yisheng shouce*, 1972). These are presented in the context of the drastic sociopolitical upheavals of the time and the almost complete demise of the Lhasa Mentsikhang. While after 1966 many Tibetan medical practitioners, institutions, and books were violently attacked as one of the Four Olds and suffered the consequences, regard for certain aspects of Tibetan medicine, especially its plant-based knowledge, began to change in 1974. Some Tibetan medical knowledge and practitioners were incorporated into China's "health care revolution," and "Tibetan medicine and pharmaceuticals" (Tib. *bögi sorig dang menrik*) were held to be part of the "motherland's medical treasure house" (Lhasa City Mentsikhang 1975: 1–2). Until then, Mao had singled out only Chinese medicine and pharmacology (C. *yiyao*), on October 11, 1958, as immortalized in "the Little Red Book," or *The Quotations of Chairman Mao* (Scheid 2002: 70; Taylor 2005: 120–23). Some Tibetan medical practitioners were invited to work in government county hospitals and newly established clinics, and some became barefoot doctors (table 4.1).

THE RED GUARDS ATTACK THE MENTSIKHANG

Mentsikhang activities were consolidated and expanded in the early 1960s, according to Janes (1995: 16–19). A new class of fifty Tibetan medical students was enrolled and various departments and in- and outpatient facilities created. In January 1963 the Mentsikhang was producing complex precious pills (*rinchen rilbu*),[3] as Jampa Trinlé, the director of the Mentsikhang at the time, recalls in his *Recollections*: "The concern that some knowledge was about to die in today's society was gone" (2006: 32). Hopes for the survival of the Mentsikhang as a socialist health care institution were high. When the Tibet Autonomous Region (TAR) was officially established in 1965, a first Tibetan medicine exhibition was staged and *First Study of Tibetan Medicine and Medical Materials* was published, cowritten (in Tibetan and Chinese) by Jampa Trinlé, with three Tibetan medical experts, one biomedical specialist, and one Chinese medical colleague. They presented it to visiting representatives from the Central Ministry of Health, who, according to Trinlé, "praised the characteristics and rich medical materials" (2006: 29–35) of Tibetan medicine.

The Four Clean-ups, another name for the Socialist Education Movement (SEM, 1962–66), then began, aimed at cleansing "reactionary" and "corrupt" elements in political, economic, organizational, and ideological fields. The SEM demanded that students and their teachers engage in agricultural labor in addition to their medical studies and work. Many were sent down to the countryside, a move meant to curb bourgeois tendencies among the intellectual elites, making it difficult to continue teaching the newly enrolled Tibetan medicine class. The SEM was in many ways a precursor to the Great Proletarian Cultural Revolution, as the first reform implemented without concessions to the situation in central Tibet (Shakya 1999: 292–93).

The Mentsikhang's situation changed drastically in August 1966, after the revolutionary Red Guards from Qinghai Normal University began to target the Lhasa Mentsikhang. The Red Guards climbed above its main entrance to remove the original Institute of Medicine and Astrology sign, renaming it the People's Labor Hospital (Trinlé 2006: 36; Union Research Institute 1968: 605). This was one of numerous changes in the name and appearance of public streets, parks, and institutions in the city that summer.[4] Yet given the scale of human loss and physical destruction to follow, these were perhaps some of the more benign acts of the Red Guards and "revolutionary masses" carrying out Mao's Great Proletarian Cultural Revolution.[5] Its landmark campaigns included the destruction of the Four Olds and attacking remaining counterrevolutionaries in artistic, literary, and political circles, now understood by many historians as a way to purge Mao's political opponents (Shakya 1999: 314).

Although written nearly fifty years later and to a large degree following the CCP interpretation of recent Tibetan history, Jampa Trinlé's *Recollections* (2006) provide a relatively detailed account of Red Guard activities at the institution, including the class struggles and vandalism.[6] Given his earlier optimism, the Red Guards' attacks came as great shock to Jampa Trinlé, as to others who had cooperated with the Communists or joined the party in the 1950s.

Already in May 1966 Mao had intensified his revolutionary policies and called on people to "completely criticize the reactionary bourgeois thought in academic, educational, press and literary-art, and publishing circles and seize the leading power in these areas" (Goldstein, Jiao, and Lhundrup 2009: 11–12). Goldstein, Jiao, and Lhundrup (2009) offer a detailed account of rapidly changing movements of the time, here summarized in broad strokes.

Tibet's Regional Party Committee, under the leadership of Zhang Guohua as TAR CCP party secretary, initially tried to take a slightly different approach to enacting Mao's so-called May 16th Notice of 1966. In contrast to other parts of the PRC where the "masses," especially young students, were encouraged to "search the capitalist-roaders who had infiltrated the Party, government, army and all cultural circles," in Tibet these activities were to be carried out under the leadership of a specially formed team under the control of the Regional Party Committee. Zhang Guohua, its leader, had served in Tibet and knew the local situation well. The earlier Democratic Reforms, the SEM's intensified campaigns against religion and "superstition," as well as the threat of introducing communes in central Tibet, had left the position of the CCP far from secure. Zhang was wary of further destabilizing the region. According to Trinlé (2006: 36), a work group of the Regional Party Committee, rather than the Red Guards, took charge of investigating the Mentsikhang for counterrevolutionary elements in June 1966.

Zhang Guohua's strategy soon collapsed, however, when students of the Lhasa Middle School, in collaboration with incoming Han Chinese Red Guards, became increasingly emboldened to follow directives from the "center" and Mao rather than the local CCP "power holders." In July, they began to attack key offices in Lhasa, in a search for counterrevolutionaries in the Regional Party Committee itself. As elsewhere, so also in Tibet: from August on, following Mao's extreme directives, destruction of the Four Olds and class enemies was delegated to the masses. For the first time, Jampa Trinlé and the Mentsikhang's two vice presidents, Kunga Phuntsog and Ngawang Chödrag, were exposed to public struggle sessions, or *thamzing*, where they were abused as "representatives of scholars" and their "offenses" published in the local newspapers (Trinlé 2006: 36). A revolutionary group of Red Guards was permanently stationed in the Mentsikhang and the institution's three-person leadership dismissed.

Then began the annihilation of the Four Olds. The Mentsikhang's library, the wooden block prints, and the thankas were either burnt or thrown into Lhasa's Kyichu River (Trinlé 2006). Similar actions took place in the homes of Trinlé and his colleagues. With the whole of Lhasa heaving with the destruction of the Four Olds, even the Jokhang and Potala became targets of the zealous young *marsuma*, literally "red army," in the terminology my Tibetan informants used for the Red Guards (Gyurme Dorje 2010: 23–25; Woeser 2006). According to Trinlé's account, there had been a directive from Zhou Enlai in Beijing, passed on to Zhang Guohua sometime in 1966–67, that the PLA should protect the Jokhang and the Potala from further damage (2006: 36–37). The *Recollections* state that Zhang Guohua himself added to this directive that classic medical texts should not be destroyed. This protected at least some works at the Mentsikhang, and "therefore the complete 80 color medical paintings and the leftovers of medical texts could be saved" (Trinlé 2006: 36–37).[7] Thereafter, the Mentsikhang was largely embroiled in class struggle rather than carrying out medical work (Janes 1995: 20). Nonetheless, its staff also cared for victims of factional and PLA fighting and the ongoing class struggle in Lhasa, including the Tibetan victims belonging to the Gyenlok faction, attacked during the PLA's June 7 massacre in the Jokhang (Paljor 1977: 35).[8] The Gyenlok faction (*gyen log*, "rebels") was one of two major political groups formed at the time, the other being the Nyamdre (*mnyam 'brel*). On this occasion, Mentsikhang staff compiled a report on the brutal ways Gyenlok members had been killed. As punishment for this report, Khandro Yangga, one of the Mentsikhang physicians, was exposed to *thamzing* (Paljor 1977; Hofer 2011d: 114–15).

THE VIRTUAL DISAPPEARANCE OF TIBETAN MEDICINE?

The increasing revolutionary fervor took over the whole of Lhasa City, soon extending to rural areas. This is described in a number of autobiographical and historical works, but most of these works focus on urban areas, with the notable exception of Pema Bhum's account from eastern Tibet (2001).[9] By 1973 the Cultural Revolution–related activities would cause, according to Janes, "the virtual disappearance of the institution of Tibetan medicine" (1995: 20). Indeed, during the early years of the Cultural Revolution there was hardly any possibility of negotiating once one had been made a target of the Red Guards. This applied as much to government workers, such as the Mentsikhang's doctors, as it did to private intellectuals, scholars, and many ordinary people, including several physicians.

Tibetan writer Tsering Woeser's book on the Cultural Revolution includes a harrowing photograph taken by her father of a violent struggle session in Lhasa against a medical doctor and his family. They were mock-garlanded with leather medicine bags and foreign money as signs of their reactionary thinking, and forced to wear paper hats stating their "crimes" (figure 4.1; Woeser 2006, 2000: 150–51). The situation of Tibetan medicine in this period cannot be understood without taking into account the impact of CCP directives and demands. Nevertheless, some *amchi*s managed to survive, and some even continued to practice and participate in transforming Tibetan medicine during this time. Such spaces existed in some rural areas, which became the new focus of official health-related

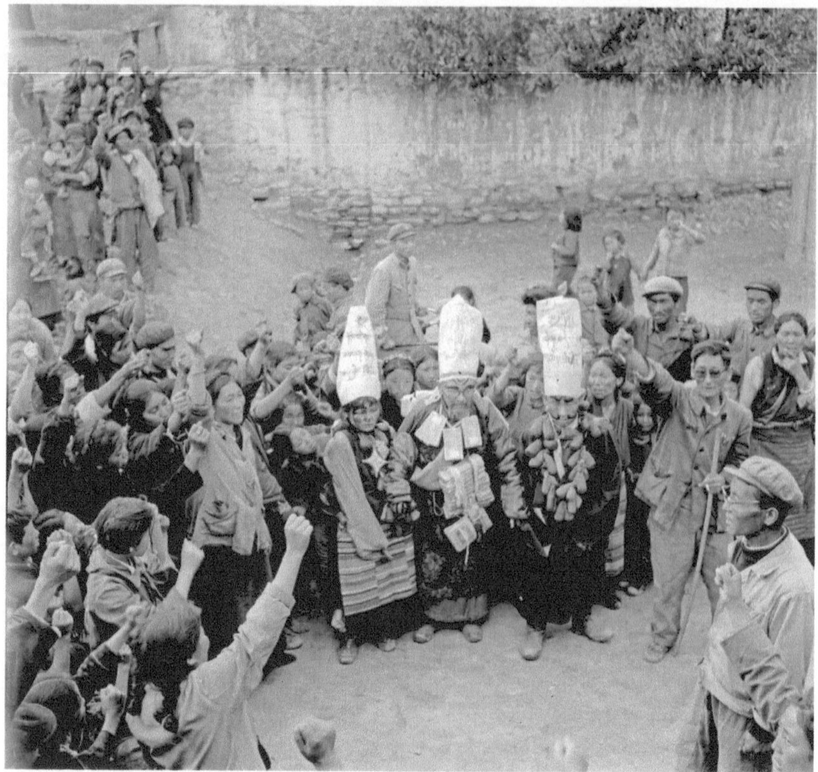

FIGURE 4.1. A Tibetan medical doctor and educator and his family during a struggle session in Lhasa. Photo by Tsering Dorjé, courtesy of Tsering Woeser.

work in the late 1960s and early 1970s. Tibetan medical practice and pharmacology began to occupy a space in this work, small as it was.

Persecution of Tibetan medical practitioners was initially just as harsh in parts of rural Tibet as it was in Lhasa, with its severity dependent on the previously established class labels and their associated punishments. Nevertheless, some *amchi* in Ngamring were able to continue their Tibetan medical work.

THE CULTURAL REVOLUTION IN RURAL TSANG

While the Lhünding Mentrong's library and its Buddhist and medical objects were saved during early attacks, in the summer of 1966, the Red Guards destroyed the physical buildings of the Mentrong and Lhünding

Monastery. Fired with zeal following a local meeting at the township headquarters (in Tarkyü) where the new party line had been announced and the local masses encouraged, the *marsuma* came first to the Mentrong, then to the monastery. For several years, Rinchen Wangyal (who described the events to me) was struggled against "very hard," and he and his family were reduced to poverty. They were denied food rations, which were based on the so-called *karma*, or work points, that had become integral to earlier mutual aid groups (*rogré*) and were now carried over to production teams, the lowest administrative level of the commune (*mimang künhré*).[10] A similar fate befell the Nyingkhang, the members and household of the locally powerful *ngakpa* clan, whose two oldest male members had served sentences in local prisons and labor camps in Kongpo and who were given as many as three "hats" at any one time. Such experiences were recounted numerous times during my fieldwork by those assigned unfavorable class labels during the Democratic Reforms. The attacks and denigrations were very harsh, which we can perhaps discern from Yonten Tsering's repeated assertions that his father had died a "natural death," rather than dying from Red Guard attacks or suicide.

Preserving Tibetan Medical Works

Few lay Tibetan medical practitioners escaped the personal attacks and destruction of medical text collections. Some hid their texts and were fortunate to discover later that the texts had survived the rains and fervent Red youths. This was the case for doctor Sonam Drölma from the Nyékhang at Tsarong and Amchi Tsewang in Ruthog. Tsewang's wife managed to hide a print copy of the *Gyüshi* and their family medical compounding work. Tsering secretly trained their two sons, Pema and Lobsang, as *amchi*. Thus despite commune obligations and the only permitted "literature" being Mao's *Quotations*, this family managed to transmit Tibetan medicine during that time (Hofer 2012). They also obtained the first modern edition of the *Four Treatises* as well as one of Yonten Gyatso's medical works, both published in 1976 in the PRC (Yonten Gyatso 1976).

An exceptional case was Yonten Tsering, who managed to save his entire medical and Buddhist text and thanka collection. When the Red Guards appeared at the doorstep of his one-room clinic on the ground floor of his former home, the Térap, he described all the texts as "medical works," though some were Buddhist texts. He added that they were necessary for his medical work helping the "People." Combined with his seemingly smooth relations with Communist cadres and villagers—he used to say that "everyone was my friend"—the strategy worked. The Red Guards did not touch him or his family's medical collection, and the physical building of the Térap remained intact.

However, according to elderly monks of the area and some textual records, not a single established monastery or nunnery in the county survived the destruction (Hofer 2012; Penpa Tsering 2013; Sherab Dorjé 1994). Buddhist medical practitioners, such as the Nyingma Chaug monastery's Tutop or Dewachen's Ani Pema Lhamo and her teacher, were physically attacked by the *marsuma* in repeated attempts to turn their thinking from "old" to "new." Most if not all of their texts and medical instruments, including materia medica storage boxes and spoons, and any leftover raw materials were burned or thrown into rivers. Only a few items could be saved. It was "a dark phase in Tibetan history, like when thick black clouds cast dark shadows everywhere," writes Jampa Trinlé in an official college history textbook on that time. "Like everything else in Tibetan culture and education, so also Tibetan medical theory and all precious cultural objects were destroyed" (2004: 135). This situation was aggravated by the lack of Tibetan medical students, until eventually "almost all hope for Tibetan medicine was lost. It was like a verdant tree drying out" (133). Tibetan medicine largely receded into the realms of silent knowing and secret practice and transmission. Doctors like Tutop and Ngawang Dorjé, who had been monks, practiced medicine covertly and with extreme caution. Tutop exchanged treatment for medical herbs that local people picked for him; Ngawang Dorjé did farmwork and assisted a barefoot doctor. Until 1972 he was unable to use his Tibetan medical skill.[11]

Continuing Tibetan Medical Work within New Parameters

At least two doctors in Ngamring County managed to gain partial approval from the local production team and commune leadership to continue their Tibetan medical work, although in greatly simplified ways. Yonten Tsering continued making and prescribing medicines as well as applying some external therapies from the ground floor of Térap House and on rounds to other villages. Due to the demands of his cadre responsibilities of registering harvests, participating in agricultural work, and working as a doctor, he made medicines mainly at night with the help of his wife. All the foreign medical ingredients had been used up, so he relied on local herbs and minerals, only making three kinds of medicines in the late 1960s. Yonten Tsering was not, however, officially a health worker or barefoot doctor, probably due to his previous class background. His medical practice was tolerated but not supported, apart from his receiving work points even when absent from agricultural work. He did not like to dwell on this time and always highlighted the positive aspects of his personal history and experience of reform.

The Bon monk Rabgyal provides a remarkable story of cooperation and negotiation with county and township cadres as well as unique circumstances. He had studied medicine in the 1940s and early 1950s at a Bon monastery near Lake Dangra Yumtso. Because Rabgyal was a monk when his parents died, their wealth was distributed among his brothers and he inherited nothing. He officially left the order to travel as a mendicant monk for several years, but his life took an unexpected turn in 1960, when Democratic Reforms came to Ngamring's pastoral areas. Rabgyal was made a local work team committee member (*u yon*) and commenced working as an administrator for the Communists in nomadic Tsatsé Chu. At that time a new administrative center was being established. During a trip to Sakya on official business to purchase grain for his nomadic area, he discovered that he could buy a large quantity of medicinal raw ingredients via a middleman. These had formerly belonged to three doctors who had been labeled "high-class reactionaries" and imprisoned. Their medicines were confiscated and renamed "reactionary's medicine" (*lokchö men*). With these newly acquired medicinal ingredients Rabgyal began his career as an *amchi*, compounding all his own medicines. From 1961 to 1975 he worked at the Tsatsé health clinic, with only one major interruption in 1969. He told me that adherents of the Gyenlok faction attacked Rabgyal's clinic that year. He referred to this event as a "great uprising."[12] Rabgyal was not harmed and resumed his work shortly afterward. He relied almost exclusively upon Tibetan medicine and was never formally trained in biomedicine, only learning rudimentary diagnostic techniques from a colleague at the health post. Partly due to his age and difficulty in communication, I was unable to understand better how he navigated the requirements of relating to the state and times past.

Prior to 1969 few Tibetans had been trained as Communist health workers. I interviewed several of them, including some colleagues of Rabgyal, also from Ngamring. One was Ngawang, who had retired from long-term service as a health worker and the head of the Ngamring County Hospital. Another was Tashi, who in the 1960s had been sent to work in Tsatsé, initially as a veterinary health worker, and in 2003 was a retired government worker.

Ngawang came from a family doing farmwork in Ngamring County with no prior connection to medicine. When a Communist work team came to his village in 1960 promoting the new reforms, they offered Ngawang a place in an eight-month training course at a PLA First of August military base in Shigatse. He accepted. The Great Leap Forward's communalization of agriculture and its focus on industrial production were not implemented in central Tibet due to the gradualist approach of the 1950s. However, Mao's core principle during the Great Leap Forward of 1958–61, to catch up with the British in industrial and agricultural production, permeated other domains in central Tibet. This principle was widely promoted for medical and scientific learning, and through the country-wide official CCP and PLA propaganda. Ngawang and others in the training course were told they had to complete their study of medicine within months. He described the approach: "What you learn in eight years from textbooks, you will now learn in eight months from practice." His training included little theory, focusing mainly on practical observation and hands-on learning with senior Han Chinese doctors. He referred to the system he had learned using the term *chiyi*, an interesting compound word made up of *chi* (*phyi*), the Tibetan word for "outsider," "foreign," or "vast," and *yi* (*yi*), the Chinese term for "medicine," thus yielding "outsider medicine."[13] This was a basic course in biomedicine, but because Mao and the national Ministry of Health promoted combined versions of Western and Chinese medicine (Taylor 2005), this training included exposure to basic Chinese medical ideas about the body and simple Chinese acupuncture.

When Ngawang returned to Ngamring County in 1961, he was dispatched with a medical kit and a dozen biomedicines to Tobé Xiang. He called his work that of a "barefoot doctor," referring to the campaign and massive paramedical health worker movement that began formally in 1968–69. Visiting patients in remote pastoral areas on horseback, he acted as both health worker and party clerk, recording information on harvests and numbers of livestock as well as dispatching government propaganda. He did this throughout Tobé District from 1961 to 1965, when he was transferred to a Tsatsé township health post to work in three capacities: civil administrator, secretary/clerk, and "barefoot doctor." That year the Ngamring health post was transformed into Ngamring Hospital and its doctors increased to six—three Han Chinese and three Tibetans.

While at Tsatsé township clinic, Ngawang acquired some Tibetan medical knowledge. The barefoot doctor campaign was gathering momentum in the autumn of 1968, characterized by self-reliance and experimentation with folk medicine (cf. Fang 2012). In Tibet, it began to open up opportunities, albeit at first limited, for experimentation with Tibetan medical therapies, mainly compounded herbs. Ngawang learned about these from exchanges with Amchi Rabgyal, who was then based at the Tsatsé township health post. In 1973 Ngawang was transferred back to Ngamring, where the hospital had become a "People's Hospital" and the doctors increased to nine. He served as the hospital director that year and in 1974 instituted a separate section for Tibetan medicine, with two government-appointed Tibetan *amchi* and its own two-room facility within the hospital. We can see this as an instance of the early integration of Tibetan medical doctors into the rural Communist health bureaucracy.

Tashi, who had been trained in Tibetan medicine by his maternal uncle in Shigatse during the 1950s, also received the PLA's First of August military medical training in 1960, following a combined biomedical and Chinese medical training, the latter mainly focused on acupuncture. After work at the county seat, he was posted to the Tsatsé township clinic in the late 1960s. He recalled the collaborative spirit in which he worked there with *amchi* Rabgyal and health worker Ngawang. He had acquired a Bon medical manuscript from Rabgyal in exchange for a thick sheepskin *chuba*, the trade exemplifying the value medical works had at that time, as texts were rare due to the widespread destruction. Although he depended mainly on about twenty "outsider" biomedicines, Tashi also used a smaller number of Tibetan medical compounds as part of his treatments, which met with the approval of local Chinese and Tibetan cadres.

In contrast to the limited medical exchange between lay medical doctors and their Medical Houses in the pre-reform period, Communist health work fostered collaboration and knowledge exchange between practitioners. *Amchi* and health workers shared a socialist health clinic that was funded by the local administration but relied on local people for medical work and gathering plants. This shared workplace bringing together doctors who were not related through kinship or religious affiliation, along with the political circumstances of the time, changed the way Tibetan medicine was transmitted. Departing from largely vertical axes of transmission from teachers to disciples, horizontal peer education was introduced and became part of the ethos of the barefoot doctors. In addition, at least at the health post in Tsatsé township, there was some experimentation with treatments from biomedicine, traditional Chinese medicine, and Tibetan medicine. In Tsatsé, even in the 1960s, Tibetan medical resources were integral to the work of the township health post. This was probably due in no small part to Rabgyal's forceful character, his connections with other leaders, and quite likely his ability to navigate the political requirements of the time.

His situation seems to be unusual, however, as the interviews I conducted suggest that Tibetan medicine and its practitioners were generally unwelcome in governmental health work prior to 1974. Rather, there was a brief but curious period during which a simplified version of Chinese medicine, as practiced in the China-wide barefoot doctor campaign, was seen as the politically safe option for Tibet—safer than relying on Tibetan or "folk" medicine. This new strategy is exemplified in *Chinese Herbal Medicines Common in Tibet* (1973a, 1973b).

THE BAREFOOT DOCTORS

One of many paradoxes of the modern history of Tibet and the PRC is that at the same time as the Cultural Revolution's propagators inflicted horrendous destruction and suffering across China, government health workers for the first time began to provide basic public and clinical health care to many rural village residents. At the core of this development was a massive public health initiative focused on the rural areas, its centerpieces being the barefoot doctors and the communal Cooperative Medical Services (CMS) scheme. These initiatives began in earnest in September 1968, the Chinese national newspaper *People's Daily* reporting favorably on the work of the barefoot doctors and the CMS scheme as "newly emerging things" (*xingsheng shiwu*) practiced in two "model communes": the Jiangzhen Commune, Chuangsha County in Shanghai Municipality, and the Leyuan Commune, Changyang County in Hubei (Fang 2012: 30–33). As in education and agriculture,[14] the work of model communes was publicized and propagated by the CCP, the unquestionable political demand being that the rest of the PRC learn from and emulate them.

Historian Xiaoping Fang's 2012 study of the barefoot doctors in the context of medical modernization in a rural Chinese village provides a uniquely rich study of the campaign in Jiang Village, in Zhejiang in eastern China, from the bottom up rather than relying mainly on campaign texts or official reports. It is based on in-depth oral history, as well as anthropological and archival research carried out between 2003 and 2011.

In Jiang Village the new policies meant that health workers formerly attached to the so-called union clinics, which had been set up in most Chinese villages during the 1950s and operated on a system of fees for services, individual accounting, self-responsibility for profits and losses, and democratic management (Fang 2012), were converted to a system of barefoot doctors. The purpose of the barefoot doctors was to provide health care yet also work in the fields, contributing to production. As they were thought to be working on the paddy fields, they acquired the name "barefoot doctors." According to Fang, their overall numbers were vastly increased to meet the official target of one barefoot doctor per production brigade. Primary and middle school students were therefore selected and given short, two- to six-month training courses in basic Western and Chinese medicine, usually in local county hospitals. These Chinese women and men, and girls and boys, were then sent back to the production brigades with medical kits. Their main work involved prevention, including the promotion of sanitation and hygiene, rudimentary reproductive health advice, and service as a bridge to higher-level care at clinics, for instance accompanying patients and caring for them en route. At the same time, they provided low-cost medical treatment of common diseases of the rural masses by means of "one silver needle and a bunch of herbs," in the words of a popular saying of the time (Fang 2012: 2).

Based on their experience and training as well as exchanges with colleagues and use of *The Barefoot Doctor's Manual*,[15] barefoot doctors tended to use several treatment modalities at one time. Their range of therapeutic options initially included biomedicines (painkillers, analgesics, antibiotics, etc.) and what were called "new techniques" (including seven-point acupuncture) and Chinese herbs. In due time, in Jiang Village a range of ready-made Chinese patent medicines replaced the compounds and decoctions made from Chinese herbs, which were often beyond the expertise of barefoot doctors. Incomes for the doctors were miniscule. Through an annual contribution made by commune members to the CMS, some of the barefoot doctors' expenses and a large part of the cost of their medicines could be covered.

The revolutionary, and indeed globally unique, barefoot doctor campaign grew out of preceding educational reforms, especially the SEM, which focused on practical learning and applicability. They combined with Mao's now famous attack on the Ministry of Health in June 1965, when he said: "The Ministry of Health is only able to serve 15 per cent of the total population, and this 15 per cent is made up of mostly the privileged. The broad ranks of the peasants cannot obtain medical treatment and also do not receive medicine. The Ministry of Health is not a people's ministry. It should be called the Urban Health Ministry, the Ministry of Health for the Lords, or even the Urban Ministry of Health for the Lords. . . . Stress rural areas in medical and health work!" (quoted in Fang 2012: 30). This became known as the June 26 Directive and informed all aspects of health work during the Cultural Revolution, with the last sentence—"Stress rural areas in medical and health work!"—also featured in the *Quotations*.

In the United States and Europe, a flood of reports in the early 1970s pointed to the successes of China's rural health campaigns, especially the barefoot doctors. Many uncritically repeated official PRC discourse, deftly spread through the Foreign Languages Press and Western journalists with access to party sources.[16] Such coverage, along with China's admission to the World Health Organization (WHO) in 1974 and the English translation of *The Barefoot Doctor's Manual* (1977), made the barefoot doctor model widely known. It featured prominently in discussions at the WHO's 1978 conference in Alma Ata, a meeting henceforth hailed as having returned the focus of international health to preventive medicine and primary health care, not least through incorporation of traditional medicine practitioners in resource-poor regions, as demonstrated in China.

Despite this international fame, little scholarly work has been done on the social history of the barefoot doctor campaign across rural China. Many international and domestic reports were heavily influenced by Chinese official accounts and restrictions on research in the PRC. Others were inflected by the appeal of Chinese medicine in the wake of rising interest in Oriental medicine, especially in the United States. While there has been some notable anthropological work (Farquhar 1994; Hsu 1999; Scheid 2007), the study by Fang (2012) not only is the most in-depth but also advances a compelling argument. Fang argues that rather than serving as a vehicle to promote Chinese medicine in rural areas during the Cultural Revolution, or to spread the tradition more broadly within China, the barefoot doctors' work spread Western pharmaceuticals to a much wider population than had been the case. Along with the purge of established physicians and institutions of Chinese medicine, this contributed to the proliferation of, and ultimately preference for, biomedicines among rural Chinese today—with traditional medicine, in reinvented forms (as increasingly also in India and Tibet), in use mainly by the middle classes.

There are few references to barefoot doctors in the Tibetan biographical accounts (e.g., Dhondub Chödon 1978: 24–25) and few visual depictions (see figures 4.2 and 7.1). We have no in-depth study of the barefoot doctor campaign in Tibetan areas of the PRC to help us evaluate how it played out in rural Tibet and whether Fang's argument pertains there. However, we can find useful evidence of the campaign in works that were published in the early 1970s in Tibet.

Classical Tibetan medical works, including the *Gyüshi*, had been identified as reflections of "old" thinking and destroyed along with Buddhist and other Tibetan medical literature in lay and monastic libraries and collections. This was thought to make way for "new" thinking, fostered mainly through compulsory study of Mao's *Quotations*.[17] This situation left health workers of any tradition and level with a dearth of study materials, the gap filled mainly by government publications of the barefoot doctor campaign.

Most prominent and epitomizing the campaign was *The Barefoot Doctor's Manual* (*Chijiao yisheng shouce*), produced by the newly established Revolutionary Committee of the Beijing Health Bureau in 1968–69 (SCMC, ZCMC, and ZCMRI 1969). An official Tibetan language translation was published in a Chinese/Tibetan bilingual edition in March 1972, titled *Chijiao yisheng shouce: "Rkang rjen sman pa'i" slob deb* (QTMCRCWTG 1972, figure 4.3). The publisher of the work was the Qinghai Tibetan Medical College Revolutionary Committee Writing and Translation Group, with the work widely distributed in the TAR, where apparently several Chinese editions of the work also circulated.

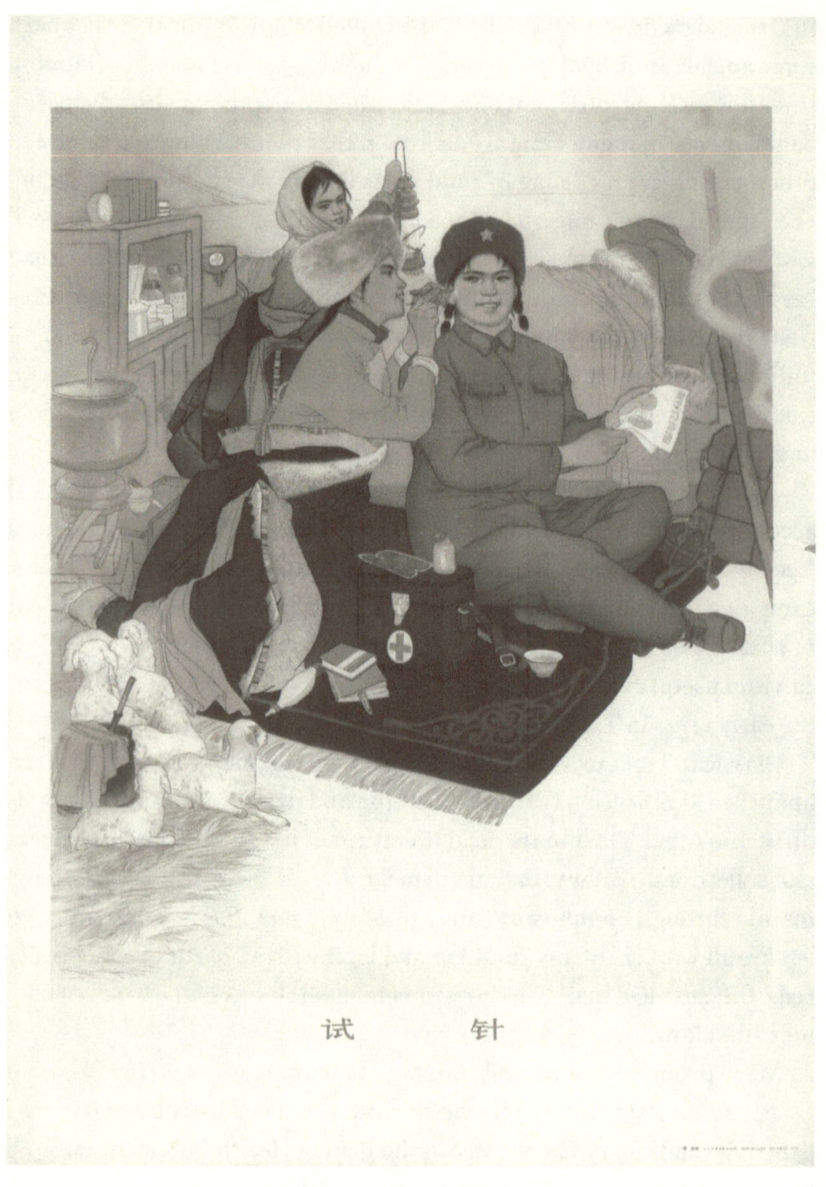

FIGURE 4.2. *Practicing Acupuncture*, by the artist Shao Hua, 1973 (77 × 54 cm). Courtesy of the International Institute of Social History, University of Leiden, Stefan R. Landsberger Collection, BG E15/230.

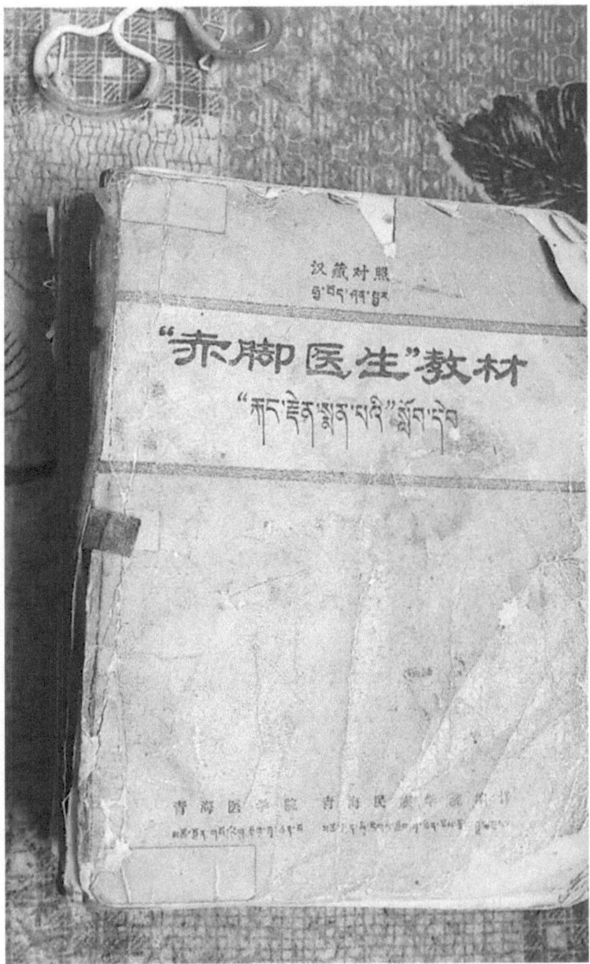

FIGURE 4.3. Cover of the bilingual Sino-Tibetan edition of *The Barefoot Doctor's Manual*, 2010. Photo by Chaksham.

The Tibetan *Barefoot Doctor's Manual* is a faithful translation of the earlier Chinese editions and hence features no Tibetan medical content. At the point of publication, no efforts were made to adjust the manual to the Tibetan situation, and not even the use of Tibetan materia medica was endorsed. This changed when *Chinese Herbal Medicines Common in Tibet* (1971–73; henceforth *The Sino-Tibetan Herbal*) and the Tibetan medicine-specific *Barefoot Doctor's New Tibetan Medical Compounding Manual* (1975; henceforth *The Tibetan Medical Manual*) were published. While the

Tibetan-Chinese bilingual edition of *The Barefoot Doctor's Manual* was, with one exception, no longer in the possession of people I worked with in Ngamring, health workers in Tsang used the other two throughout the 1970s, and some still refer to them today.

What was the officially conceived role for Chinese medicine and Tibetan medicine in the barefoot doctor campaign in Tibet as espoused in these two works? How did Tibetan medical doctors contribute to or benefit from them? Exploring these questions is crucial to examination of *amchis*' ability to work with and transmit their own tradition around the time these works were produced. The purge of the Four Olds, including many Tibetan medical practitioners and their classical works, continued unabated.

THE SINO-TIBETAN HERBAL

What we will call *The Sino-Tibetan Herbal* is essentially an exposition on revolutionary Chinese pharmaceuticals addressed to Tibetans in the Tibetan language. It covers many Chinese herbs and plants named in *The Barefoot Doctor's Manual* but diverges in one important respect: this work uses only Tibetan materia medica to compound the revolutionary formulas of the barefoot doctors. In the spirit of self-reliance, revolutionary health work in Tibet was intended to avoid importing Chinese herbs from great distances, instead using local materials proven in pharmaceutical research and having similar properties.

The Lhasa Health Bureau's Revolutionary Health Committee devoted considerable resources and research to this work. The results from early collaborations between Mentsikhang doctors and Chinese medical experts in the 1950s in Lhasa likely influenced the work. It is uncertain how long their research had been going on and who exactly was involved.[18] The foreword to the book had already been written in December 1971, with the finalized *Sino-Tibetan Herbal* published in May 1973 in Tibetan (RCTARHB 1973a), followed by a Chinese edition in July 1973 (RCTARHB 1973b).[19]

The Sino-Tibetan Herbal was effectively the first modern work on Chinese medicine in the Tibetan language and was produced in European book format (figure 4.4). The Tibetan-language edition was distributed to health posts and barefoot doctors to promote the combined biomedical and Chinese medical work of the barefoot doctors. Several of my informants in Ngamring had used this work in the past.

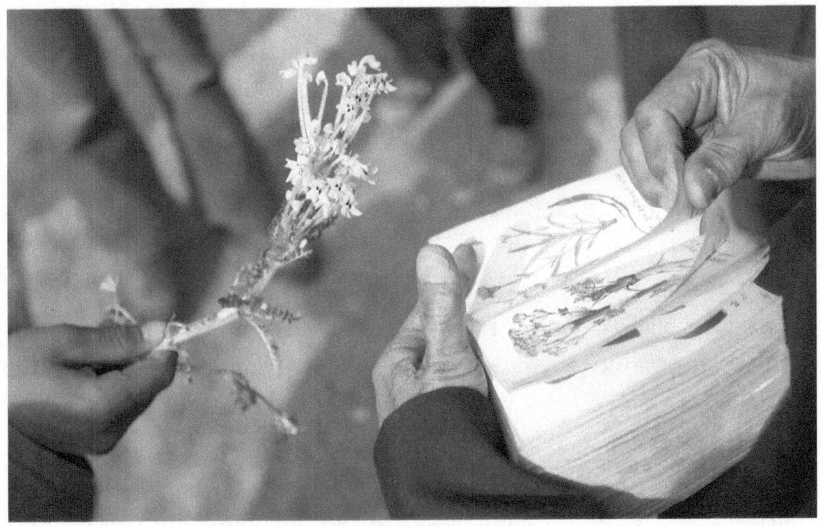

FIGURE 4.4. *The Sino-Tibetan Herbal* in use, 2007. Photo by Meinrad Hofer.

The following offers a description and outline of the Tibetan edition. I retain as much as possible of the book's language and style, quoting liberally to give the reader a flavor of the revolutionary language of the time as well as the Tibetan neologisms reflecting the political landscape of the time. The work is analyzed with regard to the position of local medical, especially plant, knowledge and how this was conceived of in revolutionary health care between 1971 and 1973, as a "newly emerging thing" rather than one of the Four Olds.

Brief Summary and Outline

The full Tibetan title of the work is *Bod ljong rgyun spyo krung dbyi'i sman rigs*. It includes the Tibetan term *trungyi* (*krung dbyi*),[20] a Tibetanized rendering of the Chinese term *zhong yi* (Chinese medicine). *Trung* (*krung*), the first part of the compound, was the new, politically correct term for the People's Republic of China, in contrast to Gyanag (China); while *yi* (*dbyi*) was directly imported from Chinese into Tibetan and used as a loan word, together making *trungyi*. The literal translation of the Tibetan title of the work would be "Chinese Medicines Common in Tibet." The title of the Chinese edition, *Xizang changyong zhong caoyao*, uses the term *zhong caoyao*, which specifically means "Chinese herbal medicines." As there are only a few medicines derived from animal origins in the book, I translate the Tibetan term *menrik*[21] (types of medicines) as "herbal medicines," even though it technically can include other kinds of materia medica. The same reasoning informs my choice of *Herbal* as an abbreviation of the title. The attention of the work's editors and Mao himself was focused on material, herbal substances rather than on other kinds of expensive ingredients and theoretical sophistication.

The Sino-Tibetan Herbal is a small (15 × 10 cm) but thick work with 1,276 pages, making it almost as thick as it is wide. Its main feature is a section of 424 color plates depicting plants and a couple of animals, using a technique that combined the use of color lithography and photography. This technology was used here for the first time in the context of Tibetan pharmaceuticals. Previous illustrations of Tibetan medical simples had been drawn by hand, or were carved in wood and used in block-printing illustrated texts.[22] Importantly, the term *trungpé*, previously used for medical simples in the Tibetan medical tradition, is not used in this revolutionary work.[23] Instead it employs, starting in the introduction, the new Tibetan combined term *sorig dang menrik*,[24] literally meaning "healing and types of medicines." Here this term is not specifically used for Tibetan medicine. This new compound term probably translates the Chinese term *yiyao*, "medicine and pharmaceuticals," used in the Chinese edition. It reflects the new emphasis on the material substances of traditional medicine and refers to the then widely used Chinese term *yiyao*, eternalized in the 1958 Mao slogan "Chinese medicine and pharmaceuticals are a national treasure house."

The work avoids mention of individual authors, commonly seen at the time as "bourgeois individualism" (unless of course one's name was Mao Zedong or Lin Biao), instead crediting the Revolutionary Committees of the TAR Health Bureau and of Tibet's Military Region (the precursor to the Tibet Autonomous Region, established in 1965).

The Sino-Tibetan Herbal's first page features three quotations from Chairman Mao:

> Prepare for war. Prepare for emergencies. Serve the people.
>
> Stress rural areas in medical treatment and health.
>
> Chinese medicine and pharmaceuticals are a great treasure house, they should be diligently explored and improved upon.

This placed the work immediately within the political mission of the time and foregrounded its foremost exponent.[25]

> Under the guidance of Chairman Mao's path of the Proletarian Revolution, medical workers and health staff in our Autonomous Region follow the unity of the Ninth National Party Congress and choose the victory route. Using Marxism-Leninism and Mao Zedong thought as weapons, further exposing and critiquing such liars as Liu Shaoqi,[26] we promote class struggle, line struggle, and consciousness of continuous revolution.
>
> Respecting the instructions of the great leader Chairman Mao "Chinese medicine is a great treasure, we should diligently explore and improve upon it," to implement Chairman Mao's strategy of "Prepare for war. Prepare for emergencies. Serve the people," [we] thoroughly explore and use the source of Chinese herbal medicines in our region to prevent diseases.
>
> Through actively developing the public work of self-collection, self-growing, self-cultivation, self-manufacture of herbal medicines, we serve workers, peasants, and soldiers better, [we] serve the Socialist Revolution, promoting the construction of society and [stressing] medical treatment and health care for rural and nomadic areas. To support these [activities], we have edited the book called *Chinese Herbal Medicines Common in Tibet* and provide this book for all the health workers and barefoot doctors as a reference.
>
> This book is published in both Chinese and Tibetan, and it includes 367 kinds of medicines, 424 colored pictures, [information] on the prevention and cure of widely encountered illnesses, and medical prescriptions of Chinese herbal medicines for prevalent illnesses. As we have not studied the works of Marx and Chairman Mao enough, and given the shortage of knowledge and time, there are surely mistakes. Comrades, please do criticize and point them out.

Here we can see that the work's purpose is stated in full revolutionary style, relying as much on Maoist thought generally as on policies espoused by the CCP in their seminal Ninth Congress of April 1969 (at which Lin Biao, the most influential figure in promoting Mao's personality cult, became China's second-in-charge).

The first part of the work (1–57) presents European-style botanical classificatory systems for plants and their parts, followed by basic Chinese medical ideas on collection and processing of herbs. It introduces key Chinese medical ideas such as the four characters[27] and five tastes.[28] There follows a general introduction to basic diagnostic and therapeutic ideas of revolutionary Chinese medicine, mainly the four diagnostic techniques (seeing, smelling and listening, questioning, and feeling the pulse) and eight medical principles (of diseases being inside or outside, hot or cold, *xu* or *shu*, and *yin* or *yang*; 51–53).

Under eighteen symptomatic headings (for instance, medicines to cure fevers, digestive conditions, diarrhea), hundreds of individual herbs and a few animal products (medical simples rather than compounds) are then listed (59–658). Every plant profile follows roughly the same form, covering approximately two to five pages each: name (often complemented with its Chinese name); appearance; location of growth in Tibet and particular habitats; time for collection; the item's "character," "taste/flavor,"[29] and "effect";[30] its chief application; and in some cases, additional notes.

The bulk of the book features the color images with Tibetan, Chinese, and Latin identifications given underneath (659–1082). The final section comprises another two hundred pages on the prevention and treatment of common diseases (1083–226), followed by an alphabetical list of herb names in Tibetan and Latin (1227–76). This last part is divided into nine subsections that categorize diseases into those that are *göné* (contagious),[31] those caused by *nöbu* (viruses),[32] internal diseases, external diseases, women's diseases, children's diseases, diseases of the five sense organs, dermatological, and those caused by *sinbu* (bacteria).[33] Within each category, common conditions and diseases are listed. The categories and names of individual diseases and conditions are listed here much like those in the latter part of *The Barefoot Doctor's Manual* (QTMCRCWTG 1972). However, in contrast, where both Chinese and many Western medicines are listed, *The Sino-Tibetan Herbal* features only nonbiomedical, plant-based drugs found in Tibet. Several recipes are offered, combining the illustrated herbs and some animal products into compounds, stating ratios and preparation. Herbs are frequently also given as single-ingredient drugs.

No Tibetan categories of medical disease or diagnosis appear in this work. Only some physical symptoms common to Tibetan medical theory are included, for example that of *chuser*, which is, however, defined here in its biomedical physiological sense, whereas in Tibetan medicine the meaning is broad and multivalent.[34]

The Sino-Tibetan Herbal attests to a phase in which reliance on Chinese medicine was hailed as an important part of the barefoot doctor campaign in Tibet. In the spirit of self-reliance, using knowledge of local plants and materia medica derived from Tibetan medicine was seen as positive, even though Tibetan medicine is not referred to as such. The work's use of biomedical and Western botanical classification combined with Chinese medical and pharmacological frameworks with Tibetan ingredients demonstrates a kind of experimentation that sat squarely with Mao's call to bring medicine and health care to the rural masses.

In line with the revolutionary reforms to the Tibetan language at the time (cf. Pema Bhum 2001), *The Sino-Tibetan Herbal* abandons the use of many features in Tibetan. For instance, the intersyllabic point, or *tshek*, is omitted; instead a small round circle is used, reminiscent of the English period. The work also omits Tibetan numerals and traditional paragraph flourishes.

Tibetans' Use of The Sino-Tibetan Herbal

In Ngamring during the 1970s, *The Sino-Tibetan Herbal*, along with *The Barefoot Doctor's Manual*, was issued free of charge to township health posts, production brigade medical stations (in other words, the barefoot doctors), county hospitals, and county epidemic disease prevention stations (the latter two receiving larger numbers for training purposes). I found *The Sino-Tibetan Herbal* commonly preserved in Tibetan medical *amchis*' libraries to this day.

Yet prescription and compounding of Tibetan simples using Chinese techniques, as presented in the last part of the book, never really caught on in Ngamring. Instead, according to elderly health workers and doctors I interviewed, when the use of local herbal medical resources was considered, it was easier to use them in a Tibetan medical way, simply consulting with those who had been *amchi* or were now working in the government system. Namgyel and Tashi did this with Rabgyal at the Tsatsé health post. Moreover, starting in 1974, Yonten Tsering and Ngawang Dorjé, the doctors then appointed to the People's Hospital's newly opened Tibetan medicine section, taught cohorts of younger health workers and barefoot doctors to prepare Tibetan medicines. They used the color section of *The Sino-Tibetan Herbal* to instruct their students and help with identification of local materials during field trips. But they did not compound or use them as *The Sino-Tibetan Herbal* (or indeed *The Barefoot Doctor's Manual*) intended. They used the collected materials only to make Tibetan medicines for diseases and conditions defined according to Tibetan medical parameters. It was, in other words, a popular visual guide for students of *Tibetan medicine* to identify plants for use in Tibetan medical compounding. This remained so throughout the 1970s, and even into the early 1980s, given the almost complete lack of textual resources on Tibetan medicine, especially color illustrations of materia medica.[35] Interestingly, this work was used in exactly the same way by exiled Tibetans in India.[36] More evidence on the use of *The Sino-Tibetan Herbal* is required to assess if Chinese medical compounds were actually made in other parts of rural Tibet, based on local ingredients.

TIBETAN MEDICAL MANUAL

The introduction to *The Barefoot Doctor's New Tibetan Medical Compounding Manual,* for short *Tibetan Medical Manual*, also employs the mandatory overarching discourse of the Great Proletarian Revolution. It aligns itself closely with Mao's quotes and policies on Chinese medicine, rural health care, and public health, again beginning with the same three quotations on its first page. In addition to the title and name of the publishing house, the title page declares that the work is a "gift on the occasion of the ten-year anniversary of the establishment of the Tibet Autonomous Region" (iii).

Interestingly, the first sentence of the introduction adapts Mao's famous 1958 treasure-house slogan to one saying that "the Tibetan science of healing and pharmaceuticals [*Bögi sorig dang menrik*] are a part [*chashé*][37] of the great treasury of the motherland's medical science" (1). While *The Sino-Tibetan Herbal* only restated Mao's slogan that "Chinese medicine and pharmaceuticals are a great treasure house," this work, for the first time since at least 1966, refers explicitly to the *Tibetan* "science of healing and pharmaceuticals" being a part of this treasure house. In common with *The Sino-Tibetan Herbal*, the name given to "medicine" in this text combines again the Tibetan terms for "healing/medicine" (*sorig*) and "pharmaceuticals" (*menrik*), continuing the new emphasis on material, tangible substances.

The introduction goes on to laud Tibetan medicine's contribution to the health of the Tibetan people. Tibetan medicine's development was based, we read, on Tibetans' experience in "struggling with all sorts of diseases," absorbing "the essence[38] of Chinese medicine [*trungyi*] and adding the great achievements made in medicine abroad"[39] (1). In confident tones, it asserts that Tibetan medicine nevertheless has several advantages compared to Chinese and Western medicine: one needs less of it, it is more effective, and it costs less. Tibetan medicines are identified as easily portable, hence particularly convenient for remote rural areas. Tibetan medicine[40] is reported to have contributed to the "(public) health revolution,"[41] and specifically the consolidation and development of the barefoot doctor units (4). The authors and their institution then state their alliance with the party line of the Tenth Party Congress, second plenum, Mao's key instructions, and the wider political demands of the period by "promoting among the medical workers of our hospital class struggle, path struggle, and continued revolution" (3).

As for health-related political campaigns, the work aligns itself with Mao's instruction that "Chinese medicine and pharmaceuticals are a great treasure house, which should be explored and diligently improved upon" (printed in bold letters) and the June 26 Directive that rural areas should be stressed in medical activities (3). Guided by these two instructions, the authors write, "we quickly organized public activities to bring about changes to the fact that there are 1. no medicines, and 2. fewer doctors in farming and nomadic areas. We worked very hard based on [the principle] of self-reliance,[42] making efforts to produce what we need by ourselves, promoting ways of overcoming difficulties, and ourselves collecting medical materials, compounding and using them" (3–4).

The *Tibetan Medical Manual* defines specific aims: to improve the health care of farmers and nomads, serve the Tibetan socialist revolution and construction, and provide a reference for barefoot doctors and medical staff in rural areas, "so they can study and move forward by carrying out research in their daily practice" (4).

The editors state that they followed Mao's instructions, "discarding the old, absorbing the essences,"[43] "using the good of the old [medicine] today" and "using the good from foreign in Chinese treatment"[44] (5). Based on these principles, the 480 formulas are said to rely on a combination of textual and practical sources, including Ju Mipham's medical compounding work[45] and "many other medical works." This indicates a certain relaxation in official policy on medical research and classical texts. With regard to practical sources, they specify the "practice, research, and experience" of the staff of the Lhasa Mentsikhang and Shentsa Hospital in Nagchu (5). They highlight the politically correct experimentation and "sharing of experiences," relying on practical exchanges and outcomes rather than emphasizing textual or "theoretical" study. All ingredients for the compounds "are found in Tibet" (5).

The introduction ends on a note similar to *The Sino-Tibetan Herbal*, with the authors excusing themselves on account of their "incompetence in understanding Marxism-Leninism and Maoist thought, their shortage of practical experience, limited theoretical and political understanding, lack of intellectual and medical works, and lack of editing experience" (6), a standard disclaimer in publications of the time. The introduction by "the editors" is dated June 26, 1975, surely chosen to align the work with Mao's June 26 Directive of 1965, which criticized the Ministry of Health for its urban biases, aiming to redirect it and to "stress rural areas in medical work."

Structure of the Book

Following a detailed table of contents, the *Tibetan Medical Manual* begins with a tripartite general section. The first part describes five (of the seven) classic Tibetan medical "limbs" of making (herbal) medicines; in the second, the remaining two limbs are considered and four of the ten classic forms of medicines introduced, adding also "medicinal baths" (*chum*); the third part details methods of processing medicines and their main forms, namely liquid, powder, and pill medicines, with further information on dosage and timing in prescription.

The main body of the book is made up of medical compound names, listed under thirty-seven broad disease categories, which range from "*lung* disorders" to "infectious fevers," "*tripa* disorders" to stomach disorders, headaches, organ disorders, pediatric, gynecological, and sexual disorders, as well as a vast section on miscellany. The book ends with a comprehensive formulaic list of 374 medical simples (266–89), stating the name, one of six tastes, character[46] (either warming [*drö*], cooling [*sil*], or neutral [*nyom*]), effect/benefit (*pennü*), and page numbers where they occur as part of the formulas in the main body of the text.

Names of authors are not mentioned in the work, and only the book's last page reveals the Lhasa City Mentsikhang as editor, indicating that this institution had again been renamed after the Red Guard designation as People's Labor Hospital in 1966.

Simplification, Renaming, and Reformulation

In the naming of medical compounds and the number and kind of their ingredients, we see a general simplification compared with earlier, widely used Lhasa Mentsikhang publications on medical compounding, for example Khyenrap Norbu's works, written before his death in 1962, such as *Excellent Vase of Elixirs* (reprinted by Tashigang in India in 1974) and *Effect of Medical Compounds* (n.d.).[47] The work is also less complex than classical works such as the sections on compounding in volumes 3 and 4 of the *Gyüshi*.[48]

Many names of medicines have been greatly simplified and are drawn from the compound's major ingredient or the function of the medicine. In contrast, pharmaceutical works such as those by Khyenrap Norbu frequently employ poetic names for medicines, for example Trinsel 25 (Vermillion Voice 25) or Zhijé 11 (Pacifier 11). The more complex medicines were, the more "secret" and poetic their names.

Furthermore, the manual includes none of what are currently considered the most basic or classic medicines for each of the three core constitutions of the *nyépa*, such as Agar 8 for *lung*, Tigta 8 for *tripa* (although recipes for Tigta 5 and Tigta 9 are given), or Sendu 5 and its derivatives for *béken*. This absence needs to be interpreted in the context of the requirement for low-cost medicines made from local ingredients. For example *Agar konyon*[49] is grown in India and *sendu* (pomegranate) is available in eastern but not central Tibet. To make Agar 8 was therefore difficult to impossible, hence the medicine is not mentioned in the work.

Tibetan Medical Manual compounds also feature far fewer ingredients for each compound, typically between five and seven. Only a handful of formulas feature as many as twelve ingredients.[50] Often the work suggests using just one medical plant to treat a disease. In the pre-1962 texts, Tibetan medicines combined *at least* three ingredients, and the properties of just one medicinal would not have been discussed in the compounding literature (*ngojor*); these would have been discussed in the *trungpé* literature. But the use of a single plant or herb to treat diseases was the mainstay of *The Sino-Tibetan Herbal* and revolutionary Chinese medicine, and this seems to have rubbed off on the *Tibetan Medical Manual*. Only a few medicines in the text are supposed to be made in the form of butters (*menmar*) or baths (*chum*), which were probably considered expensive and wasteful.

While a majority of the medicines in the *Tibetan Medical Manual* are produced as powders and some as pills (*rilbu*), many were prescribed as liquids (*thang*), that is, boiled in water. The unusual preference for boiling herbs in liquids is easily explained, as it was one of the most common ways of using herbs in revolutionary Chinese medical practice.

While the *Gyüshi* categorizes eight kinds of source materials (Clark 1995: 131), the ingredients in the manual derive mostly from the herbal medicines category (*ngomen*) and, as such, are found mostly on the Tibetan plateau. The manual also includes some substances from common domestic and wild animals, but notably absent are the "precious ingredients" (*rinchen*), as well as many foreign ones from India (usually classified as "medicines from the plains" or "tree medicines"; see Hofer 2014b, 2014c). The political requirement of the day was low-cost Tibetan medicines made by and for peasants and nomads; such choices were in line with the spirit of self-reliance.

The standard structure for recipes here is statement of the names of ingredients and their ratios, followed by description of their "properties" (*pennü*). For example, *Semde* 5 (Peace of Mind 5) medicine requires: 5 ounces (*sang*) of *ba spru*, 5 ounces of *tang kun gi 'bru gu* (plant *tang kun*), 4 ounces of *lca ba*, and 3 ounces of *go snyod 'bru gu*, which should be ground and then made into either powder or pills and divided into six portions (20). This medicine's properties are described as helping "unhappy mind, dizziness, ringing in the ears, pains, blurry vision, and all *lung* diseases" (20–21).

There are few continuities between this revolutionary compounding manual and earlier Tibetan medical compounding texts such as those by Khyenrap Norbu or Ju Mipham. And there is also little in common with the kinds of medicines in common use in Ngamring prior to 1959 found in local medical text collections. The discontinuity lies mainly in the simplification and rationale of the *Tibetan Medical Manual*.

With its focus on low-cost, locally sourced, simple medicines, the *Tibetan Medical Manual* surely met official requirements for socialist primary health care in rural Tibet during the Cultural Revolution. The conditions of resource-poor settings and the limited means of the CMS scheme had to be considered, as well as the barefoot doctors' low levels of education and rapid medical training. And above all, the work was to serve the political purpose of fostering the "Tibetan socialist revolution and construction."

Any work of Tibetan medicine in the new regime clearly needed to escape the many accusations its practitioners had endured. Authors needed to create a rhetorical distance between their own work and assertions about the "old medical system," in which Tibetan medicine, according to the party line, had produced remedies too expensive for patients and containing "superstitious" ingredients, or preparations that "simply didn't work."[51]

Interestingly, in contrast to *The Sino-Tibetan Herbal*, few conditions in the *Tibetan Medical Manual* are classified in Western medical terms. Why would this work, which included "barefoot doctor" in its title, follow Tibetan medicine's disease classification and ideas of how the body worked? The *Tibetan Medical Manual* shows how in just a few years after publication of *The Sino-Tibetan Herbal*, Tibetan medicine had moved away from being one of the Four Olds. Tibetan medicine and pharmaceuticals were now becoming the much-hailed Communist health care revolution for nomadic and farming rural areas.

NEW BEGINNINGS?

Though well-known scholar-physicians at leading Tibetan government institutions, such as Tenzin Chödrak and Troru Tsenam, remained in prisons and labor camps until 1979–80, the early 1970s saw mounting efforts to rebuild a small but ever-growing degree of Tibetan medical practice, research, and education in government facilities. Although the exact impetus and timing of these shifts in Tibet is not yet clear, it was probably related to a wider trend across the PRC. In the early 1970s in the PRC, new allowances were made for a fuller practice of Chinese medicine compared to what had been incorporated into *The Barefoot Doctor's Manual* and related literature. Many Chinese medical academies, for example, reopened their doors, and private practice in some cases resumed (Scheid 2007; Hillier and Jewell 1983). How was Tibetan medicine reworked during this time, when classical works and Tibetan medicine courses were reintroduced?

From the Gyüshi *to a Revolutionary College Textbook*

In March 1974, the Vocational Health School of Lhasa City enrolled two cohorts of students to study Tibetan medicine at the middle school level. There were, however, no books available for teaching use—except *The Sino-Tibetan Herbal.* Jampa Trinlé, who had not yet been officially rehabilitated and was producing Tibetan almanacs in 1972–74, was forced to produce a textbook for the Vocational Health School students. The requirement was, according to his *Recollections*, that it would "accept Mao Zedong thought and dialectical materialism and the need to clean up idealism, such as feudalism and religious superstition" (Trinlé 2006: 39–43). The conditions for producing such a textbook as well as teaching the students were far from ideal. Trinlé constantly feared another round of struggles and accusations, hence he was reluctant to write the textbook and had to be forced. It is revealing that even in 1974, the instruction from his superior was that "no details" from the *Gyüshi* should be incorporated into the new publication.[52] It meant that he had to scrap some earlier drafts he had used for the simplification of the *Root* and *Explanatory Tantra.* With the help of several remaining teachers and Mentsikhang colleagues, as well as the private physician Rinzin Nyerongsha, and based on clandestine borrowing of secretly held classical works from each other, Trinlé summarized and thus "cleaned up" the contents of surviving medical classics. His former colleague Ngawang Chödrak was largely absent from Lhasa at the time, having been struggled against, made to wear the "hat of lords," and then forced to undergo years of "education through labor" (Trinlé 2000: 456–57).[53]

Finalized in 1974, the textbook was then used in the three-year course. According to Trinlé, this work proved useful and was later officially published and distributed elsewhere in Kham, Amdo, and Inner Mongolia, where Tibetan medicine was again being officially taught (42).[54] Since Trinlé does not mention in this section of his largely chronological and detailed autobiography the creation of the *Tibetan Medical Manual*, we have to assume that he was not involved in any significant way. However, through his description of the conditions under which he worked to produce the Vocational Health School textbook in 1974, he offers us a glimpse into the difficulties likely facing the authors of the *Tibetan Medical Manual.* At the end of their introduction they might be hinting at this in describing a lack "of intellectual and medical resources" (Lhasa City Mentsikhang 1975: 6), though this also may have been a standard requirement or a protective device for writers to distance themselves from the "scholarly elite" (the same phrase also appeared at the end of the preface to *The Sino-Tibetan Herbal*).

New Tibetan Medical Institutions and Training Courses

The Health Bureau's changing attitude toward Tibetan medicine soon began to manifest in the rural health care infrastructure. In November 1974, the People's Hospital in Ngamring County opened a two-room Tibetan medical clinic, where it employed three Tibetan medical doctors: Ngawang Dorjé, Yonten Tsering, and Tashi. Such units were also established in many other county hospitals that year.[55]

According to a locally written history by Wangnam, the *Short History of Ngamring Dzong Tibetan Medical Hospital* (1999), the Ngamring Tibetan *amchi* diagnosed and treated large numbers of patients,[56] using both Tibetan pharmaceuticals and external treatments. In the beginning medicines were limited. Owing to lack of funds for medicines, People's Hospital staff, rural health workers, and local people were mobilized to pick medical plants.[57] The three doctors then compounded medicines from the bulk of these materials and exchanged the rest for more complex, ready-made pills from the Lhasa Mentsikhang factory.[58]

Wangnam writes: "We were working hard to use Tibetan medicine, and we did well to support the 'mother-line's cause,'"[59] demonstrating the kind of political phraseology required in 1999. The report states that between 1974 and 1988 eight training courses in Tibetan medicine were organized by the Tibetan medicine section, from which forty-six health workers from all over Ngamring County graduated, passing their exams with an average score of 82 percent. The document also reports that "they learned to identify five hundred different plants, so that they would be able to go to the mountain to pick medical plants and make simple medicines by themselves," testifying to an impressive degree of knowledge in the field and emphasizing pharmacology as the most legitimate way to present Tibetan medicine. As discussed earlier, the image section of *The Sino-Tibetan Herbal* was used in these courses. The report adds that two of the participating township and village doctors received *kachupa*-level degrees, part of the traditional degree system that had been previously used in Lhasa, indicating a certain reinvigoration of earlier educational practices.

The motivation behind these trainings that was stated in the document, "benefiting people in remote areas," clearly mirrors Mao's directives for stressing rural areas in health work. Although the report no longer includes extracts from the *Quotations*, it features political campaign slogans of the 1990s. The document ends somewhat predictably by stating that the Tibetan medical staff "have been greatly inspired" by the outcomes of the Third Plenum of the Eleventh National Communist Party meeting in 1978. This assembly had ushered in the most sweeping policy changes of the post-Mao era until the Third Forum on Work in Tibet in 1994. Both of these events would have a tremendous bearing on how Tibetan medicine was practiced in Ngamring and elsewhere. Although these consequences are not spelled out in the report, the outcomes of the Eleventh National CCP meeting led to the reincorporation of certain Buddhist aspects into medical work. Most significantly, according to my interviewees, it meant that doctors could once again openly study the classical works as well as return to their private Buddhist practice.

The few years that passed between the preparation and publication of *The Sino-Tibetan Herbal* (1971–73) and the *Tibetan Medical Manual* (1975) thus signaled the start of an ever-widening acceptance of and government support for Tibetan medicine and its use in rural primary health care. In the eyes of local Tibetan doctors, this support was further strengthened when the Tenth Panchen Lama visited Tibet in the early 1980s and became an outspoken supporter of Tibetan medicine. A photograph of his visit to the Tibetan medical section at the Ngamring People's Hospital was proudly hung in one doctor's home.

— · —

While almost all Tibetan medical work came to an end at the Mentsikhang between 1966 and 1973–74, in the midst of the greatest contraction of Tibetan medical practice, a few doctors in a rural part of Tsang kept up their work and, in some exceptional cases, did so even in government facilities. Tibetan medical doctors began to employ Mao's revolutionary discourse to relegitimate Tibetan medicine as a valid health resource, especially for rural areas.

Although doctors in Lhasa still had to be cautious in 1974 in compiling a medical textbook for a Tibetan medicine course, and presumably also when working on the *Tibetan Medical Manual*, their efforts continued. Together, the continuous work of doctors in rural areas and the production of new texts in Lhasa grew into a regionwide movement to revitalize Tibetan medicine. Until Mao's death in 1976, this took place at basic levels of clinical and pharmaceutical practice. Yet it lay the foundations for the reintroduction of more sophisticated Tibetan medical epistemologies after 1978, albeit with traces of "Mao Zedong thought and dialectical materialism," for instance in the ways many Tibetan pharmacology works are structured even today.

This situation of Tibetan medicine in the 1970s is in stark contrast to that of other aspects of Tibetan culture, particularly Buddhist religion prior to the significant Eleventh Party Congress in Beijing in 1978 (Goldstein and Kapstein 1998), but also to some extent with regard to the Tibetan opera, or *ace lhamo* (Henrion-Dourcy 2005, 2017)—although it is perhaps more difficult to draw comparisons here—and to the Tibetan visual arts (Harris 1999; Tsewang Tashi 2014). Comparisons of Tibetan medicine with these domains are particularly worthy of exploration in future work. As for Tibetan medicine, the government made much earlier allowances, starting in 1974 and in some cases unofficially even earlier. The greater continuity that resulted enabled Tibetan medical scholars, when they gathered in Lhasa in the early 1980s, to "recollect and recover what had been lost and disappeared during the Cultural Revolution" (Trinlé 2004: 134), relatively swiftly recuperating many aspects of their tradition. They began to write and to reprint medical works.

In terms of margins and centers of Tibetan medicine, it is from the widespread distribution of *The Sino-Tibetan Herbal* and the *Tibetan Medical Manual* in the 1970s and the increased numbers of students trained in Lhasa and then posted in rural Tibetan areas that Lhasa, as a center for government health care, for the first time comprehensively reached remote rural areas to provide health care. In the words of Veena Das and Deborah Poole (2004), these are instances when "the state inscribed itself" on the margins, using state welfare and political campaigns to affect the lives of doctors and ordinary citizens.

Accepting the currently limited source and archival materials, the extent of this development seems to exceed earlier efforts of the Lhasa Mentsikhang and the Tibetan government to extend their influence, for example through the child health campaign of the 1920s. And they of course occurred under radically different circumstances. The revolutionary political circumstances could not have been replicated elsewhere, even in the PRC of the 1980s, when the mass mobilizations and campaigns characteristic of the Cultural Revolution ended.

While the Cultural Revolution saw notable achievements in the realm of Chinese medicine, it was after Mao's death in 1976 that traditional medicine and qigong gained momentum in the PRC (Hsu 2009: 475). This also applies to the Tibetan situation. The start of the Vocational Health School training in Tibetan medicine, the efforts of Tibetan medical doctors working in rural health facilities, and the publication of the *Tibetan Medical Manual* provided the first-aid and survival measures for the severely damaged Tibetan medical tradition. In the spirit of the revolution, the *Tibetan Medical Manual* tried to simplify medical recipes and drugs but could now acknowledge that the research included study and distillation of classical works. This is reminiscent of the extensive combing of Chinese pharmaceutical texts described by Hsu (2008: 475–76), which eventually led to the "discovery" of the antimalarial drug artemisinin, or *qinghaosu* (Hsu 2006).[60] Yet a full-scale rehabilitation, in particular of Tibetan medicine's more complex theoretical, philosophical, and Buddhist aspects, occurred only after 1978 and especially during the 1980s. Tibetan medicine was then revived in select monasteries, and leading Buddhist scholars got involved, such as Troru Tsenam, Nalanda Tsultrim Gyentsen, and Tenzin Chödrak, who had by then been officially rehabilitated.

Xiaoping Fang asserts that the barefoot doctor campaign in rural China contributed in the longer term to ousting Chinese medicine as a prime health care resource (2012).[61] The situation for Tibetan medicine in Tibet was rather different. In the early 1970s, while the region relied mainly on Western medicines, the rhetorical praise of local medicines, both Chinese and Tibetan, as being a part of the nation's "treasure house," and their role in rural health as espoused during the barefoot doctor campaign, helped to rekindle Tibetan medicine at a crucial time. Even highly simplified publications such as *The Sino-Tibetan Herbal* and the *Tibetan Medical Manual* were important, and impressive on a scholarly level. They aided the practice of Tibetan medicine in various localities. Nationally they promoted Tibetan medicine as a functional heritage, establishing it as a part of the nation's "treasure house" and helping the tradition gain political support on local, regional, and national levels.

CHAPTER 5

REVIVING TIBETAN MEDICINE, INTEGRATING BIOMEDICINE

> Tibetan medicine should improve relations between the nationalities and develop the economy and the culture of [minority] nationality areas.
>
> —*Short History of Ngamring Dzong Tibetan Medical Hospital*

A SMALL place for Tibetan medical practice, publishing, and teaching had opened up after 1974, and the first classic texts were soon republished, albeit with "religious elements" cut out. Following the Third Plenum of the Eleventh CCP Central Committee in Beijing in December 1978, which ushered in religious freedom alongside economic and other reforms, Tibetan medicine was able to expand more fully. State policies allowed Tibetan medical doctors to revive the tradition's own epistemologies in government clinics and schools, paid them salaries, and recruited new students. Doctors tried to revive and adapt their practices to the new circumstances over the ensuing two decades. During the 1980s and 1990s, state-sponsored Tibetan medical infrastructure and personnel grew rapidly in urban centers, expanding in county hospitals. Tibetan medicine was practiced in selected township clinics, which took in former barefoot doctors who had benefited from exposure to simple Tibetan medical techniques. The former three-tier primary care system of brigade health stations, commune health center, and county hospital was reorganized along the lines of the new administrative units, changing to the three tiers of village-level health worker, township clinic, and county-level hospital. Following decollectivization and the (re)introduction of the "household responsibility system" in 1981–83, the commune-based Cooperative Medical Services (CMS) scheme, on which the lowest level of care had depended for income, collapsed. The barefoot doctors in many cases became village health workers but had great difficulty sustaining their work and stocking medicines.

STATE-SPONSORED REVITALIZATION OF TIBETAN MEDICINE

Fundamental to government support for and expansion of Tibetan medicine in the 1980s were what Janes calls "Chinese State interests" (1995: 23). We need to place these in a wider context of growing freedom in social, cultural, and religious practices paired with increasing market-driven economic development fostered throughout China under Deng Xiaoping, and in the TAR through a six-point plan announced by party secretary Hu Yaobang in May 1980.[1] Chinese state interests were, according to Janes, primarily concerned with Tibetan medicine as an arena where the state could show overt respect for a select aspect of local culture and customs (23–24), with the added benefit of providing locally appropriate primary health care for rural populations. Both interests contributed to central government efforts to relegitimate itself after the devastation wrought during the preceding years and to help counter the ongoing challenges posed by the reluctantly participant minority populations. In renewed attempts to co-opt minority populations, "Tibetan medicine likely represented a reasonably safe and apolitical forum" (Janes 1995: 23).

Janes has shown in detail how the state, through central, regional, and local governing mechanisms, orchestrated the expansion of Tibetan medicine—for instance, by setting up higher-level education in Tibetan medicine at Tibet University, and later establishing an independent Tibetan Medical College. Most contemporary Tibetan and Chinese works on Tibetan medicine published in the PRC in the postreform period necessarily highlight the role of the state in promoting Tibetan medicine.[2] Such state-led imperatives, like those that created traditional Chinese medicine (TCM), would seem to lend themselves to analysis through the "invention of tradition" theory (Hobsbawm and Ranger 1983). Janes and Hilliard (2008) employ this line of analysis for Mongolia, where after seventy years of persecution, traditional medicine needed to be "reinvented" when democracy was established in 1990. There were no longer any practitioners to transmit and revive medical practices.

For the TAR in the 1980s and 1990s, due to the shorter period of attacks on Tibetan medical practitioners, Janes and Hilliard speak instead of a "revival" of Tibetan medicine: by the mid-1980s, "the institutions of Tibetan medicine—the hospitals, clinics and medicine factories—had been restored to their formerly integral position in Tibetan society" (35). In fact, Tibetan *amchi* established frameworks and institutions for Tibetan medicine that had not existed previously. The state was not interested in rebuilding destroyed Medical Houses or funding practitioners in their homes or monasteries. They wanted Tibetan medicine to fit into the recently built-up health infrastructure, and thus at least partially integrate it with biomedicine. Thus the theorizing, practice, and funding of Tibetan medicine had to change.

From the 1980s onward, new laws regulated and legitimated what was variously called nationality or ethnic medicine and pharmaceuticals (*minzu yiyao*), in ways similar to Chinese medicine. The latter was enshrined in the constitution of the PRC in 1982–83, precipitating a host of "nationality medicine"-specific regulations and laws on national and regional levels.[3] In marginal areas such as Ngamring in Tsang, TAR-specific policies were thus easily promoted and enacted. A cohort of government servants and local cadres at the county level in Ngamring, for example, firmly established Tibetan medicine in government facilities. Some of them were at the forefront of Tibetan medicine's local revitalization but avoided challenging the hegemony of the post-Mao PRC state and party line.

At the same time, a range of private *amchi* in Tsang pursued their own projects and actively sought to reestablish meaningful social and medical networks and practices. Some of these did not overlap with those the state was eager to promote in government clinics and colleges, where a tendency to standardize knowledge transmission and practice was inevitable, as was the integration with biomedicine. Multiple advocates and initiatives emerged in and across two main currents of Tibetan medical revitalization during the 1980s and 1990s: that led by the state and that embodied by local private *amchi*.

The first current of Tibetan medical revitalization was promoted through government cadres and institutions in urban settings and to some extent in the rural primary health care system. High levels of financial and often personal investment persisted here until 1994, when new market-led health reforms began to be implemented in the TAR in earnest, almost twenty years after the rest of rural China. Reforms eliminated much of the funding previously available for building Tibetan medical institutions and providing rural primary health care. The second current, which began later and continues today, has been the revival of Tibetan medicine in private family homes, clinics, and schools, as well as monasteries—at times with the support of international nongovernmental organizations (NGOs). Some of these initiatives aimed to fill gaps in primary care provision that persisted or became apparent in the wake of medical privatization after 1994 for poor rural patients.

The lives of some of the actors encountered in this chapter straddle governmental and private medical domains, as well as the pre- and postreform periods, which experienced radically different forms of sociality and politics.[4] How did private initiatives and practitioners relate to state-funded Tibetan medical institutions and initiatives? Where and how did private *amchi* reestablish their work? In what ways did their practices differ from *amchi* who trained in the state system, not least in relation to the continuously reshaped government policies regarding the integration of Western and Tibetan medicine? What was the role of women *amchi* in the postreform era?

The parallel development of state and local medical institutions and practices resembles similar processes in Chinese medicine during the same period. The CCP's endeavor to abstract, standardize, and fully institutionalize Chinese medicine as TCM was far from complete (Scheid 2007). This was despite prominent CCP involvement in the creation and use of TCM in revolutionary discourse and health work in the 1950s and early 1960s (Taylor 2005), the barefoot doctor campaign (Fang 2012), and the postreform period (Farquhar 1994, 1996; Hsu 1999; Scheid 2002, 2007).

Through accounts of attempts to reestablish Tsang's Tibetan Medical Houses, revive medical work among Buddhist monks and nuns, and establish a private Tibetan medical school, this chapter analyses revitalization of Tibetan medical cultures and the ways these operated outside of governmental Tibetan medicine institutions and state-sponsored initiatives.

REINSTATING MEDICAL HOUSES

As we have seen, Tibetan medicine's authority as well as the social and physical aspects of the lay Medical Houses were successively dismantled during socialist and Communist reforms and campaigns in Ngamring and Sakya. In the postreform period, with its more open political context, to what extent could Medical Houses be rebuilt? Could private medical practice be revitalized?

Rebuilding the Mentrong

For the first half of the twentieth century, the Mentrong was a *gerpa* household with landholdings and several *yokpo* (servants). Its high social standing and economic and ritual power derived from family connections to the western Tibetan Ruthog kings and the royal and medical lineages of Ngamring's past rulers. This position also conferred ritual responsibilities from the local monastery. Classified in 1959–60 by Communist work teams as "serf owners" and "exploiters," members of the Mentrong were punished harshly during the successive reforms and campaigns. Despite its initial loss of most of its material wealth and its almost complete destruction near the beginning of the Cultural Revolution, parts of the physical building survived for another three years. Rinchen Wangyal and his wife continued to live in a ground-floor room with a makeshift roof. This accommodation was porous to the summer rains, but the couple had nowhere else to go.

These remnants of the house were finally destroyed in 1969, when it became, according to Rinchen Wangyal, a casualty of the government's crackdown on widespread local protests.[5] Rinchen Wangyal and his wife then moved to a one-room shed, where they lived for the next thirteen years, under no better circumstances. They were later permitted to join the commune and subsisted largely on official barley and butter rations calculated on the basis of their labor contributions to the local production team. They were given land in early 1980–81, when the newly introduced Household Responsibility System (*gentshang lamlug*) was implemented in Ngamring. This system redistributed previously communalized land. The amount depended on the kind of land available and the number of household members above a certain age.[6]

With no surviving children, Rinchen Wangyal and his wife had adopted her younger brother, Kunsang. He was apparently too young to be eligible for consideration in the system, so the family received a very small plot on which they could barely subsist. When Kunsang came of age, he started a small business, and in the late 1980s, the Mentrong began to earn a modest livelihood. Kunsang married Yeshe Wangmo of the Nyingkhang around 1984, and they produced three children, two boys and a girl. Once Kunsang's business became profitable and the family had enough money, they constructed a small single-story house on the new land. By 2001, this had been extended to two stories. The house was not as large as the previous one, but it was hard won. The newly rebuilt Mentrong featured few aspects of what had previously made it a medical house. The family established an elaborate altar room, but otherwise it looked much like other two-story houses in the area.

These circumstances made it impossible for Rinchen Wangyal to recover his medical practice and work again as an *amchi*. Substantial means (financial and temporal) were required to obtain the medical raw materials necessary to an *amchi*'s work. Furthermore, practitioners had to depend to varying extents on family wealth and tax benefits rather than income from seeing patients, and that family wealth was no longer there. Rinchen Wangyal had to take up farming to feed his family. Due to his class background, he had never been considered for training as a barefoot doctor, which would have not only helped with the family's material situation but probably enabled him to maintain at least some of his medical skill. Nevertheless, he attempted to reinvigorate symbolic, social, and occupational features of the Mentrong.

In 1982, Jampa Trinlé, by then reinstated as director of the Lhasa Mentsikhang, visited Lhünding to conduct historical research and search for medical classics to restock the Mentsikhang library. To everyone's disappointment, not a single book from the Mentrong library remained. Rinchen Wangyal, in the meantime, had recovered a large medical bag that he had given to the Nyémo Lama in anticipation of Democratic Reforms. The Mentsikhang representatives asked if it could be displayed in Lhasa, and Rinchen Wangyal agreed to donate it. In gratitude to the historical Jang and Lhünding medical traditions, Jampa Trinlé arranged for a statue of its founder, Jangpa Namgyel Drazang, to be made for the Mentrong. The gilded statue was presented to the family and installed in the their new *chökhang*. It forms the centerpiece of their altar in the (now expanded) Mentrong House (figure 5.1), the only reminder of the Jang medical tradition

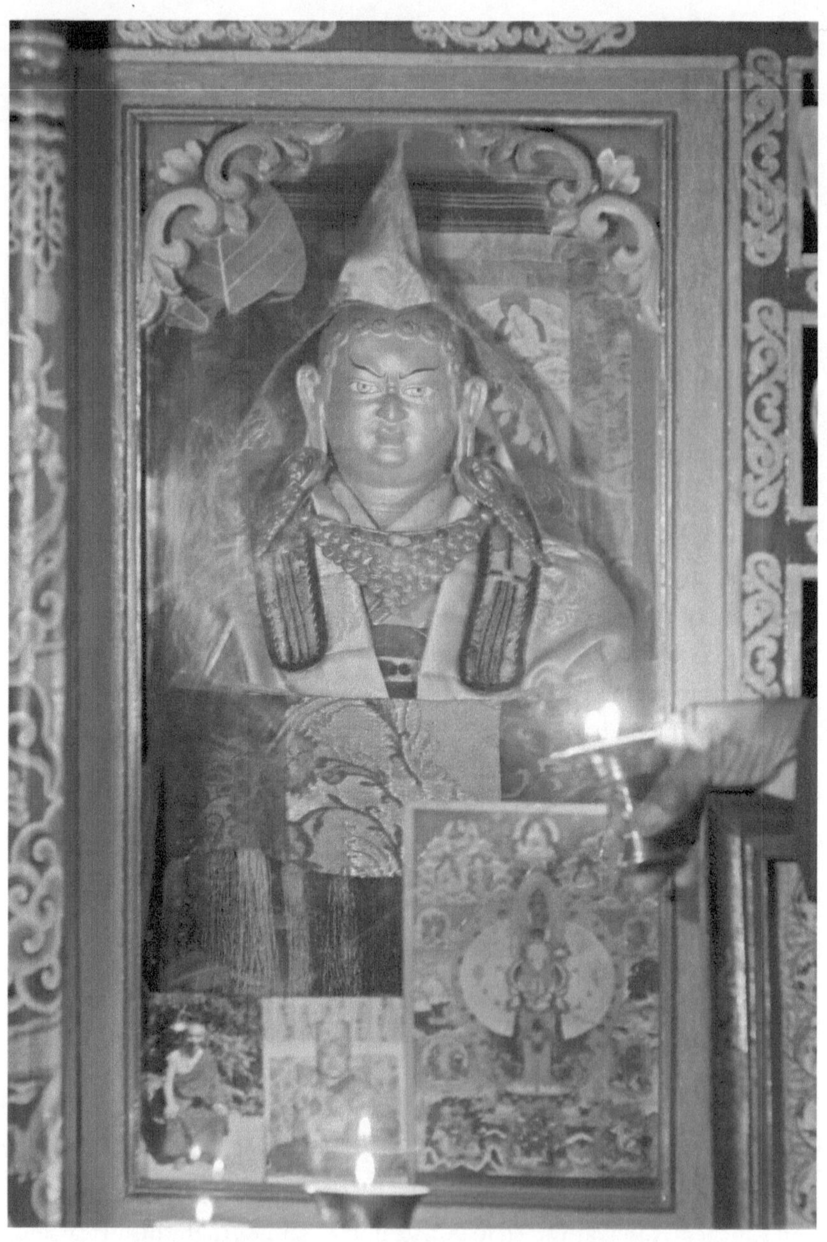

FIGURE 5.1. Reinstated statue of Jangpa Namgyel Drazang, Mentrong, 2007. Photo by Meinrad Hofer.

with which the Mentrong had been so intimately linked. In the 1940s, the material items kept in the Mentrong's *menkhang* and *chökhang*, along with Rinchen Wangyal's training in Phuntsoling, had made possible the reestablishment, however brief, of the Mentrong.

When I visited in 2003, I heard hopes that members of the Mentrong could restart the practice of medicine. It was, therefore, a happy surprise to hear from Rinchen Wangyal in 2007 that the youngest grandson, then twelve, had been sent to Lhasa to apprentice with a close disciple of Jampa Trinlé, who was then retired. In the capital, the boy benefited from extended family, including Kunsang's retired uncle and aunt, Ngawang Dorjé and Ani Payang of the Nyingkhang, Ngawang Dorjé having kept up his medical practice at his new Lhasa home.

Rinchen Wangyal commented, "Now the inheritance of the bone lineage[7] entirely depends on the boy," his face expressing both hope and anticipation. That he used the expression *bone lineage* testifies again to the emphasis and value placed on the rhetoric of patrilineal descent in the transmission and continuity of Medical Houses. The erstwhile *amchi* clearly considered his adopted son Kunsang, from his late wife's side of the family, to hold the "bones" of the Mentrong's patrilineage by virtue of membership in the house. This was a way to make up for their lack of biological children, which was possibly related to the harsh circumstances in which Rinchen and his wife had spent the years of intense reform.

Memorizing the "Communist Gyüshi*": The Ruthog* Amchi

These recent efforts to return some of the old medical authority to the Mentrong differ significantly from what happened to the village *amchi* in Ruthog, a slightly lower-lying farming village by the Tokshung River in southern Ngamring. Here Tibetan medical practice did not entirely stop, yet due to changed socioeconomic circumstances, the practice has of late not been easy to maintain.

Tsewang was known as the Ruthog village *amchi* and practiced in the fourth generation. During my first fieldwork in 2003 he was in his seventies. His son Pema (b. 1964) had succeeded him in the family occupation. Another son, Lobsang (b. 1969), had also been taught medicine, but after taking orders as a monk at Ngamring Gonpa in 1987, he stopped his medical training. The continuity of the medical tradition in the practice of Tsewang and Pema was the result of fortuitous circumstances and timing, not least that Tsewang and his wife had seven children who had survived into adulthood and that classical Tibetan medical works were accessible.

Tsewang was already an experienced doctor when the Democratic Reforms began in Ruthog, and his *trelpa* household (which was similar in status to Yonten Tsering's Térap) was labeled "middle-off farmers"[8]—between rich and poor categories. Like Yonten Tsering, they had lost almost everything during the land reforms. Their wooden medicine box, the medicine bags and instruments, and books that had been passed down the generations were at first kept in the house while the family moved to the ground floor. At the start of the Cultural Revolution, these items were said to be "poisonous roots of the landlords,"[9] as Pema's seventy-year-old mother recalled. She described how the people throwing things out of their home were undecided about burning the bags and boxes and wondered whether they could find any "safe" use for such "poisonous roots." They finally decided to use the bags and boxes for salt and other household goods, but there was no doubt that the books had to be destroyed. Pema's mother recalled feeling sorrow at what was happening, her wish being for the family medical tradition to continue. She managed, at great personal risk, to hide two of their Tibetan medical books and thus saved them from being thrown in the river. One of the texts was a print edition of the *Four Treatises*, the other a family medical compounding book (*menjordeb*) where previous generations had added their own recipes and annotations (figure 5.2). The family subsequently moved to other accommodation and the house was locked, then finally destroyed.

Tsewang had by then been recruited to work as a secretary for the new government owing to his literacy. He hardly ever applied his medical skills beyond his own family during the early reforms and almost completely stopped during the Cultural Revolution. Saved to some extent by his secretarial role, the most severe beatings were endured by his mother-in-law, Pema's grandmother, whose family was related to the royal family of Ruthog in western Tibet. Despite these difficult circumstances, Tsewang managed to homeschool Pema in the early 1970s by practicing Tibetan letters using coal on a wooden board. Tsewang decided Pema and his baby brother would stay at home and become *amchi*, while the older brothers and sisters would be married out. He was often criticized for not sending Pema to the government school, where only Chairman Mao's works and songs were taught and the sole textbook was the *Quotations*.[10] Others

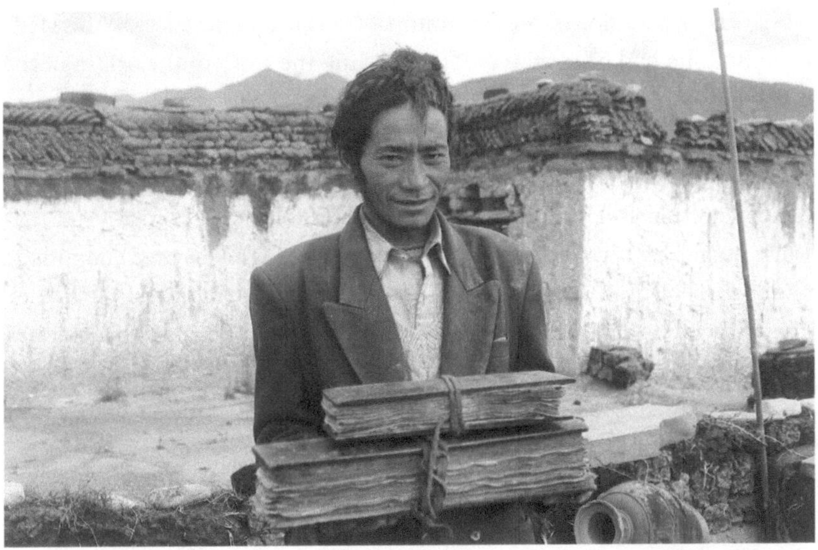

FIGURE 5.2. Amchi Pema presents his family's *Four Treatises* and *Menjordeb*, 2003. Photo by the author.

accused the family of keeping the children out of school so they could earn more work points, called *karma*. It was in 1976, Pema recalled, that he began memorizing the *Gyüshi*; he also attended school by that time, where other books had slowly started to reappear: "There were two lessons: one in the morning and one in the afternoon. At lunchtime when I came home. I did not do homework; I just studied and memorized the *Four Treatises*. In the evenings too, I kept on studying the *Four Treatises*. I didn't do well in school, but I learned the *Four Treatises* by heart!"

Pema did not memorize the *Gyüshi* from the printed *peja* that had been saved by his mother. He explained that its lettering was much harder to read than what the family referred to as "the Communist *Gyüshi*" (*Tangi Gyüshi*).[11] I subsequently discovered that this 1976 Communist *Gyüshi* was the first modern, European-style printing of what was mainly the content of the *Gyüshi*, but it had been thoroughly reedited under duress by Jampa Trinlé in 1974 and then published as a Tibetan medical textbook. Yet the family considered this close enough to call it the *Gyüshi*. The printing, possession, or teaching of classical block-printed works was considered one of the Four Olds, and only a very few books with Tibetan medical content had been published in the previous decade, by revolutionary committees and under the heavy influence of Maoist thought.

In this 1976 edition of the Communist *Gyüshi*, all references to the Medicine Buddha had been edited out, including the story of the origin of the medical teachings. Also gone were the formal requests of the student to the teacher of the *Gyüshi*, found prior to 1976 at the beginning and end of each volume and each chapter of the work, which gave the text its typical dialogic format and Buddhist authority. Pema continued to memorize that work during the coming years. At the same time he learned diagnostic and therapeutic techniques from his father and assisted him with patients. The family did not acquire later reprints of the *Four Treatises* (which reincorporated sections on the Medicine Buddha). Yet they clearly considered the Communist *Gyüshi* the teaching of the Medicine Buddha, whom they revered highly, placing his statue in the family's current altar room.

While his father used the family-owned medical compounding manuscript in traditional Tibetan book format, Pema did not. Again, citing easier legibility, he studied what he referred to as the *Sorig Zintig*, a reprint of work by the nineteenth-century Rimé master Jamgon Kongtrul Yonten Gyatso,[12] republished in Xining in April 1976 (Yonten Gyatso 1976).[13] In most cases, however, he followed his father's practical approach and his compounding methods and techniques, only later studying the family compounding work, more out of interest than necessity.

While Pema still practices, as the only *amchi* in the village, the Ruthog *amchi*'s medical techniques, especially moxibustion and bloodletting, as well as the family medical compounding, the Medical House could not be fully reestablished in the postreform era. When the family reacquired land in the early 1980s, they could only afford to construct a single-story house. Their absolute reliance on farming and the lack of extra cash income made the family medical practice financially precarious, to the point that the house has never been extended. Tsewang, who once assisted with the Ngamring Dzong's Tibetan medical doctors' herb collection trips and kept up good relations with the county civil servants, never entered government service, as it would have left the village without a doctor. Thus the household did its best to maintain an active medical practice, although the physical house was effectively no different from most other farmhouses in the village.

Here the uninterrupted medical practice in the bone lineage, that is, its social continuity, was made possible by the fortunate situation of Tsewang and his wife having had several surviving children and their somewhat lighter punishment compared to those in the Mentrong (Tsewang, for example, had not been banned from working for the Communists). This allowed them slightly better material circumstances, and meant that Tsewang could secretly maintain some of his medical knowledge and skill, which he also taught to his sons at home.

Medical Practice: The Ruthog Amchi

The Ruthog *amchi*'s rebuilt home, though simple, has become the site of medical practice once again, the days of covert practice having ended in 1974. Upon my visits, I found books, instruments, and medicines kept in the altar room,[14] and patients consulted in the kitchen-cum-living room, where medicines were ground and compounded as the need arose.[15] On average, Amchi Pema saw a couple of patients every day while continuing to work the fields and perform a variety of other jobs in the household. Although people called Pema a private *amchi* or a *gergyi amchi*,[16] his home was very much a public space, and family members were frequently called to assist in consultations and treatment. This was particularly the case for his daughter, then his only child, as Pema hoped she would become an *amchi* herself. Whether he would have the same willingness if he had sons, I am not sure.

Although Amchi Pema compounded medicines, he did not collect the necessary medicinal herbs or other materials. This was largely because collecting herbs required longer absences from home. He relied on people bringing plants and minerals from nomadic areas or, when raw materials could not be found in his area, purchased them from traders in Lhasa. Amchi Pema spent considerable money on medical substances, especially those collected in high mountain locations that are rare or difficult to find and those imported from India or Nepal. Some patients offered raw medical materials in exchange for treatment. Whatever the source, all the medicines he gave to his patients were prepared in front of their eyes, sometimes with their assistance, freshly ground on a large stone and prescribed as fine powder (figure 5.3). The patients were instructed to take them with boiled water, as he believed medicines prepared this way to be more effective. Because each was compounded in accordance with a particular diagnosis, a medical prescription was never repeated precisely, which probably accounts for his vague answer to my question about how many different medicinal compounds he typically made.

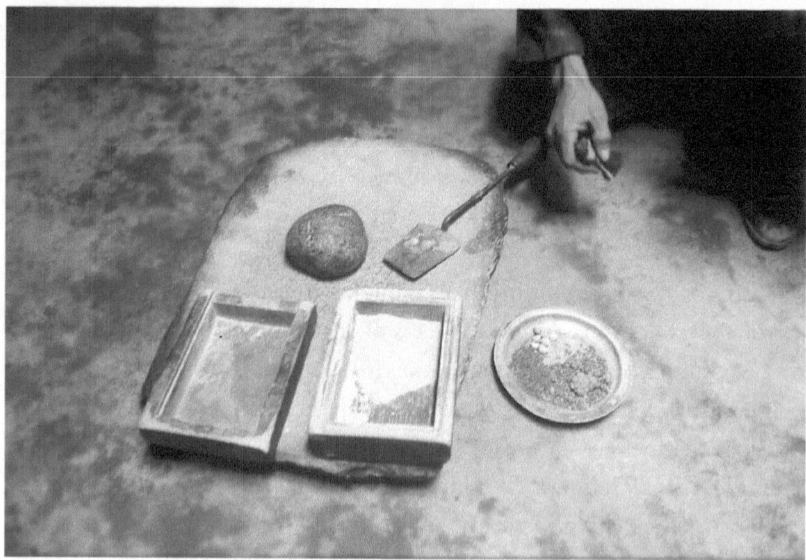

FIGURE 5.3. Ingredients being ground on a large stone and prescribed as fine powder by Amchi Pema, 2003. Photo by the author.

Because of Pema's method of producing medicines, the family spent a lot of money on raw materials but received hardly any remuneration for the medicines and consultations. "Being an *amchi* today means losing money," Pema said repeatedly. He seemed uncomfortable with the idea of charging for his services: "This has not been the tradition in our family. To start it now is very difficult—people have become used to it." His mother added, "If people had a feeling of shame [*ngo tsha yod pa*], they would give something anyway, but most people these days are shameless [*ngo tsha med pa*]." These comments illustrate the social role of *amchi* (cf. Kloos 2004) as well as social dynamics in the village that prohibit Pema from asking for or receiving payment.

One of our conversations was interrupted by a patient who had sprained his ankle a few days earlier. Amchi Pema prepared some dried artemisia, forming cones for moxibustion, a kind of *mégyap* practice, meaning literally to "apply fire." After inquiring about and feeling the location of the pain, he placed a poultice of wet barley grain on a specific point of the patient's ankle with the moxa on top. Everyone was quiet as the moxa cones burned slowly toward the skin before making a popping sound, after which the leftover ashes were brushed off the skin. Following this short consultation and a chat, the patient left. Amchi Pema then picked up our conversation about the remuneration of his practice:

> We have a saying in Tibet: "When you have crossed the river, you forget the bridge; and when you have recovered from an illness, you forget the doctor." That's how I feel when I treat my patients these days. When they recover from their illness, they don't need me anymore and they forget me. Then later they might tell me, "You have really helped me," and give me a cup of *chang*—that's all. They always say, "I will give you money," but never act. They forget and instead I get a cup of *chang* and that's it. I lost lots of money like this.

Despite radically changed social and economic circumstances, making medicine and treating people is still a not-for-profit enterprise, an approach to medicine that, in the words of members of this household, makes a "real *amchi*" (*amchi ngönné*). In our conversations Amchi Pema and his mother used this term to distinguish him and his father from the government "*amchi*," in fact the local village health worker and largely an "injectionist" (*khap gyapnyen*) who uses exclusively Chinese biomedicines, especially injected ones. But I also take his use of "real *amchi*" to refer to an *amchi* who embodies an alternative economy and morality of treatment, and does not ask for payment due to religious considerations. The fact that this *amchi* continues to compound his own medicine, as they have done in his lineage for generations, has exacerbated his precarious financial situation, but his approach is related to ideas of medical work procuring religious merit.

The Dispersal of Térap

The Térap building survives to this day in Gye Village, its *menkhang* and signature medical mural intact (see figure 1.3). The social, symbolic, and occupational aspects of the Medical House, however, only partially survived into the postreform era. Its material and immaterial wealth, its medical instruments, bags, and books and a member's medical knowledge and skill, have been dispersed over time. Yet hopes to reunite at least some aspects of its pre-Communist assemblage were high. Plans to restore the Térap's physical building and transform it into a Tibetan medical clinic, a new kind of Tibetan medical institution, for the village and the valley's population, were well underway in the summer of 2007. In the meantime, the building was used by villagers to make and store the *tsatsa* that were being prepared to be interred in a new stupa built in the village (figure 5.4).

Before turning to other aspects of the dispersed legacies of Térap in the postreform period, we shall briefly revisit what happened after 1959, when it was taken away from Yonten Tsering's family during the land reform. Four previously landless farmers' and servants' families were given deeds to the house, moved in, and divided the doctor's belongings. The *amchi* himself, along with his parents and his wife, moved to a shed. The medical equipment and library of Térap were transferred to a downstairs room. After initial loss of access, Yonten Tsering was then allowed to use that room as a "clinic space," in addition to his work as a secretary for the local government. He managed to preserve books from destruction by the Red Guards, who left the building itself unscathed. After moving briefly into another home in Gye, Yonten Tsering finally relocated to Ngamring town in 1974, having gained a permanent position in the Tibetan medicine section of Ngamring's People's Hospital.

Despite having taken up residence there, between 1980 and 1982 he and his wife reacquired farmland in Gye and built a small house in the location where they had last lived in the village. With the new policies, each of the four families who were living in the Térap building also received farmland at that time. Eventually they established new homes in other parts of the village and sold their shares to Tashi's father, Gyatso. Gyatso owns the house, but during my 2006–7 fieldwork he no longer lived there. With the exception of the medical mural and the ground-floor room belonging to Yonten Tsering, which he visited from time to time, the Térap had long ceased to be a Medical House.

Like Rinchen Wangyal and his wife, Yonten Tsering and Yeshe Lhamo had no surviving children. This is perhaps striking, given their knowledge of medicine, particularly maternal and child-related medicine, and the continued emphasis on bone lineage, at least rhetorically posited as the ideal for medical lineage transmission. Yeshe Lhamo, Yontan Tsering's wife, told me in a private conversation many years after my main fieldwork, when I asked her specifically, that she was unable to become pregnant because they did not have enough to eat and had to work so hard. This clearly hints at a challenging situation even for this family during

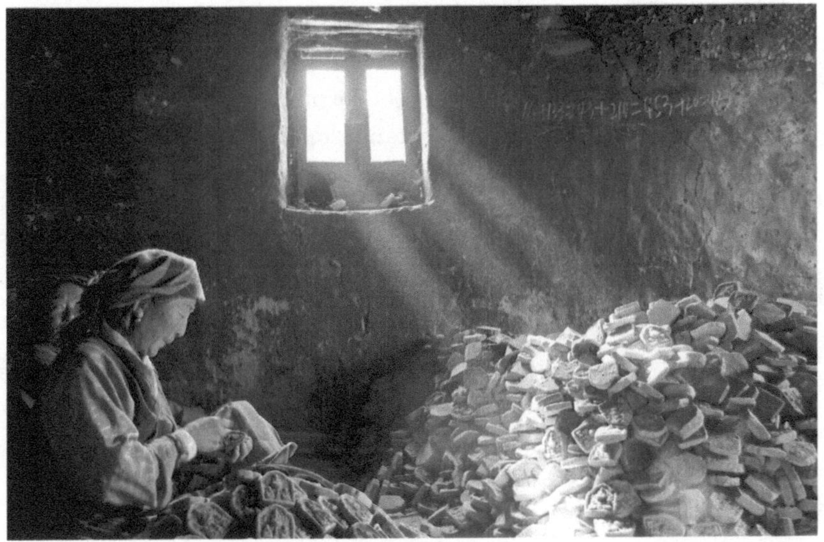

FIGURE 5.4. Térap being used for making and storing *tsatsa* for a new stupa in the village, 2007. Photo by Meinrad Hofer.

the Democratic Reforms, when they lived in the shed, and all the years afterward, despite very different accounts given by her husband.

They eventually adopted Tenpa, one of the sons of Yonten Tsering's younger sister, who had married and lived in Phuntsoling. Tenpa attended regular school in Ngamring and, since he showed no special interest in medicine, did not apprentice with his father. Instead, Yonten Tsering taught students from other backgrounds according to the various governmental health campaigns: first, in the 1970s and 1980s, the barefoot doctors and village and township health workers; and later, in the 1980s and 1990s, younger colleagues who had graduated from Lhasa Mentsikhang and the Tibetan Medicine College but had little practical skill. The techniques in which he trained younger doctors included pulse and urine diagnosis, pharmacological and external treatment methods, and importantly, the compounding of medicines. Most of the medicines were produced at the Tibetan Medicine Section of Ngamring's People's Hospital, using medical materials jointly collected in the summer months, thus keeping medicine quality high and expenditures low.

Yonten Tsering did not pass on his medical knowledge and skill within the bone lineage or the Térap, nor in classical teaching lineages (*lobgyü*) with one or all of the three core aspects of traditional learning (*wang*, *lung*, and *tri*). However, he eagerly shared his knowledge with numerous groups of students, amounting over his lifetime to several hundred individuals. Only in special cases did his teachings take on the qualities of what were known as teaching lineages. For instance, one doctor from Tobé township stayed with him for some months, and similarly, after Yonten Tsering had retired, two teenage boys lived with him and his wife for three years, with him teaching them medicine and giving them the *lung* to study the *Four Treatises* prior to memorization.

Whether mere serendipity, the influence of Yonten Tsering, or any of the remaining powers of the Térap in which he grew up, Tashi Tsering, the youngest son born there to Gyatso's wife, as a teenager developed an interest in Tibetan medicine, for which he had the strong support of his parents. Tashi Tsering was admitted to the Tibetan Medical College in Lhasa in 2004, and in 2008 was due to graduate and embark on the usual year of practical training and internship at a Tibetan medical and biomedical government hospital. He spent his holidays as a volunteer at the Tashilhunpo Monastery clinic, helping to give injections, make Tibetan medicines, and hand them out at the pharmacy.

As things stood in 2007, it was the elders' plan that Tashi Tsering would start a private medical clinic in the Térap building after completing his training. He would be married locally and work with another young *amchi* graduate from the village, who had been to Pelshung and then the Lhasa Medical College. An international donor was close to agreeing to pay for the renovation and expansion of the house as well as an initial stock of medicines. During the first months after the clinic opened and summers thereafter, Yonten Tsering would further instruct the young *amchi*, focusing on the therapeutic specialties of his family medical tradition. Patient fees could, it was estimated, be kept low through on-site medicine collection and compounding, potentially supported by local and international donations I would raise. Yonten Tsering vowed to donate to the new clinic in the Térap building his collection of medical equipment, including a wooden box for medical materials, the grinding stones, medical bags, and his precious medical texts and thankas.

Other Medical Houses and Monastic Amchi

Other medical houses had also been only partially reestablished, their transmission as yet unsecured. One of these was Sonam Drölma's Nyékhang.

Though its rich collection of medical texts had been saved from destruction and the building partly rebuilt, her practice remained very limited and exceedingly difficult after the Cultural Revolution. Her training with her grandfather had been cut short by his death and attacks on the Four Olds, and in the 1980s it was hard to extract any surplus from subsistence farming. For her medical work, mainly for the people of the local villages, she relied on local medical resources, yet had limited time to collect and prepare them, and her family lacked financial resources. At the same time, she was bringing up children, running the household, and doing farmwork. Despite her hope that her son might become an *amchi*, the household's continued poverty and her son's middle school education limited this prospect. As of 2006–7 this level of education was no longer enough to enter the Tibetan Medical College in Lhasa without passing extra exams. The entry requirements in Chinese language had been raised, disadvantaging graduates from rural primary and middle schools, like her son, where Tibetan was still the medium of instruction. Yet government-approved institutional licenses were increasingly necessary to work in a government clinic—or to be permitted to work at all. The continued practice, however limited, of this long-standing household lineage (*khyimtsang gyü*) and the possibility of its transmission were therefore uncertain. Lack of funds was clearly a major obstacle, compounded by Sonam Drölma lacking government or monastic support, living in a poor area, and having to do all the things expected from a lay woman.

Some private *amchi*s managed to start independent private practices even without previous family history in medicine, particularly those who either had a foot in the government bureaucracy or were connected to the newly reestablished monasteries and nunneries. This was the case with the former Bon monk Rabgyal, who had served as resident health worker at Tsatsé township clinic for almost fifteen years.

Rabgyal left the clinic in 1975 and, with his wife, set up a new home in the extremely remote pastoral Nyingu township. There they lived with their children, Rabgyal practicing as an *amchi* among pastoralists and teaching medicine to two of his sons. A repayment of several thousand Chinese yuan (CNY) from the government had enabled this move. The sum, paid after he obtained an official license and the Tibetan medical degree of *rabchampa*, made up for what he successfully argued had been underpayment in earlier years. After initially relying on the pastoral economy,

Rabgyal began to make a substantial income from his medical practice and soon was widely sought out in the area, as many already knew him from his days at the Tsatsé township clinic. With the help of family members, they compounded all the medicines used in his practice, and by the time of my fieldwork the sons were practicing independently in a nearby township in Nyima County, Nagchu Prefecture. They all charged considerable fees for their medicines but were still sought out by many people in the area. Cheaper and also very desired was cauterization, another kind of *mégyap*, or "fire" treatment, particularly suited to treat the many "cold" diseases common in this windy and cool high-plateau environment of the Changthang.

What of the monastic medical practitioners? Could they restart their medical work once Buddhist practice was again officially allowed? Many of the monks and nuns mentioned in chapter 2 returned to a more open and complete medical practice once the CCP congress of 1978 had introduced limited freedom of religious practice. Tutop, the abbot of the Nyingma Chaug Gonpa, was one of the first to resume medical practice, training a monk in the late 1970s. He had kept up some of his practice while riding out the harshest reforms by basing himself in a remote cave. There patients sometimes came to him for treatment and in exchange brought medical plants.[17] At the time of my research, patients often sought him out for healing rituals as well as medicines, the balance tipping more and more toward ritual treatments rather than medicine as he grew old and had difficulty picking plants and the monk he had trained in medicine was no longer there to help.

The nun Ani Pema Lhamo was valued for her treatment skills, often sought out by lay patients in the valley and the older monks at Pangyul, some of whom had learned to make simple medicines and upon her death inherited her text and medicine collection. She had tried to reestablish Dewachen Nunnery, above the monks' monastery at Pangyul, but in 1983 moved to Thölung, near Lhasa.

Ani Ngawang, the student of Khyemen Rinpoche, rebuilt the Chiu Tekcholing nunnery in Nyémo, where she passed on her teacher's medical legacy—including the preparation of *tsotel* for simple *rinchen rilbu*—to several nuns and monks. Ani Ngawang and her nunnery were highly regarded for an eye medicine compounded there, which according to her main disciple contained homemade *tsotel*.

Extensive rebuilding of the monasteries in Ngamring only started in the mid to late 1980s, proceeding initially in small stages. Some were never reestablished, and some villages and hamlets are still saving up to rebuild the stupas and *lhakhangs* torn down through revolutionary fervor or violent political pressure. As of 2016, none of the local monasteries in Ngamring County had started any formalized clinic arrangements. Those monks and nuns with medical knowledge simply treated patients from their residences, sometimes combining, as was the case with Tutop, medical treatment with healing rituals and Buddhist prayers. The great exception in the wider region was Tashilhunpo in Shigatse.

— • —

The laborious and often painful process of trying to reunite the violently dispersed parts of Medical Houses and monastic medical practice is ongoing, with long-term viability uncertain. This contrasts with what Janes and Hilliard assert was by the mid-1980s a "restoration of the institutions of Tibetan medicine—the hospitals, clinics and medicine factories—to their formerly integral position in Tibetan society" (2008: 35). Neither the Medical Houses nor the monasteries had at that point been truly recovered, yet *amchi* from Medical Houses and monasteries had constituted the majority of medical practitioners prior to the reforms. They had a much harder time restoring and securing the continuity of medical practice on their own terms and under new socioeconomic conditions. After the early 1980s, they had exactly as much land as everyone else and received no tax exemptions in recognition of their work.

State-funded institutions set up in the postreform era, by contrast, typically established Tibetan medical institutions as partial replicas of biomedical institutions, and in such cases received impressive state funding (Janes 1995; Trinlé 2004, 2006). In total these new places for Tibetan medical practice far exceeded the previously formalized governmental Tibetan medical institutions, spreading Tibetan medicine funded by the government to counties and even townships. In the process, they replaced many of the diverse practices of Medical Houses and monasteries that had been the institutions of Tibetan medical practice on the margins. Following Janes and Hilliard's logic, it seems to me that only the Mentsikhang in Lhasa, as a traditional Tibetan medicine institution, had truly been reinstated to its "formerly integral position in Tibetan society"—at least in outer appearance, if not with its earlier ethos of practice and teaching. Otherwise, Tibetan medicine in government facilities was established within new institutional, social, and medical frameworks.

In the oft-heralded integration of Tibetan medical and biomedical institutions and practices, which was happening everywhere in the 1980s except perhaps at the Lhasa Mentsikhang, governmental Tibetan *amchi* had to develop entirely new frameworks for Tibetan medicine. This may explain why some *amchi* were not content to participate in this process; instead they envisioned a less "diluted" version of Tibetan medicine, characterized by continued production of their own medicines (Pema and Rabgyal mainly), integration of certain Buddhist elements in healing (Tutop), and application of manual techniques not routinely learned or applied in state colleges and clinics (Rabgyal, Pema, and Sonam Drölma). Although the last years of the Cultural Revolution allowed for small expressions of Tibetan medical practice, this most extreme phase of modern Tibetan history had taken a huge toll on the continuity of the Tibetan medical tradition. In many cases it has taken years to make up for the damage, economic impoverishment, gaps in the transmission of medical knowledge—and even the lack of progeny—that resulted.

A prominent initiative aimed at restoring some of the losses due to the Cultural Revolution in Tsang, which strove to complement the limited and largely biomedical government primary health care in the area, was the establishment of Pelshung Tibetan Medicine School.[18]

PELSHUNG TIBETAN MEDICAL SCHOOL, THE SWISS RED CROSS, AND THE STATE

Following the Tenth Panchen Lama's release from prison in 1978, he became a figure of great importance for Tibetans striving to reestablish Tibetan cultural and Buddhist institutions in the 1980s. He worked actively to support the limited freedoms regained through the creation of government laws, policies, and commitments that he hoped would give Tibetans and other nationalities lasting institutional guarantees for the survival of their culture, religion, language, and to some degree, a genuine regional autonomy (Barnett 1997: xii). Among the Panchen Lama's activities was the start of Tibet Development Fund (TDF). The first modern charitable organization in Tibet, it was specifically designed to attract and manage foreign aid for development projects (Barnett 1997: xiii).[19] In 1986 the Panchen Lama officially invited the Swiss Red Cross (SRC) to Tibet as the first international aid organization there.

The Panchen Lama's wish had been for the SRC to open a biomedical hospital in Shigatse, but the organization's International Cooperation Department (ICD) proposed instead to support the rural health care system, which it considered to be in poor shape.[20] Between 1988 and 1992 the first delegates from the SRC provided basic biomedical training for newly recruited Tibetan students and refresher courses for rural medical personnel with prior biomedical training, such as township doctors and village health workers. This instruction was subsequently subcontracted to the local Vocational Health School and county hospitals (1992–2002).[21] Shigatse Health Bureau then made a formal request to the SRC to establish a school of Tibetan medicine. The charity agreed, and the school was inaugurated in 1991 in Pelshung, about ten kilometers outside of Shigatse Town, on land previously donated by the Panchen Lama but otherwise wholly funded by the SRC (Swiss Red Cross 2005).

A main aim of the training at the Pelshung Tibetan Medicine School, according to SRC documents, "was to contribute to the improvement of the health care situation of poor communities in remote parts of Tibet via the comprehensive training of young men (women were not yet admitted) to become traditional Tibetan doctors" (SRC 2001). A later document introduced a range of SRC programs and activities, including what is here termed Traditional Tibetan Medicine (TTM):

> At the request of the late Panchen Rinpoche, SRC agreed in 1991 to support the creation of a private school for TTM. Students are selected in remote and underserved villages of the 19 counties; the studies last five years and are entirely free. The first batch graduated in 1996, and the second batch will finish its studies at the school proper in 2003. The graduates will then take another year at the Shigatse Health School, in order to learn elements of Western Medicine, Obstetrics, Pediatrics, Nutrition, Health Education, Sterilization and Hygiene, etc. (Swiss Red Cross 2003: 9)

That support for TTM fitted well within the World Health Organization's guidelines for supporting primary health care through inclusion of traditional medicine practitioners, as pronounced in the seminal Declaration of Alma-Ata from 1978, as well as other SRC documents. One SRC document written by a long-term delegate to Tibet asserts that "what concerns Public Health [is that] there currently exists a pluralistic system. Western medicine and Tibetan medicine can benefit each other. . . . Therefore, we contribute not only to the survival of a culture threatened with extinction, but also equally improve long-term health care in rural areas" (Swiss Red Cross 1998: 6). In addition to Tibetan medicine supporting primary health care for rural areas, the support for TTM is also thought to counter cultural decline.

SRC partnered in the Pelshung School project with Jampa Trinlé, the local senior *amchi*, who was behind the Shigatse Health Bureau's official proposal for the Pelshung Tibetan Medicine School. He was a rehabilitated doctor and graduate of the Tashilhunpo's Kikinaka School, later head of the Shigatse Mentsikhang Hospital. To distinguish him from Lhasa's Mentsikhang director, who incidentally has the same name, I will refer to him as Shigatse Jampa Trinlé.

The timing of the opening of the Pelshung School is relevant, as it shows how all three parties involved—SRC, the Shigatse Health Bureau, and rural medical students—considered Tibetan medicine an important part of the health care system for the rural TAR. This view shifted dramatically with the introduction of the New Cooperative Medical Services (NCMS) scheme, an updated rural medical insurance scheme aimed to reduce rural populations' healthcare costs that began in a few pilot townships in Tsang in 1998 and was implemented in the entire region in 2003 (Janes 2002; Hofer 2008a, 2008b).

Shigatse Jampa Trinlé's personal motivation and influence regarding the ethos and curriculum of the Pelshung School should not be underestimated. Initially a monk at a monastery in his home district, Namling, in 1954 he enrolled at Kikinaka Medical School (alongside Yonten Tsering and Ngawang Dorjé). Following his final exams during the Democratic Reforms, Jampa Trinlé left the order to work as a farmer, secretly continuing his medical practice. In the 1970s he was officially reinstated as a health worker, gradually climbing the ladder of health-related civil service while continuing to see patients on a daily basis (Trinlé 2000). In 1982 he became director of the new Shigatse Mentsikhang Hospital, a facility that attracted several thousand patients every year. Like the Lhasa Mentsikhang, it shifted toward providing "integrated care," offering both "Chinese" (the local term for biomedical) and Tibetan medical treatment. Since the mid-1990s, more patients received biomedicines than Tibetan medical treatments at this hospital.[22] Shigatse Jampa Trinlé's support for the Pelshung School, given his official position and local influence as well as support from the prefecture-level Health Bureau (led by Dr. Puntsok, a former student at Kikinaka), must not be overlooked. He was, for instance, crucial in defending the choice to invite only male students to the school, a policy the Swiss Red Cross accepted only with great reluctance.

Medical Training at Pelshung and Making a Living Back Home

After Shigatse Health Bureau had sent an invitation to rural communities to bring forward male candidates for the Tibetan medical training at Pelshung, Jampa Trinlé traveled the prefecture visiting and interviewing those who seemed most promising and had good written Tibetan. He also recruited monks from distant monasteries and a few from Tashilhunpo Monastery. There the monks had wanted to add Tibetan medicine to their existing clinic, which since the early 1980s had been providing Chinese-style biomedicine and TCM acupuncture, its last Tibetan medical practitioners (who returned after the Cultural Revolution) in the meantime having passed away. Jampa Trinlé also selected a few boys from either active or historical Medical Houses.

When this first cohort of thirty-eight students joined the school, they were in their early teens and had received, in most cases, a basic primary school education, though a few had some additional monastic or family-related medical training. Upon entry, students were obliged to take three vows to their teacher: to go back and practice as an *amchi* in their home village or home monastery after graduation; to work as a private *amchi* and not join government service; and to not change profession (Heimsath 2003: 4–5). The thirty-eight young men received what could best be described as a monastic-style education. The day began with prayers to the Medicine Buddha and Manjushri, the bodhisattva of transcendental wisdom. A large part of the day was devoted to memorization of the *Four Treatises* (figure 5.5) and study of the *Moon Jewel of the Body's Measurements*,[23] the *Essence of Medical Compounding* by Khyenrap Norbu,[24] and some popular commentaries on the *Four Treatises*. There was also some classroom teaching and practical instruction in medicine making. The students learned about diagnosis and a wide range of therapeutic techniques, including external therapies[25] and bonesetting (albeit mostly theory only) as well as how to recognize Tibetan materia medica—both wild and dried forms—and how to compound some basic Tibetan medicines. They had no exposure to biomedical ideas, as a result of insistence by the school's director and the SRC's attempt to be culturally sensitive.

After graduation, this first group returned home with a certificate from the school, medical instruments, and a bag of 90, 100, or 150 types of Tibetan *rilbu*, depending on the student's final grade. The SRC and Jampa Trinlé thought of these medicines as the young doctors' start-up capital, from which they could make their initial income, allowing them to thereafter replenish their stocks of materia medica. When planning the project, the idea was that the graduates would enhance the economic viability of their practice by making their own medicines.

The reality encountered by the first group of doctors, once they returned home, proved to be different—and difficult. The doctors had limited practical training in Tibetan medicine; their own and others' confidence in their ability to heal was minimal (cf. Craig 2007). They were in their late teens and early twenties, whereas Tibetans generally trust older, more experienced doctors. The idea of the power and trustworthiness of doctors coming from a medical lineage or a Medical House was still strong, and only a few of the first cohort had such a family background.

Furthermore, like Pema and Sonam Drölma, they were confronted with predominantly subsistence economies in their remote nomad and farming areas. Jampa Trinlé had advised his student doctors to set a price of ¥1 for three doses of Tibetan medicine taken three times a day. His students soon found that payments generally came in kind, if they received remuneration at all (none came from poor people or relatives). They sold whatever goods they received to have cash and replenish their stock of medicinals, but in most cases they were unable to fully replenish their stock.[26] In addition, most graduates had to balance their medical practice with work as a farmer or nomad. In a first evaluation of the program, the external consultant to the SRC, Professor Meyer, wrote that "only one of the graduates visited in 1998 could make some profit from his medical skill."[27]

Meyer found that many of the doctors had started to administer biomedical treatments. Given the widespread use of biomedical drugs in rural Tibet, in particular injected ones or those administered through

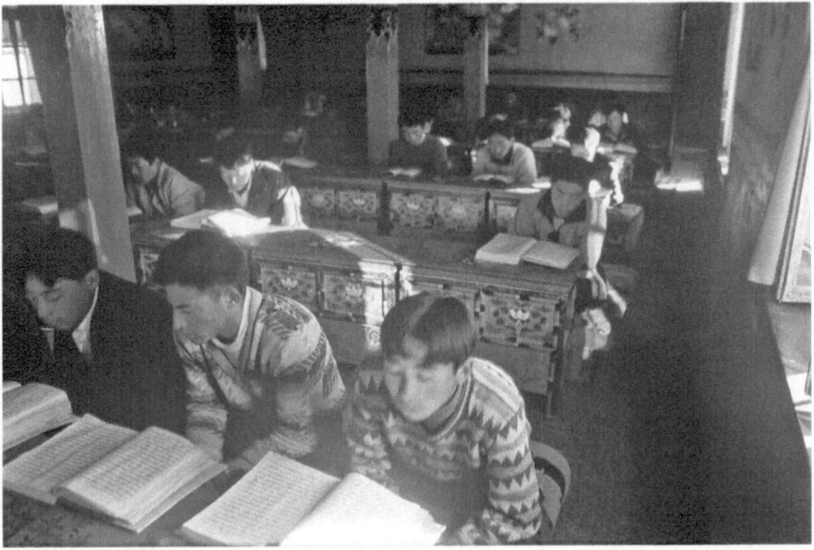

FIGURE 5.5. The Pelshung students memorizing the *Four Treatises*, 2003. Photo by the author.

intravenous drips by doctors and village health workers in clinics, it is hardly surprising that rural patients would ask the Pelshung doctors for similar kinds of treatment in their homes as well. As one did not absolutely need a medical license to sell or purchase biomedical drugs, the doctors could easily stock these. If they did not have them, at least they could deliver medicines people had bought. This saved their patients the delivery charges in the newly part-privatized rural health care facilities.

Meyer's recommendations included that the Pelshung *amchi* be given biomedical training to reduce the risk of medical malpractice—a very real risk given their insufficient training. The first group of students was called back to Pelshung in 1999 for a six-week intensive course in basic biomedicine, including lessons in hygiene, sanitation, mother and child health care, and the safe use of injections.

That same year, in October, a second cohort of fifty-six students (again exclusively male and selected by Jampa Trinlé) started training. Forty-two of them hailed from rural backgrounds, their studies financially covered by the SRC, while twelve were from more affluent families, including some from urban areas who could pay their own costs. The training was shortened to four years, and the school's headmaster, Jampa Trinlé, was the primary teacher, with some teaching support from previous graduates.

Compared with the first graduates, the second group received a more realistic training. After four years of Tibetan medical education (and following the closure of the school), the SRC sponsored three-month internships for them at the Mentsikhang in Lhasa and its branch in Lhoka Prefecture. Here they often came in contact with biomedicines, despite the fact that these are nominally Tibetan medical institutions (cf. Adams and Li 2008). Then they all attended the Vocational Health School in Shigatse for nine months' biomedical training, with fees and subsistence paid by the SRC. It was more common for doctors among the second intake to speak and write Chinese, knowledge they had acquired in primary school, at the vocational school, or since graduating.

In 2003, a second evaluation of the first cohort of students was carried out in their home villages, which showed the adverse effects of the vows students had taken to remain private Tibetan medical doctors in their home villages or monasteries.[28] Later, when the vows were lifted, doctors of both cohorts were free to set up clinics and practice in places other than their home regions, to join government service, and even to change their profession. This development left them better equipped to make decisions in the midst of the challenges of practicing Tibetan medicine in remote areas, at a time when rural health care provision was beginning to change radically. Since the second batch began training in October 1999, the NCMS rural insurance scheme had been introduced, later spreading throughout Tsang. Tibetan medical care, which was not reimbursed under this scheme, almost completely ceased to be provided through government channels, and people increasingly chose the reimbursed biomedical therapies (cf. Hofer 2012: 176–80; Hofer 2008a, 2008b). Although the majority of graduates from both cohorts have remained private *amchi*, some have chosen to join government service, including a larger percentage of the second group.[29] Some saw government service as an opportunity to see patients more regularly, some to have an ongoing exchange with biomedical health workers and learn new skills, some for the status of working in a government institution, and some because they found it difficult to continue to practice at home. The majority, however, joined because they were granted a small but stable income of on average ¥200 a month. Despite having undergone shorter training, their biomedically trained colleagues in the township clinics usually earned substantially more than the Pelshung graduates, accounted for by the fact that they had official graduation certificates from a government school.

The lack of official recognition of the Pelshung degrees by the Shigatse Health Bureau, which, as we should recall here, had proposed establishing Pelshung School, contributed to the decision to close the school in 2003. One report cited a long-term delegate who had coordinated the activities of the school, who attributed the school's problems and long-term viability to three factors: "A section for TTM has opened at the vocational school in Shigatse, which trains 40 TTM doctors a year," offering students an official government-approved certificate[30] while TTM Pelshung school diplomas were not recognized by the official health care bureaucracy; and he considered that "TTM was incapable of tackling the major public health problems" in the prefecture.[31] Why this change of attitude toward TTM's capacity to make a difference in primary rural health care provision?

The assessment of the SRC delegate questioned one of the two main project aims for the establishment of the Pelshung Tibetan Medicine School: the support of the rural health care system through TTM. TTM's inability to tackle major public health problems should be understood in the context of the dominant biomedical health care paradigm that pervades both primary and public international health care initiatives and which has abandoned efforts to incorporate traditional medicine practitioners based on the Declaration of Alma-Ata. The move toward biomedical interventions rather than reliance on indigenous medicine also represents attitudes that are now more prevalent, especially among biomedically trained development workers and international NGO delegates, not just in Tibet. The Health Bureau's unwillingness to provide official certificates, on the other hand, reflects the state's changing outlook on Tibetan medicine in primary rural health care and state control over the legitimacy and authority of private Tibetan medicine practitioners and private education more broadly in Tibet.

TIBETAN MEDICINE, RURAL PRIMARY CARE, AND NATIONALITY POLICY ON THE MARGINS

At the same time as these private initiatives were taking place, Tibetan medical care was being incorporated into PRC-government institutions, as discussed by Janes and others. In Ngamring, this current of revitalization mainly comprised the establishment of a Tibetan medicine section at the biomedical People's Hospital in 1974 and then the independent Tibetan Medicine Hospital, established between 1993 and 1996.

Wangnam's *Short History of Ngamring Dzong Tibetan Medical Hospital*, written in 1999, reports on both developments in tightly confined political rhetoric and structured mainly by two nationally important events.[32] The first is the Third Plenum of the Eleventh CCP Central Committee in 1978, which, according to the author, writing on behalf of the senior physicians, "inspired us to further expand medical services to people living in remote rural areas." This was achieved, as the report quotes expanding patient numbers between 1974 and 1988. Intimately linked to this growth, the report states, was a structure in which most medicine production was carried out locally with medical materials picked by doctors and health workers during the summer months. The senior doctors offered courses in Tibetan medicine to barefoot doctors, village health workers (as barefoot doctors were called after 1983), and township-level health workers, whose workforce added to the efficacy and volume of medicines collected in the wild.

Tibetan medical work in Ngamring is then said to have substantially expanded in 1993, when the three senior doctors of the Tibetan medical section of the People's Hospital managed to secure extra funds from Lhasa and from a sponsor from China proper to establish the separate Ngamring Tibetan Medicine Hospital. The substantial building—featuring a reception and pharmacy area and several treatment rooms—was completed in 1994.[33] The facility increased its staff, keeping the three senior doctors and adding three graduates from the Lhasa Mentsikhang and Tibetan Medical College. Only one was a woman.

Both the *Short History* and doctors' accounts of this period clearly show that the work of Ngamring Tibetan Medicine Hospital in many ways was a continuation of the Maoist call to "stress medical work in the rural areas," with traditional medicine playing a significant role in this endeavor. Rural patients using the Tibetan medicine facility increased, and the thirty medicines they prepared were considerably more complex than the *Tibetan Medical Manual*'s recipes of the barefoot doctor era. For instance, they made Agar 8 and traded locally collected ingredients for foreign ingredients that the Lhasa Mentsikhang imported in bulk.

The second political event structuring the *Short History* is the Third Forum on Work in Tibet, held in Beijing in 1994, which, according to Barnett, entirely reversed the liberal policies of the 1980s (Barnett 2003). In 1992 hard-liner Chen Kuiyan became party secretary of Tibet after condemning the 1980s liberalization as a failure, claiming it had indirectly fueled the large-scale protests in Lhasa between 1987 and 1989 (Barnett 1994). In line with the usual requirements for political reports, the *Short History* describes the Third Forum on Work in Tibet as a wonderful milestone opening up new opportunities. It repeats the newly emerging government discourse regarding Tibetan medicine: that it would "improve relations between the nationalities." The report further describes Tibetan medicine as a means to "develop the economy and the culture of nationality areas." In so doing, "Tibetan medical treatments have to fit the market economy as well as fundamental Communist principles" (Wangnam 1999). This indicated how significantly Tibetan medicine was now to depart from its main mission of providing primary health care through low-cost local means.

The *Short History* clearly demonstrates the changing nature of "Chinese state interests" in the wake of the 1994 forum (cf. Janes 1999, 2002). While economic liberalization had already started in the rest of the PRC during the 1980s, such measures were delayed for the TAR—partly due to major protests of 1987–89. After the Third Forum they were implemented in the TAR, in what Barnett (2003) termed a "marketization of politics," with at their core Chen Kuiyan's "grasping with two hands" of "economic development" and "security." Under the umbrella of these policies came restrictions on the practice of religion, which also manifested in the field of Tibetan medicine—for instance, in 1995 a ban on the performance of the annual medicine empowerment ritual that the Lhasa Mentsikhang had revived in the 1980s. Under the rubric of development, specialized industries were singled out as "pillar industries" for the TAR, including mining, tourism, and Tibetan medicine (Barnett 2003).

Despite these developments and the financial cuts that came with the following five-year health plans, the cohort of older government servants and local cadres in Ngamring managed to challenge financial cuts by the health bureau and kept patients' expenditures for health care as low as possible. They were able to minimize the impact of Chinese state interests and maintain the socialist-cum-Buddhist health care ethos that they had upheld for two decades.

— · —

The reemergence of private Tibetan medical practice in rural Tsang, despite long odds and substantial growth in governmental Tibetan medicine institutions, shows that in addition to the state-led policies and support for Chinese and Tibetan medicine between the 1970s and the mid-1990s, an alternative sphere reopened for the practice and teaching of Tibetan medicine. Here much medical, if not economic, power remained in the hands of those who possessed lineage affiliations, the associated medical techniques, and increasingly, international networks. Some senior *amchi* actively drew on these to foster the revival and transmission of Tibetan medicine knowledge in rural areas. Internationally sponsored schools were established, such as the Kailash Projects School in Darchen in Ngari and the NYIMA Foundation–sponsored school in Lhundrub.

Sometimes these initiatives, although sanctioned by the state and even carried out in addition to government jobs by senior cadres, can be read as a partial resistance to the wholesale co-opting of traditional medicine practitioners by Chinese state interests, especially the pharmaceutical commercialization that was to follow. To (re)establish or continue private practice in rural Tsang was, however, often a precarious undertaking. Through the postreform period, the region remained the "poorest relation" of the TAR. The few new government job opportunities in Tibetan medicine and biomedicine were highly desired and in many ways socially prestigious.

Rural private *amchi*, whether trained prior to 1959 or in the Pelshung School in the 1990s, often lacked the means and social standing characteristic of many urban practitioners, both in Lhasa and in other parts of the PRC among Chinese medicine physicians (Scheid 2007). The socioeconomic order in which Tibetan Medical Houses and monasteries had functioned and flourished in the pre-Communist period was gone forever. During the introduction of the household responsibility system in the TAR, nothing in the land and benefit allocations benefited *amchi* practitioners who provided the medical care for their local communities.

After government health care was privatized beginning in the mid-1990s (Janes 1999, 2002), rural *amchi* were sought out, especially by poor patients, but therefore often faced severe economic challenges in keeping up their practice, as these patients were unable to pay for services. When the newly introduced NCMS did not reimburse Tibetan medicines in the early 2000s, these medicines, though available in government clinics and hospitals, became more expensive and had to be paid out of pocket (Hofer 2008a, 2008b). Many private initiatives to revitalize medicine in the private domain, like the Pelshung School and home training for *amchis*, had completely disappeared by the early years of the new millennium. Those from Tsang desiring to study Tibetan medicine, like Gyatso's son Tashi, now had to take courses at Lhasa Tibetan Medical College. However, access, educational, and financial requirements were usually beyond the means and local possibilities of many rural Tibetans who were interested in pursuing this career, as we saw for Sonam Drölma's son.

Those who wanted a medical career of sorts were often forced to enroll in the Shigatse Health Vocational School, as only a middle school leaving certificate was required. This school offered a few Tibetan medicine modules, but in effect produced biomedically trained health workers and nurses. These courses were often chosen by women who would have liked to study Tibetan medicine but for various reasons could not attend the Tibetan Medical College in Lhasa.

The revival of private medical work between the mid-1970s and the mid-1990s was much slower and more limited than medical work funded and promoted by the state in governmental institutions. When the state began to pull back its funding for the rural provision of Tibetan medicine in the 1990s, and in 2000 excluded it from reimbursement through the NCMS, this seriously threatened the Tibetan medical practice of both governmental and private *amchi* in rural areas. It also further consolidated the hegemony of Chinese-biomedical pharmaceuticals in the Tibetan villages and pastoral townships, a process that had begun with the barefoot doctor campaign, as Fang (2012) has argued.

The shift toward government training provoked by various legal and economic factors (cf. Hofer 2011d) means that newly standardized Tibetan medical diagnostic and therapeutic techniques spread more widely, leaving little room for the diverse medical cultures that were embodied and transmitted in private and monastic domains. Government training and practice openly embrace the integration of Sowa Rigpa with biomedical ideas, standards, and practices.

One of the main differences between private and governmental Tibetan medicine practitioners, even in the younger generation, is the former's ability and confidence in Tibetan medical diagnostic and therapeutic methods, as well as their capacity to prepare at least some of their own Tibetan medicines. By contrast, government Tibetan medicine practitioners trained in the Tibetan Medical College in Lhasa rely to a greater extent on Chinese biomedical pharmaceuticals and almost exclusively on manufactured Tibetan medicines. They are in the process losing some of their Tibetan medical clinical and pharmacological skills and knowledge, and this inevitably weakens the sustainability and efficacy of Tibetan medicine.

CHAPTER 6

LOOKING AT ILLNESS

> When I look at the way society is going now—you know they say that today everyone can do business and can become rich—then I also have to think about medical fees or moving to Lhasa. In my mind I am not happy about the idea, because people are poor here and there would be bad talk about us in the village. Also, there would be no real *amchi* left in the village.
>
> —Amchi Pema, 2003

AT the opening of this book, two monks from Tashilhunpo Monastery in Shigatse visited Yonten Tsering, who diagnosed the older of the two with *lungné* (wind disorder). After they had "looked at illness" and shared some tea with us, the monks left with three Tibetan medical compounds and a couple of *hormen* (nutmeg-and-*tsampa*-filled cotton bags), a cross between a home and professional remedy to be warmed in oil or butter and applied every evening. No money changed hands; the monks simply thanked the doctor profusely.

As the year progressed and the end of my longest stretch of fieldwork approached, the officially retired doctor had looked at the illnesses of over 2,500 people in similar circumstances.[1] This took place in his Shigatse home and during several day- or weeklong medical rounds to rural villages in the prefecture. I attended many hundreds of these encounters, acting as a participant observer, lending a hand, and filming some. Whether in town or in the countryside, I observed that the *amchi*'s medical encounters and his medicines were given entirely free of charge and that many of his patients were monetarily poor and little involved in the cash economy. Only government employees and business people typically offered a donation in return for treatment. The elderly doctor covered most of the expenses for medicines and his travels from his generous government pension, while two foreign sponsors donated money for medicines. I had helped to recruit the donors, one of them agreeing on the basis that Yonten Tsering charge a flat fee of ¥2 per patient, so as not to disadvantage private doctors in the area. With these three sources of cash, Yonten Tsering's funding differed from Pema, younger doctors, and graduates from the Pelshung Tibetan Medicine School.[2] That said, several retired government *amchi* from Ngamring and elsewhere also carried out a lot of medical work without remuneration, one of them saying, "It's okay to ask for money from patients in this life, but it's not for the next life."

The *amchi* and pharmacists of the Tashilhunpo Medical Clinic in Shigatse offer Tibetan medicines—if not entirely for free, at least at a low rate made possible by local, small-scale production on a noncommercial basis—drawing patients from the most deprived strata of the economically poorest region of central Tibet. In what ways do *amchi* in Tsang engage in a Sowa Rigpa moral economy, and what is at stake in the pan-Chinese and TAR-specific political economy of primary health care? Exploring instances of a Sowa Rigpa moral economy contributes a localized perspective to current debates on the broader trajectories of Tibetan medicine in the PRC. In particular, this perspective may illuminate the diminishing presence of Tibetan medicine in governmental primary care and the repercussions of large-scale industrialization of Tibetan pharma for smaller producers across the Tibetan plateau.[3]

In his monograph *Manufacturing Tibetan Medicine and the Moral Economy of Tibetanness* (2013), anthropologist Martin Saxer focuses on the nature of the relationship between the "moral economy of Tibetanness" and the current industrialization and commercialization of Tibetan medicine production. The classical studies of peasants' resistance to market-driven transformations of traditional modes of production and distribution in eighteenth-century Great Britain (Thompson 1971) and in Southeast Asia (Scott 1976, 1985), from which the moral economy argument derives, posited that physical survival was at stake when peasants stated the moral illegitimacy of certain capitalist practices and demanded minimal subsistence and food rights. In contrast, Saxer argues that what is at stake in the moral economy of Tibetanness "is not physical but rather cultural survival, for which Tibetan medicine has become an important realm"

(2013: 14). To show how the moral economy is similar in structure but different in form and scale from classical cases of moral economies, Saxer explores the practices and discourses of a retired government servant who set up a private NGO-sponsored school and noncommercial Tibetan medicine factory as well as those of big traditional pharma companies like Cheezheng and Arura. He draws on global attempts and engagements in "saving Tibetan culture," convincingly showing that local expressions of the moral economy of Tibetanness are intimately linked with the global moral economy of the "Tibet question."

The medical work of people like Yonten Tsering and the doctors at Tashilhunpo Monastery (as well as Pema in Ruthog and the Pelshung *amchi*) evidences the need to bring back material and physical survival, bodily health, and well-being into our analyses of the moral economy of Tibetanness. The Sowa Rigpa moral economy needs be studied in the context of both industrialization and privatization of primary health care. When we look at the kinds of diseases treated and patients' lack of access to medical care that addresses these in the long term, either due to high cost or a shortage of *amchi*, we are drawn back to some of the original moral economy arguments.

Rural patients of the doctors discussed here depended on their bodies for work on land on which they depended economically, socially, and morally. They benefited directly from doctors' principles and practices of Buddhist and Tibetan medical ethics, meaning they were able to access health care and sustain their livelihoods. Tibetan medicine often made a tangible difference in their physical subsistence, their very ability to work as farmers and pastoralists in Tsang. Colleagues' work on *amchi* in Amdo, eastern Tibet, and Mustang, Nepal (Craig 2012), as well as in Ladakh, India (Blaikie 2013a), provide similar instances of the Sowa Rigpa moral economy. A morally informed medical practice appears to be a necessity on the margins, where government health care and internationally driven "Save Tibet" projects rarely reach.

The political economy of Tibetan medicine and health has profoundly affected how *amchi* offer treatments and medicines and the chances patients have to benefit from these encounters and therapies (Hofer 2008a, 2008b). Both *amchi* and their patients have been exposed to "unhealthy health policies" of global and national kinds (Castro and Singer 2004). The increasingly large-scale production and national marketization of Tibetan medicines affect the everyday life of the poorest sections of Tibetan society, in the form of further restrictions on accessing health care, at least partly due to cost. This is in addition to economic marginalization and exclusion, especially in rural areas of the TAR (cf. Fisher 2014).

It is from the vantage point of rural and economically marginalized Tibetans, many of whom come to see Yonten Tsering in villages or combine a visit to Tashilhunpo Monastery or Shigatse with a visit to its medical clinic, that we need to reconsider the moral economy of Sowa Rigpa and Tibetanness. Yonten Tsering and Tashilhunpo's moral economy is not mainly a matter of cultural survival; for many it is a question of physical survival and bodily fitness. By examining certain *amchis*' selective, practical resistance to the increasingly capitalist-driven government primary care and Tibetan pharmaceutical industry, we can see how this moral economy of Tibetanness works in the service of the health and well-being of Tibetans with few other means to access medical care.

THE POLITICAL ECONOMY OF PRIMARY HEALTH CARE IN TSANG

With some delay compared to other parts of the PRC,[4] governmental health care funding in the TAR was transformed in the 1990s. Within one decade, the socialist model of health care, imperfect as it was, had to adopt liberal market-based values featuring a narrow, vertical approach to primary care that profoundly limited the access of poor and rural patients to care and essential medicines (cf. Tibet Information Network 2002; Fisher 2002). This development fundamentally challenged the ethics and economies of many governmental hospitals, clinics, and doctors in Tibet (Janes 1999a; Hofer 2008a, 2008b); it also posed particular problems for the continuity of Tibetan medical primary care in rural areas. In these circumstances, the revival of Tibetan medicine continued to be an often hard-won and drawn-out process.

In the early years of the new millennium, funding for rural primary and secondary health care in the TAR was further revised. The budgets of county hospitals, township clinics, and village health workers for upkeep of facilities, salaries, and medicines were now to have three sources: central government, the TAR government, and people's contribution to the newly introduced New Cooperative Medical Services (NCMS). Given this insurance scheme's insufficiency, fees for services and medicines had to be collected, even though by 2003 over 90 percent of the rural population of Shigatse Prefecture and the TAR had signed onto the NCMS insurance plan.[5] As out-of-pocket expenses for services and medicine had risen significantly in the wake of the first wave of market-based revisions of socialist health care during the 1990s, the NCMS would help rural people afford and hence access medical services—and prevent them from financial ruin and poverty in the case of catastrophic illness. However, in the TAR as in China proper (Carrin et al. 1999; Liu and Hsiao 1995), patients' health care costs saw only a small reduction. Even after adjustments and increased central government contribution to the scheme in 2003, out-of-pocket expenses remained high (Wagstaff et al. 2008). Regional health inequities across rural populations in the PRC continued unabated (Qian 2010)

Nevertheless, national and regional health bureaus' commitment to a largely neoliberal model of health care persists in China (Qiang and Blomqvist 2014), fully supported by large global funding agencies such as the World Bank and Asian Development Bank (Janes et al. 2006). In the TAR's rural government health facilities during my fieldwork, few health care services were provided for free, mainly comprising contraception and family planning services, basic birthing assistance in clinical facilities, vaccination, and epidemic disease control measures. Family members who brought women to clinics for childbirth were rewarded with ¥50.

It is now well documented that health inequities in low-income countries (or regions) and even in high-income countries that feature great inequality and income disparity (such as the United States), having undergone or currently undergoing neoliberal health reforms, have widened the gap between those who can access and afford health care and those who cannot.[6] Poor patients therefore frequently delay health care or sink deeper into the "medical poverty trap" (Whitehead, Dahlgren, and Evans 2001), or what is colloquially referred to in the United States as "medical bankruptcy." They often die from conditions and situations that could have been avoided (Farmer 2015). As the ability to work, to survive childbirth, and to raise healthy children are all influenced by access to health care, this development has contributed to rising social and economic inequality in many areas over the past twenty years (Nguyen and Peschard 2003; Samuel 2010: 321–22). It has also, in many places (but not the United States in this case), had an especially detrimental effect on women's health and empowerment, as women tend to be more vulnerable, less mobile, and generally more negatively affected due to the vagaries of human reproduction and harmful patriarchal values and practices (Ward 1998; Inhorn 2006).

Due to increased political sensitivities and international researchers' diminishing access to the TAR, the latest developments in health care funding and adjustments to the NCMS and their combined impact on health care access in the TAR are poorly researched and understood compared to other postsocialist countries with similarly neoliberal health policies (Janes and Chuluundorj 2004; Janes et al. 2006). Nonetheless, we can get a fairly good picture from reports by international NGOs, government statistics, and ethnographic work.

By 2010 health-care costs for poor, disabled, and otherwise disadvantaged households in rural Tibetan areas of the PRC remain obstructive, preventing even basic health needs from being met in a timely or satisfactory manner (Sagli et al. 2012; Hofer 2012; Nianggajia 2011). Care in remote rural areas is often inadequate. Village health workers in the early 2000s earned only about ¥50 a month. Though such workers usually have knowledge and skills in the administration of about twenty biomedical drugs, they have no specialized training to manage childbirth or emergency complications. The latter almost always require referral to higher-level facilities, such as county or prefecture hospitals, often too distant to be reached in time, of little use, and more expensive yet covered to a lesser extent by the NCMS. Such referrals are thus often ignored by patients or are difficult to realize. Furthermore, Tibetans in Amdo have been reported as frequently mistrusting medical personnel, perceiving them as prescribing unnecessary diagnostic tests and medications to increase the income of a facility or doctor (cf. Nianggajia 2011).

There has been a pronounced increase in for-profit health care in Tibetan towns and cities, in line with the rest of the PRC (Schrempf 2011; Hofer 2012). Here all expenses for medical care are paid directly by the patients; still, they often prefer this route, as procedures there are considered less bureaucratic and more accessible than in government clinics. To make matters worse, social inequities between urban/rural and government/private employment sectors have increased dramatically, and the economy of the TAR has been characterized by pronounced social exclusion and economic marginalization of Tibetans (Fisher 2002, 2005, 2014). PRC state subsidies are given as a "gift of development," in return for which

Tibetans are expected to accept the terms set by the state: most importantly, not getting involved in "politics" (Yeh 2013). Hence there is no open opposition or civil rights protest, even by educated Tibetans.

Tibetan medical practitioners on the margins have experienced the manifold impacts of this political economy of health and medicine. Many have found it extremely challenging to continue to adequately address rural patients' illnesses, and Tibetan medicine has been sidelined in government rural primary health care. At the same time Tibetan medicine is becoming an increasingly widespread option in urban areas, and Tibetan pharmaceuticals are commoditized for urban Tibetans and middle- and upper-class consumers across the PRC.[7]

THE PRECARIOUS PLACE OF TIBETAN MEDICINE IN PRIMARY CARE

Alongside dramatically increased health inequity in the wake of privatization and market-based reforms in the PRC starting in the late 1970s, there has also been a pronounced and documented reduction of TCM services in the governmental health care sector at large, particularly in rural areas since the late 1990s (Xu and Yang 2009; Fang 2012). A similar trend is also visible in the TAR with regard to Tibetan medicine. Already in the 1990s this was linked to the lower profit margins associated with common Tibetan medicines as compared to biomedical diagnostic and therapeutic interventions, as a result of which many clinics across the TAR stopped stocking Tibetan *rilbu* and powders (Janes 1999a).

I have documented decreasing numbers of *amchi* and availability of Tibetan medicines in township clinics in five counties in Shigatse Prefecture.[8] Even among those officially employed as Tibetan medical doctors in such facilities, several had no Tibetan medicines in stock (Hofer 2012: 174–79). Conversely, I have seen cases where an *amchi* had Tibetan medicines in stock but did not use them, even for illnesses widely treated that way. Often patients preferred biomedical treatments, especially intravenous drips and injections. "Fast effects" aside, there was often a financial element in this, as the NCMS readily reimbursed expenses for biomedicines. Since Tibetan medicines, with a few notable exceptions, were then excluded from the NCMS scheme, patients' out-of-pocket expenses for Tibetan medicine were often greater than for biomedicines (Hofer 2008a, 2008b, 2012).

One prominent way in which large governmental Tibetan medicine institutions met the first wave of privatization of government health care funding in the 1990s was by scaling up commercial production and for-profit sales of Tibetan medicines (Janes 1999a, 2002). This approach in some cases helped maintain Tibetan medical institutions in the wake of dramatic government funding cuts.[9] Other money-making ventures were initiated by hospitals specializing in Tibetan medicine or biomedicine, such as joint ventures with Chinese medical institutions in China proper as a means to maintain work and salaries (Janes 1999a). Hospitals and clinics that made Tibetan medicines for their own patients on site, such as the Ngamring Tibetan Medicine Hospital, continued to offer the medicines at affordable prices despite the funding cuts. At this institution, the fees for consultation (¥0.5 to ¥2) and for the usual prescription of three medicines a day (¥1) meant that they continued to attract patients and even saw the number of patients increase, while the number attending the neighboring People's Hospital dropped, due mainly to the costs.

The 1994 Third Forum on Work in Tibet had further implications. Tibetan medicine was declared one of three "pillar industries" of the TAR, along with mining and tourism, entitling Tibetan medicine factories and the like to government loans and incentives. Since the beginning of the new millennium, there has been a veritable rush to commercialize and scale up Tibetan medicine production. "Precious pills," in particular, were turned into profitable products aimed at local urban and national middle classes and markets, to whom they could be sold as over-the-counter (OTC) and "preventive" medicines (Adams and Craig 2008; Saxer 2013). This is a startling development considering their great symbolic and medical value in the 1950s, when they were expensive, their production and distribution sometimes sponsored by wealthy people (see chapter 2).

The introduction of new standards for drug production, laws imposing Good Manufacturing Practices (GMP), and requirements for commercial factories to obtain drug registration necessitated and promoted huge investment by government and private businesses in the industrialization of previously smaller and sometimes not-for-profit government hospital pharmacies. Prices for common Tibetan medicines (that is, those regularly prescribed to rural patients by governmental Tibetan medical doctors) had increased, a result of the enormous investments required to meet GMP standards, often paired with rising costs of raw ingredients (Craig and Glover 2009). There have also been other attempts to modernize practices in Tibetan medicine institutions, ranging from individual doctors' incorporation of biomedical diagnostic and therapeutic means to structured institutional approaches to dual diagnosis and integrated medicines.[10]

Perhaps counterintuitively, I found many *amchi* who provide Tibetan medical care in ways that defy the capitalist logic of marketized health care. These doctors provide treatment to those rural patients most severely affected by health inequity, and they lose money in the process. I take their Sowa Rigpa moral economy as a response to the rising commodification of health care and Tibetan medicine production that contributes substantially to the physical survival and well-being of rural Tibetans.

"LOOKING AT ILLNESS"

When, on a cold February morning at eight o'clock, two women arrived at Yonten Tsering's new home in Shigatse, we were in the middle of packing. Yontan Tsering was getting ready for another trip to treat patients in rural areas in Tsang, this time in Sakya and Rinpung Counties. The aluminum cases containing the doctor's medicines stood by the door with a leather barefoot doctor's case proudly placed on top. Khaki-colored sleeping bags and mattresses made up another pile, surrounded by an array of neatly knotted plastic bags containing *tsampa*, noodles, dried meat, and vegetables in a cardboard box for a journey of several days. Yeshe Lhamo, a visiting relative, and the maid were busy between kitchen and courtyard, boiling water for tea and making breakfast. Although the driver would soon arrive, without a moment's hesitation Yontan Tsering agreed to see the two early visitors and do what he referred to as *natsa taya* ("look at illness") or *nepa taya* ("see ill people").

We sat down with them in the open courtyard, the medicine trunks were returned to their usual spots, and the doctor pulled up the sleeves of his down jacket. Both women were wrapped in thick clothes, their colorful aprons over the woolen *chuba* lending brightness to the gray, wintry scene, as did their shy smiles. He began asking their names, places of residency, and ages, writing this information in his notebook, in the space below a prefilled patient number (which was well over 9000).

"What ails you?" he asked Dawa, the older of the two women, who had come from Deling, a farming village in Thongmön County. "I have strong pains in the joints of my hands and feet," she responded, showing her hands to the doctor. He took them in his hands and gently passed his fingers over her calcified joints.

YT: How long has this hurt you?

D: Many months; it makes it quite difficult for me to work.

Yontan Tsering reached for her wrists to read her pulses—a contemplative moment as the doctor pressed three fingers on the *tsön*, *ken*, and *chak* points located along the radial arteries. As he worked quietly, taking in what he felt, the silence was broken only by a request to see her tongue, which, as usual, was inspected with a quick and practiced eye. Still holding her wrists, with empathy he said, "I can see it must be painful, but this *tsadrum* disease of yours is not too bad. Don't worry. I will give you some good medicines."

The consultation with Dawa lasted about ten minutes, by the end of which they had shared a moment of laughter and the doctor had furnished her with two Tibetan medicines to be taken every day for a month. These were in addition to a biomedical rheumatism medicine she was instructed to take each morning and which she could get more of from her township clinic. In his notebook he wrote: "Has *tsadrum* disease, the symptoms are pain in the joints and the bones of hands and feet. Continue to take Chinese medicine in the morning, and take one pill of Trinsel 25 at midday and five pills of Pökar 10 every evening for one month."[11]

It was then the turn of the second woman, Chödron, a forty-three-year-old farmer.

YT: And where are you from?

C: Also from Deling—we are neighbors.

YT: What ails you?

C: My eyes.

YT: I see, your eyes. And has the illness lasted a long time?"

C: Yes, it has.

Yonten Tsering then uttered an extended and empathic *nyingjé* (pity, compassion) before asking the patient to look toward the sun so he could examine her eyes.

> YT: Yes, I can see there are quite a few red spots. May I see your tongue please? All right, and otherwise, do you have any other problems?
>
> C: Yes, my stomach.
>
> YT: Mmh. Are you taking any *tangmen* [Communist medicines] for that?
>
> C: No, I am not. I have been to the Gonpa Menkhang [the monastery medical clinic].
>
> YT: That's good, the Gonpa Menkhang is good.

After taking some time to read her pulse, he had further questions:

> YT: And at night, can you sleep?
>
> C: Yes, I can, but I wake up early, and in the day I cannot work very hard.
>
> YT: Do you get pains in the abdomen?[12]
>
> C: Yes, in the stomach.
>
> YT: Does it bloat?
>
> C: Yes, it does.
>
> YT: I give you some very good medicines, but the pain won't go away immediately. How long have you had this stomach ache?
>
> C: Two years at least.

While Yonten Tsering wrote out her medical record, he confirmed to Chödron that he would give her two medicines, one for the stomach and one for the eyes, each to be taken for fifteen days. He went to find the medicines and then, while she held open the small plastic sachet into which he counted the *rilbu*, the consultation turned to friendly chatter. It transpired that the two women had heard that the doctor was to hold a mobile clinic in a village near theirs a few days ago, but by the time the women reached the clinic, the doctor had gone back to the county seat.

While no distinct diagnosis was provided, Chödron was given medicines to alleviate symptoms that Yonten Tsering noted in his case record book as "red spots on the eyes," "excess *lung* element," and an aching stomach. Along with the biomedical eye salve, which he explained how to use, she was given "Sendu Nyikhyil for the stomach" and "Seljé 25 for the eyes," as the notes reveal, all to be taken and applied according to his instructions. While counting out the medicines, the doctor had decided to extend treatment to twenty days in total.

These medicines, along with a small piece of paper with her patient number and the doctor's home telephone number, were placed in a bright blue bag—one of hundreds the *amchi* had ordered. The bag proudly displayed the logo of the Lhasa-based TAR Tibetan Pharmaceutical Factory, where we had purchased the Tibetan medicines.[13] He added, "Come back if the medicines help you and you need a checkup."

As he secured the bag's yellow band and handed it to the women, he passed on his oft-repeated dietary advice to both patients: limit chilies and avoid spicy foods and garlic. Turning to the older woman, he repeated that she should keep warm and cover herself well. Yonten Tsering then proudly told them that this morning we were leaving for Sakya and then on to Rinpung to treat more patients. He added that the Acha, his affectionate term of address for me, had helped secure donations, which drew a broad and grateful smile from the two women. In neither case was there any payment; in fact, the doctor had explicitly told the women, "Today I am not taking any medical fees." Dawa and Chödron were then invited to the kitchen, where Yeshe Lhamo served them steaming cups of butter tea.

Yonten Tsering packed up the medicines again and put on his large, fur-lined leather jacket, intent on keeping out the cold. Before joining him and the students loading the rest of the things into the car parked outside, I chatted with the women in the kitchen. It turned out that the express aim of their journey to Shigatse had been to see Yonten Tsering. There were several reasons why they had traveled that far—about ninety minutes on the public bus. One was the high cost and questionable quality of care at their local health facilities, although they also mentioned its business-like character. Another was that they perceived their ailments to be "old diseases," for which Tibetan medicines were widely held to be effective. And furthermore, they had received recommendations from others who had experienced the kind and effective treatments of this doctor. No direct reference was made to the medicines the *amchi* dispensed being free of charge. However, to openly mention anything in this regard would have been inappropriate, considered "shameful" and "embarrassing" (*ngotsa*).

Kindly delivered, trusted, and effective treatment drew patients from all over Tsang to the Tashilhunpo Medical Clinic, the Gonpa Menkhang, referred to by the women during the consultation. Yet, what set Yonten Tsering apart from the Tashilhunpo, or for that matter any other clinic, was that he never expected patients to pay. Some of them offered money and were able to leave donations. The doctor otherwise tried to avoid being given gifts or payments in kind, such as tea or farm products, explaining, for example, that their typically strong tea was not conducive to his health.

YONTEN TSERING'S MORAL ECONOMY

The work and expressed ethical ideals of Yonten Tsering evoke a distinctly Tibetan version of moral economy in the context of Tibetan medicine, in which medical ethics and their expression in the treatment of patients in many cases have deep historical roots in a family or Medical House tradition. Those who could afford it gave donations, while those who could not were still treated in most cases, tax relief and help from resident family members helping to reduce household spending. *Amchi* were careful not to be seen as "making money" with medicines (cf. Kloos 2004), hence they avoided going on rounds, instead working from home and visiting private homes if specifically called. More recently, among many older doctors, such Tibetan medical practices have become entwined with socialist medical ethics acquired during their decades of work in the Communist system, which also offered medicines to "the masses" for no or very low cost. Yonten Tsering's medical work in his Shigatse home and on rounds to rural villages continued along the lines of this Buddhist-cum-socialist ethics. He worked tirelessly for his patients and never explicitly asked for fees or appeared to judge anyone, whether or not they gave something. His actions more than what he said—he never critiqued the government for its health policies—were a direct response to the increasingly market-based logic of government health services. Ethical concerns contributed to his decision to retire early, along with several other senior doctors. The capitalist logic that had been ushered in with the health reforms for the rural TAR in the 2000–2005 health plan was incompatible with their medical ethics. One of Yonten Tsering's colleagues recounted his experience: "I got a good government salary but as I knew all the patients and they couldn't pay their medical fees, I paid on their behalf. So half of the salary I got from the government went back to them. [*He laughs.*] I took early retirement and now practice privately, giving Tibetan medicines to patients and practicing religion."

Based on long-term experience, doctors like this man and Yonten Tsering knew only too well that in most rural villages and townships medical care was at best inadequate and distant, and at worst available but unaffordable. Doctors skilled in Tibetan medicine with adequate supplies of the medicines were rare. The *amchi* and their patients perceived Tibetan medicines as effective for many common but debilitating ailments, especially those considered "old diseases," such as many kinds of rheumatism.

When asked why they worked this way, Yonten Tsering and others emphasized the importance of treating poor farmers and pastoralists, giving everyone an equal chance to be in the best possible health. They usually added that this was also their religious practice, and that they gained spiritual merit from their medical work, as reflected in Tashi's comment, "It's okay to ask for money from patients in this life, but it's not for the next."

In contrast to "cultural preservation" or ruthless "Chinese business culture" (Saxer 2013), many of the older doctors I worked with in Tsang stressed the importance of treating all patients no matter whether they could pay or not, and mentioned their medical work serving as religious practice.

In the encounters with Dawa and Chödron from Deling Village, a Sowa Rigpa moral economy was expressed, enabling not the survival of "Tibetan culture" or Tibetan identity (cf. Janes 1999b; Adams 1998), but crucially the treatment of these women's problems for pragmatic reasons. Being well enough meant being able to subsist on what they could make their land yield, whether through their ability to work in the fields (mostly the work of men), or with animals and in the household, such as collecting water and fuel (the primary domain of women). In other words, a link remains between the moral economy of Yonten Tsering and the ethics of Sowa Rigpa on the one hand and the physical survival and well-being of many of his patients on the other.

Others of Yontan Tsering's generation and sometimes later ones worked to facilitate affordable health care in a way that was no longer possible in government services, which were now shifting from a socialist approach to a predominantly capitalist, neoliberal mode. The costs for Tibetan medicines were on the rise as a result of the recent health care reforms and the newly created urban and national markets for traditional pharmaceuticals with whom these rural patients were now competing. The link among poor patients' quality of life, their health, and the doctors' practical morality was tangible. And to Yonten Tsering, I am quite sure it was visible when "looking at illness."

While Tibetan medicine's wider reputation is often attested in the realm of "old diseases," sometimes Yontan Tsering's medicine meant the difference between life and death. Although he never assisted directly in childbirth, many young women came to see him before giving birth and asked for medicines to help with the delivery or complications. *Zhishé* 11 is widely known to help in giving birth and preventing extensive bleeding afterward (Craig 2012: 215–52). The *amchi* always had some in stock. In most cases, *Zhishé* 11 was prescribed as preventive medicine, women taking it in case of need. Still, three times during our five weeks of medical rounds in Tsang, family members came at the last minute to ask the doctor for medicines to either stop the bleeding or help deliver either child or placenta. The notebooks speak of similar situations from earlier years: brief entries recording "a woman's stuck placenta," "difficulty in delivering the child," and "excessive bleeding." In each case, Yonten Tsering gave *Zhishé* 11 as an emergency medicine at a higher dose.

Among named diseases (see table 6.1), there are several disease categories for which he prescribed medicines that underscore the link between his medical work and his patients' physical subsistence. Most common among adult patients, especially women, from farming areas, were symptoms that Tibetan medicine classes into five types of *drumbu*, commonly translated in modern English-language Tibetan medical literature as "rheumatism" or "arthritis." Dawa, as we have seen, was diagnosed with *tsadrum*. Among both male and female adult patients, the *amchi* commonly treated gastrointestinal conditions, which he perceived as the result of poor dietary habits that included use of too much chili and repeated intake of cold or old foods, as well as issues of food hygiene. He was careful not to make too many suggestions regarding people's eating habits, all too aware that many would simply be unable to follow his advice due to their dependence on their own products and habits. In men (and some women) who had liver- and *tripa*-related problems, he was firm in reminding and encouraging them to drink less *chang* or other kinds of alcoholic drinks.

TABLE 6.1. Sample of patients seen by Yonten Tsering as recorded in his Case Record, October 2006–August 2007

Patient	*Symptoms*	*Diagnosis*	*Treatment*
1. F, 61, NGAMRING COUNTY, YAMO TOWNSHIP [MR]	Initially the disease struck for 1 month, hands and feet could not move, hard to pass stools and urine, feeble voice, always swollen stomach, presence of bile in *chur brtag pa*, upon examining the urine wind element (*rlung khams*) is found to be very strong. Stools and urine are colored white.		Three pills of Bsam 'phel Nor bu for 30 days, Zhi Gser, and 3 pills of Dra lis is 16 for 30 days
2. NGAMRING COUNTY, YAMO TOWNSHIP, 34	Heart trembling and unhappy heart for 16 years Mind not happy, sometimes finds it hard to sleep, hard to pass stools, earlier performed moxibustion at *rlung gsang* (point)		As a remedy prescribed Zhi gser and Rlung sman for 15 days, 5 pills of Srog 'dzin 11 for 15 days, and 1 moxibustion at *brang gzhung dkar nag* At the moment should also take 5 pills of medicine for a cold (*tsham pa'i glo sman*) and moxibustion (*me btsa'*) performed on *lten gsang du*
3. F, 40, NAMLING COUNTY	Pain in the joints of arms and legs, swollen joints	*grum 'bu'i nad*	Four pills of Spos dkar 10 and 4 pills of Seng ldang 25 for 20 days
4. F, 76, PHULING TOWNSHIP	Vomited blood from her stomach	*snying gyi na tsha*	Take Zhi byed 7 (noon) and in the evening Rdza ti 20 for 4 weeks
5. NGAMRING [MR]	Placenta is stuck		Zhi byed 11
6. F, 70		*khrag tshad mtho po'i nad*	Tsan dan 18, Skyu ru 25 for 15 days, 'chi med la brgyad(?) and 1 Mu tig 70
7. 48, DROMO COUNTY	Gets dizzy in head, ringing in the ears, face swells, hard to sleep, BP 130/100, reduced appetite, weak *me drod* (digestive fire)	*tsha shar*	Se 'bru drnas gnas, 3 pills of Dra lis 16 and 1 pill of Tho rangs Bla med, for 20 days

8. F, 50, THONGMÖN COUNTY [MR]		*rtsa grum* (for 15 years)	Continue with biomedicine and 3 pills of Mgrin mtshal 25 and 4 pills of Spos dkar 10 for 10 days
9. F, DELING TOWNSHIP	Pain in hands and feet	*rtsa grum*	Continue biomedicines in the evening, take Mgril tshal 25 and Spos dkar 10, in the morning and afternoon for 1 month
10. F, 43, DELING TOWNSHIP	Red spots on patient's eyes, excess of *rlung* element, stomach not happy		(Biomedical) eye medicine, Nyin bu 5 for stomach and Gsal byad 25 for her eyes
11. 40, SAKYA COUNTY, TSARONG TOWNSHIP [MR]	Has headaches, heart trembling (*snying 'dar ba*) and pain on back (*stod*), as well as high blood pressure (BP 180/100)	*mkhris rlung*	Take Tsan dan 18, Skyu ru 25 and A gar for 10 days
12. F, 45	*Rtsa nad* in legs, sometimes has swollen stomach (*pho ba sbo*). Hard work on fields, BP 110/70. Sometimes has backache.	*Rtsa grum nad*, but principal illness is *ma zhu mkhris pa'i nad*	Use 3 medicines for *rtsa grum* disease, these are Se 'bru Drangs gnas and Zhi gser for 10 days, and Seng lden 24/25 for 30 days. Use 3 pills of A gar for 7 days for backache.
13. M, 3, LHÜNDING [MR]		*Glo ba'i nad*	Blon po gsum sbyor for 10 days
14. M, 41, LHÜNDING [MR]		*Cham pa* and *glo'i nad*	3 pills of 'khrag kun for 10 days
15. F, 28, LHÜNDING [MR]		Has *rlung* and *rtsa* disease	Agar 20 for 10 days (for *rlung* and *rtsa* disease) Antibleeding medicine Kur kum 8 for 10 days
		Is about to give birth	To facilitate and ease the birth, take Zhi byed 11 for 10 days
16. M, 6, LHÜNDING [MR]		*Srin nad*	Khyung lnga for 10 days

Note. The content of this table is my translation from Tibetan. *MR* means "seen on medical rounds" in a rural area of Shigatse Prefecture. All other patients were seen at the *amchi*'s Shigatse home.

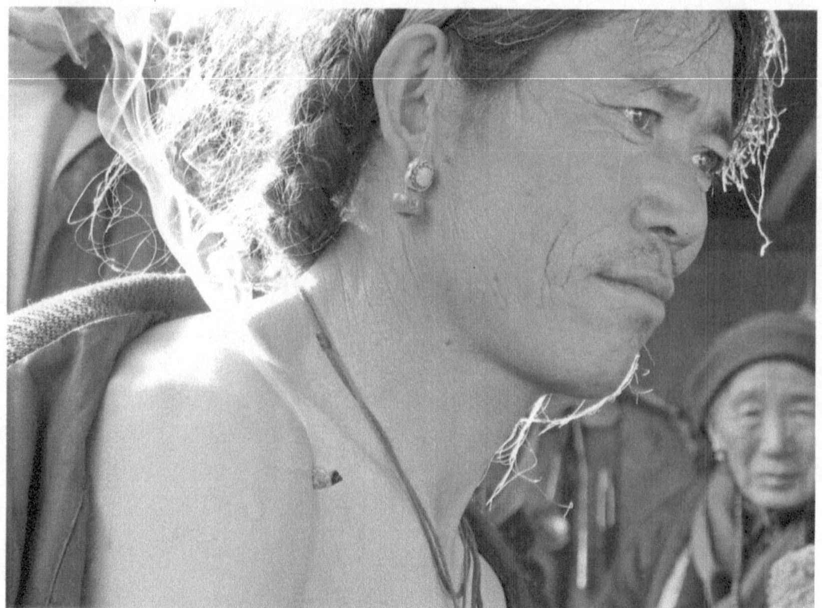

FIGURE 6.1. Yonten Tsering's treatment of a patient with moxibustion on medical rounds, 2007. Photo by the author.

Also prevalent was the vast group of illnesses related to *lung* or wind conditions (such as *lungné*, *sok lung*, etc.) and the numerous symptoms of *lung* more broadly. These range from feeling cold all the time or being mentally imbalanced, to high blood pressure (*trakshé thopo*) and *dribgyön*, a common condition recognized in Tibetan medicine and similar to a stroke in biomedical thinking.[14] In children, by far the most frequent problems were common colds, coughs, pulmonary conditions, and earaches. One of Yonten Tsering's special techniques in diagnosing children was to read the pulse not at the wrist, where it is difficult to ascertain before the age of eight, but on their ears.[15]

The full extent of the health care needs of rural Tibetans became evident to me only during Yontan Tsering's medical rounds to rural areas (figures 6.1 and 6.2). These were enormous and many times overwhelming.

On Medical Rounds

Long queues of Tibetans began to form as soon as Yonten Tsering and his accompanying students had obtained official permission to set up the mobile clinic at a local school in the county seat of Sakya, otherwise

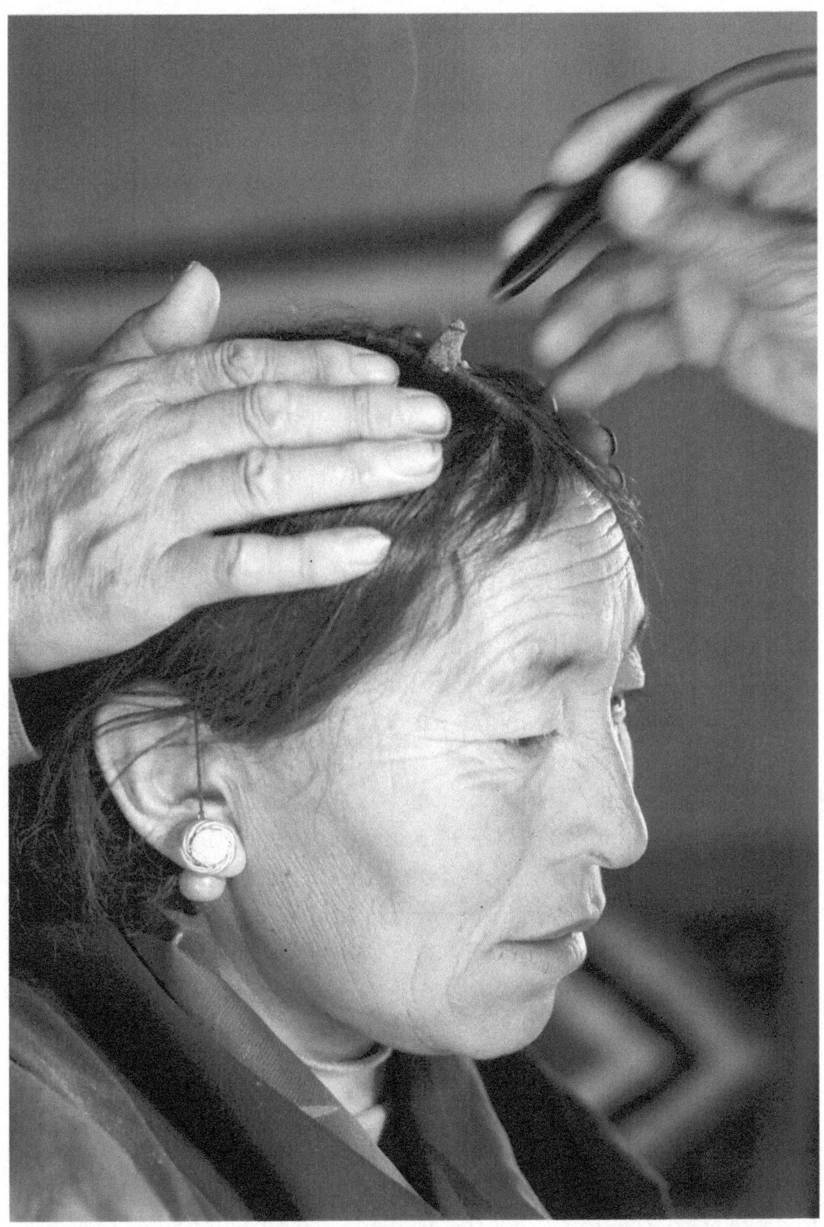

FIGURE 6.2. Moxibustion applied to a patient's head on Yonten Tsering's medical rounds, 2007. Photo by Meinrad Hofer.

mainly known for the famous Sakya Monastery. Some of the students began to hand out numbered tickets to organize the patients and allow everyone to be seen, setting off fights over these desired *passi*. This scene of evident medical need brings to mind Farmer's (2004) experience of the brimming courtyards of Haitian hospitals and his awareness that it would take him hours to cross from one side to the other as people insisted on stopping him to share their troubles, many having left conditions untreated for far too long.

That afternoon, in just under six hours of work at the mobile clinic, Yonten Tsering saw over 120 patients, most for an average of two minutes. Each consultation followed the same sequence as those at home: briefly questioning the patient, inspecting the tongue, reading the pulse, taking notes, and writing out the medicines to be taken, sometimes followed by brief additional dietary advice. The only difference here was that he never checked blood pressure (for lack of time), relying when necessary on the biomedicine students to do that for him. To speed things up, he engaged the students and myself in counting out pills into the small plastic bags, adding labels that indicated what time of day the medicines should be taken. During exceptionally busy times, he avoided applying moxibustion, as it requires more time and greater calm.

The following day 250 patients showed up, and subsequent days—in Rinpung, Tashiling, Khangsar, Phuntsoling, and elsewhere—all passed in a similar manner. The second or third day in any one place usually drew even larger numbers, as people from surrounding villages, who had heard by word of mouth about the occasion, arrived in groups riding on tractors. Hundreds of patients flocked to see the doctor. At times they risked pushing over the doctor's little school desk, despite the young students' crowd control. Some who stood in the queues, especially in the county seat, were the poorest of the poor, including several beggars; the others were mostly farmers, both men and women. They waited, sandwiched together, some carrying babies, the old and lame leaning on sticks, others spinning wool to make use of the time. After the day had been officially called to a close, still more patients arrived at the room where the doctor ate dinner or slept.

In Khangsar Village, at the end of a rough road about an hour's drive from the county seat of Rinpung, the doctor again set himself up in the central square of the village, as there was no government building to offer shelter. There was no health facility here either, except for a village health

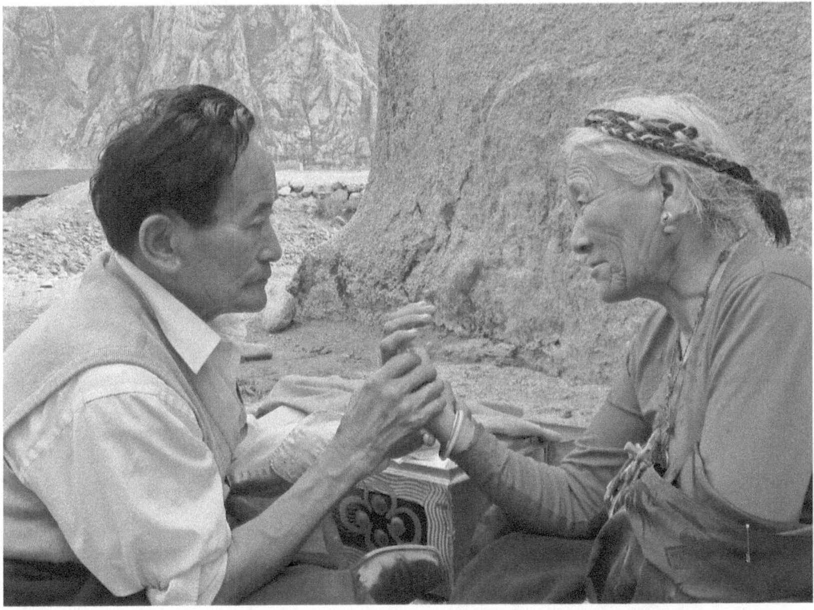

FIGURE 6.3. Tibetan medical doctor reading a patient's pulse by the side of a country road, Ngamring, 2007. Photo by Meinrad Hofer.

worker whose supply of medicines amounted to fifteen biomedical remedies, which were unaffordable to many, despite the quite reasonable prices and apparently locally implemented NCMS. The living conditions of the approximately fifty households in this village seemed quite difficult. Their very limited involvement in the cash economy was indicated by the fact that many wore clothes made from handspun wool. Both men and women in the crowd were spinning as they awaited their turn, chatting together. Here the atmosphere was more relaxed than the county seat, and although people were probably less able to access and afford health care, they were more willing to wait for the prized moment of sitting in front of the doctor and being asked, "What ails you?" The tone of his voice, though a little hoarse after several full days of work, continued to exude empathy. When the sun had disappeared behind the mountain ridge and cold descended, there were still patients to be seen.

Wherever we went, word had spread, and often patients waited on the side of the road. On one occasion an elderly woman had waited for over seven hours next to a Tibetan rug and a thermos of tea, which she offered to the doctor while he read her pulse (figure 6.3). Another time, on the

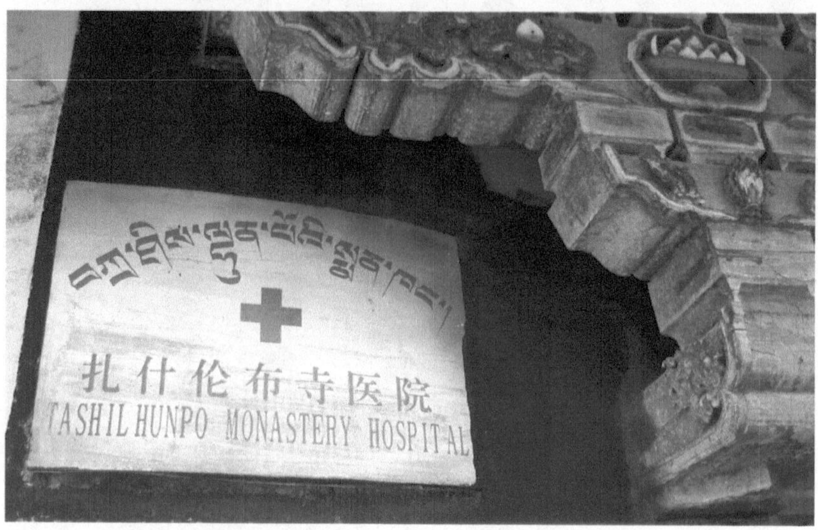

FIGURE 6.4. The Tashilhunpo Clinic entrance, 2007. Photo by Meinrad Hofer.

highway back to Shigatse, a group of women and men held hands across the road, forcing us to a halt. All told, I was overwhelmed by the scale of medical want apparent to us each day. In equal measure, I was deeply impressed by how calmly the doctor kept diagnosing patients, no matter how chaotic the situation, and by the fact that he often had no time to eat during the entire day. Aspects of Yonten Tsering's "seeing patients" and "looking at illness" reminded me of the way Tibetans flock to see Buddhist teachers. From a lay person's perspective, their encounter with lamas is usually short due to high demand; it involves eye contact and the receipt of a blessing through either touch or the receipt of or contact with a blessed substance. Buddhist teachers on their part speak of "seeing" worshippers, offering lay people a chance to come in contact with holiness, arguably continuing aspects of the South Asian Hindu tradition of *darśan*, or "vision of the divine" (cf. Eck 1998).

MEDICINES ON A SMALL SCALE

The late afternoon sun shone into the main consultation room of the Tashilhunpo Clinic, where I was interviewing Lodrö, the clinic director. Wearing a white coat over his robes, with a shaven head and a broad smile, he was the most seasoned medical practitioner here and the only monk-

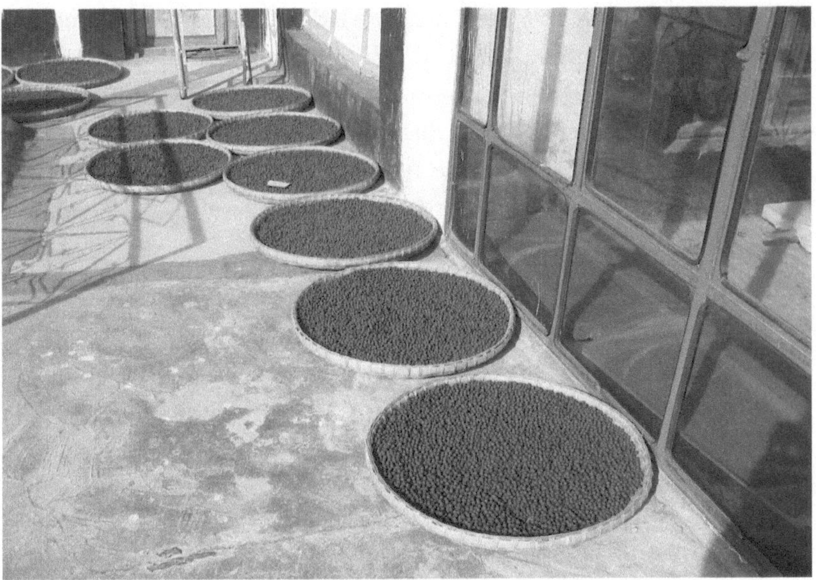

FIGURE 6.5. Medicines drying on the roofs at the Tashilhunpo Clinic. 2007. Photo by the author.

doctor who had been ordained at this monastery before the Democratic Reforms. Back then he was forced to leave, outwardly leaving the order and working as a barefoot doctor in his home region. As soon as the monastery reopened, he resumed duties as the monastery's health worker in addition to his religious commitments. In the early 1980s, with a small group of monks, he set up a tiny medical clinic in the monastery, reading patients' pulses according to Tibetan medicine and providing treatment with Western medicines and Chinese-style acupuncture. When the monks were too sick to come, Lodrö carried his old barefoot doctor medical kit to their residence, tending to them there. In 2002 the small medical clinic expanded to an impressive two-story traditional-style building. It now has thirty-five rooms located around a pleasant courtyard and is open to the public six days a week until noon, all clinic staff devoting their afternoons to the production of Tibetan medicines (figures 6.4, 6.5, and 6.6).

That sunny afternoon, as usual, the monks and other workers were still preparing and processing the raw materials for the Tibetan medical pills and powders, of which they made between thirty-five and forty types.[16] When the pharmacy's grinding machine was turned off and the lead pharmacist had presumably called it a day, other monks with their white coats now removed dropped by, eager to hear what Lodrö had to say to me. The room filled with almost all of his thirty staff members. By the time they got there, we had reached the most controversial questions. These were mainly on the future of local medical production in light of the recently introduced Good Manufacturing Practices, a set of regulations for the production of commercially sold Tibetan medicines. Lodrö responded:

> I don't really understand much about the GMP. But I am certain that our medicines are of very good quality. We have good ingredients, and the medicines are compounded carefully. It is not about what you wear and the building where you make the medicines, whether it is closed off from the outside and whether the medicines are touched or not touched with your hands. It is not at all about that. . . .
>
> Our concern with regard to GMP is mainly about cost and quality. If we were to start production [with GMP], we would need to invest ¥1 million just for the [new] building, the air conditioning, and the machines. It would make the medicines too expensive for our patients, so we don't plan to do this.
>
> In the old days we made medicines with our hands, and they worked very well. GMP is an outsider's concept that has come to Tibet. We pay so much attention to the cleaning and the process of making the medicine that I am confident to say that our medicines are very good, without GMP. We don't need GMP to make good medicines.

Lodrö's perspective on the difference in quality between medicines made according to GMP and in the "old ways" echoed views and opinions held by other Tibetans I spoke with who were involved in producing or using Tibetan medicines, at large factories or as smaller producers, providers, or consumers. There were intense controversies over the implementation of GMP and the repercussions of the large-scale industrialization of Tibetan medicine. While the application of GMP to Tibetan medicine production has raised concerns and debates over the quality and efficacy of medicines (Saxer 2012, 2013; Craig 2012), *amchi* I worked with in Tsang were particularly concerned about its impact on the affordability and accessibility now and in the future. They pointed out how the shift to GMP-regulated production, the dramatic upscaling of Tibetan medicine manufacture, and the effects on the prices of raw materials and end products would further compromise rural Tibetans' access to Tibetan medicines. How does this relate to the moral economy of Tashilhunpo Clinic and its patients, numbering annually well over 100,000, who queue up at the site six days a week?

The basic material economy of Tashilhunpo Clinic, the day-to-day costs of operations—doctors' and workers' salaries, upkeep of buildings and equipment, raw materials, and Tibetan and Western medicines—had to be covered by patients' consultation and medicine fees. The clinic received no government subsidies, and only occasionally did the monastery make in-kind or financial contributions. Larger infrastructure and human resource investments had so far been funded from external private sources. The Swiss Red Cross, for example, had paid for the education of four Tashilhunpo monks trained at Pelshung and for some of the medicine factory's equipment. The clinic building (completed in 2002) had been funded by a private sponsor from Shanghai.

Should the Tashilhunpo factory want to be certified according to GMP, the investment required would amount to more than all the combined costs from 2002 to 2007 that the monks listed for me, including expenditures associated with building and equipping the clinic and production unit, and provisions for training or staff. What had been invested in the current facilities and staff in these five years had facilitated several hundred thousand consultations, including many for economically disadvantaged patients. The total annual output of Tibetan medicines was around five tons, covering part of the treatments prescribed, others being biomedical pills, injections, and intravenous drips. The ethos of the clinic was to provide affordable health care through both Tibetan and biomedical means, and any profits were reinvested into the facilities.

Tashilhunpo's medicine production was crucial to keeping expenses for Tibetan medicines low (figure 6.6). The clinic relied on staff expertise and relatively cheap labor, thus avoiding having to buy expensive ready-made medicines from other factories. They sourced raw ingredients from local harvesters, middlemen, and abroad. Then they engaged in the laborious process of making the medicines, which in several cases had as many as twenty-five to thirty-five ingredients. Their imperative, as Lodrö and the pharmacists pointed out, was to produce high-quality medicines and to keep costs down. The introduction of GMP, so they thought, would compromise both of these values. Moreover, they believed GMP's effect

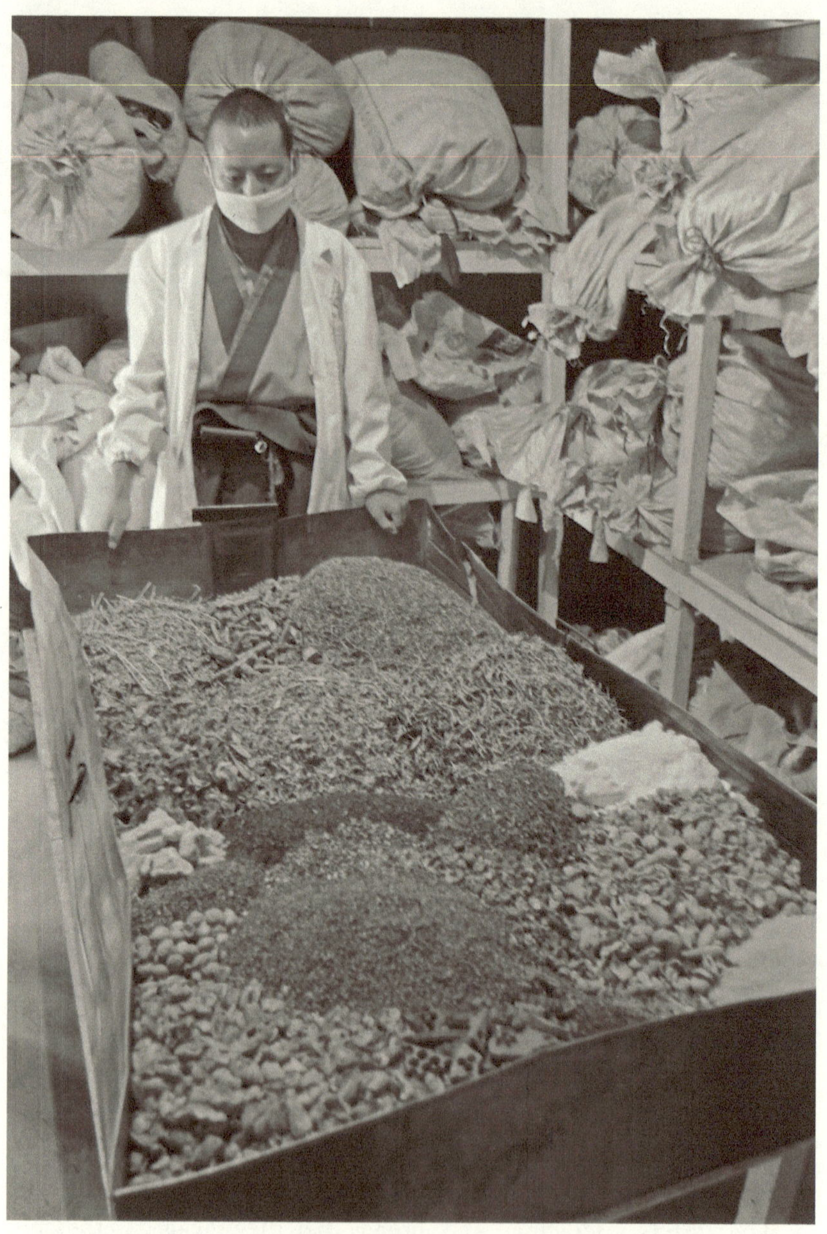

FIGURE 6.6. Medicine production at the Tashilhunpo Clinic, 2007. Photo by Meinrad Hofer.

on the quality of Tibetan medicines would decrease quality and efficacy rather than improving it. They expressed worries over carelessness in medicine production that had resulted from scaling up production and from the gap between the people who produce and those who prescribe medicines.

A medical factory attached to a large prefecture-level hospital in Ngari produced medicines for its own patients at one time. But in 2007, this facility closed as it could not comply with GMP requirements. The Tashilhunpo monks had heard about this and were worried. If GMP-certified practice was required for noncommercial factories like the Tashilhunpo Clinic, they would either have to close down production and buy medicines (inevitably raising prices for Tibetan medicines) or raise large donations or government grants to build a GMP-compliant plant and obtain the various drug registration numbers, raising enormously the costs of production and the required monitoring. That year, they had already been affected by the new laws, as they were no longer permitted to sell their medicines to independently practicing Tibetan doctors, including former colleagues from Pelshung. The clinic was not concerned, as the demand from their own clinic was large. The other Pelshung *amchi*, however, were disadvantaged by having to buy more expensive medicines from Lhasa (such as the TAR Tibetan Pharmaceutical Factory), where, unlike government-trained doctors, they were not eligible for discounts.

The Tashilhunpo Clinic's continued emphasis on and investment in training people to carry out local pharmaceutical production was another expression of a Sowa Rigpa moral economy. Their main concern was to treat those who could not easily afford medicines, thus benefiting their health and well-being. At their pharmacy, this concern was expressed in their unusually outspoken criticism of GMP and large-scale production, but also in their firmly expressed intention to keep focusing on providing good medicines for local people. While the clinic's monks sometimes spoke of how important Tibetan medicine was to helping to "preserve Tibetan culture," their discourse and medical practice made clear that they were more connected to their belief and vocation: to benefit the lives of their patients.

— · —

The sheer numbers and kinds of medical problems encountered and recounted, and the ways they have been treated by Yonten Tsering and the Tashilhunpo Clinic, show the enormous difference that affordable or free Tibetan medical services made to the poor. These *amchis*' moral economy still confronts a crisis of physical subsistence, as in the classic works on moral economies. While this is not a food crisis where barley, potatoes, or rice are lacking, it is certainly a medical crisis on the margins. Its characteristics are that economically and geographically marginal Tibetans (or, for that matter, marginal Nepalis or Ladakhis, as in Craig's and Blaikie's ethnographies from 2012 and 2013) lack access to medicines and health care that can meet their physical and mental needs to live a good-enough life, regardless of gender or income, and that enable them to work and live off their land as much as possible. The work of Yonten Tsering and the Tashilhunpo Clinic has attracted occasional funding from international donors, most likely those interested in saving Tibet or supporting the survival of a Tibetan culture they perceive as threatened by extinction, through Tibetan medicine projects, as was explicitly stated by the Swiss Red Cross. However, the emphasis of these privately practicing older *amchi* and the clinic should be interpreted primarily in terms of a moral economy, in which bodily, spiritual, and mental well-being is at stake. Here, cultural survival, if a concern at all, features only tangentially. This ethnography therefore provides an important counterpoint to framing the Tibet issue in terms of cultural survival alone, or worse still, of cultural genocide.

The accounts of Yonten Tsering and of Tashilhunpo Clinic show how *amchi* like Tsering, Lodrö, and others embody a Sowa Rigpa moral economy in their practice of Tibetan medicine, which refuses capitalist, market-based exchange standards. Instead these practitioners follow their own interpretations of the meaning and ultimate values of Tibetan medical encounters, which are deeply religious, and in some cases religious-cum-socialist.

For a study of Tibetan medicine and its role in health care on the margins, if we heed anthropologist and humanitarian physician Paul Farmer's insights for an anthropology of structural violence, we have to keep "the material in focus as a way to avoid undue romanticism in accomplishing this task" and to "give an honest account of who wins, who loses, and what weapons are used" (Farmer 2004: 307–8). "Structural violence," says

Farmer, "is embodied as adverse events if what we study, as anthropologists, is the experience of people who live in poverty or are marginalized by racism, gender inequality, or a noxious mix of all of the above." We must address in greater earnest questions pertaining to the *material* ways in which the adverse outcomes of structural violence are embodied and how people address real-world physical effects in relation to access (or lack thereof) to the most basic health care provisions.

Even if Tibetan primary care is not as desperate and unavailable as the situation in Haiti, for example, for basic health services (Farmer 2004) or in Mongolia for maternal and migrants' health services (Janes and Chluundorj 2004; Lindskog 2014), the unending, sometimes overwhelming queues of patients coming to Yonten Tsering and the Tashilhunpo Clinic comprise the ethnographically visible. Yet there is a firm link to ethnographically invisible elements: the history of forced integration into the PRC and the many violent CCP reforms and campaigns. In this book, I have attempted to bring to life some of the voices from outside the officially orchestrated silence in state narratives about these very reforms.

CONCLUSION

> It is a fact of experience which is always verified that history is made in the short term by the conquerors, who may be able to maintain it in the middle term but can under no circumstances impose it in the long term.
>
> —Reinhart Kosseleck, *Expérience de l'histoire*

TIBETAN *amchi* in rural areas of Tsang played a crucial role in facilitating the continuity of Tibetan medical practices despite often harsh and violent Communist reforms. Mao's stress on "rural areas in health work" and emphasis on self-reliance, especially during the latter part of the Cultural Revolution, created a space in which selected *amchi* and others could continue to adapt Sowa Rigpa in a changing political and economic climate. A combination of official policies and the ability of some to negotiate with those implementing revolutionary reforms and campaigns meant that Tibetan medical work continued, though in simplified form, sometimes including the teaching of Tibetan medicine to the younger generation. Paired with its subsequently recognized potential to demonstrate the government's respect for nationality culture as well as commercial profits, Tibetan medicine was swiftly revitalized, starting in the 1970s. The events and actors encountered in this book have all in their own ways shaped the current situation of Tibetan medicine. By the early years of the new millennium, Tibetan medicine became one of the most vibrant domains for the expression of Tibetan language and culture within and beyond the TAR. This is rooted in the particular trajectory of Tibetan medical *amchi*, especially their earlier revitalization of medical practice as compared to other expressions of Tibetan culture, especially Buddhism (Goldstein and Kapstein 1998) and work in the performing and fine arts (Henrion-Dourcy 2005, 2017; Tsewang Tashi 2014).

CENTERS AND MARGINS IN THE TRANSFORMATIONS OF SOWA RIGPA

A wider and deeper understanding of the trajectory of Sowa Rigpa during the communist-socialist revolution and collectivism of the Mao Zedong era, into the decollectivization, privatization, and implementation of liberal market economies after Mao, emerges from this study. It contributes to the medical and social anthropology of Tibet the theorization of so-called medical lineages in terms of Medical Houses, thus providing an analytical tool to make sense of professional and social organization, the physical structure of houses, and gender in Tsang. Going beyond central and institutional narratives and working with largely nongovernmental Tibetan medical practitioners—yet pointing out their connections to central figures and institutions—allow us to make important adjustments to accounts of the twentieth-century history of Tibetan medicine.

In the 1959–66 period, in contrast to the reforms implemented at the Mentsikhang in Lhasa, *amchi* in outlying Medical Houses, monasteries, and nunneries (constituting the majority of *amchi* in Tibet) were not visibly demonstrating their contribution to the health of the newly conceived "masses." Rather, given the ongoing wider social and economic reforms (especially the land reforms and class struggle), many *amchi* lost the economic basis as well as sociopolitical legitimacy necessary for official continuation of their medical work. The reason many *amchi* were unable to continue working in their accustomed fashion was not because of official opposition to the practices themselves, but because of official opposition to the class structures in which they were embedded. With religion seen in Marx's famous formulation as an opiate to dull people's perception of their exploitation, the work of *amchis* suffered from the connection with religion. The promotion of science and the accompanying belief that Tibetan medicine was unscientific also worked against them. Yet the new structures left an opening for those who signed onto the revolution and could use revolutionary commitment as a basis for their practice, since the practice itself was not only not prohibited but, after Mao's famous saying about the treasure house of Chinese medicine, could be legitimated as a parallel to what Mao had praised.

In the early years of the Cultural Revolution (1966 to about 1972), with few exceptions the material basis for *amchis*' work, the instruments and texts, were vigorously destroyed as belonging to the Four Olds, whether in Lhasa or in rural areas of Tsang. Depending on the class labels assigned, *amchi* were often treated harshly, in particular those who had served the Tibetan government, belonged to the higher social classes, or were monks and nuns still unwilling to be reformed. These individuals frequently served prolonged (often fatal) prison sentences or were put in "education through labor" camps. Other *amchi* were slightly more fortunate: those firmly established in Communist health posts or as cadres could in some cases continue their work, while some continued as private practitioners secretly and at great risk.

The barefoot doctor campaign and hence some of the Chinese medical techniques and recipes encapsulated in the widely disseminated *Barefoot Doctor's Manual* (first published in 1969) reached the Tibetan areas through a Sino-Tibetan bilingual edition published in March 1972. The campaign highlighted using "local resources" (especially "Chinese medicine" as well as "folk medicine"), creating a new space for Tibetan *amchis*' knowledge, medical training, and practice. The *Sino-Tibetan Herbal*, a work on botanicals and animal products growing in Tibet identified for the use in basic Chinese medicines, which had been outlined in the *Barefoot Doctor's Manual*, became a key resource for teaching Tibetan medicine. Such diversion from the official purpose makes a lot of sense, as no other classical pharmacological texts and illustrations were available and allowed. In 1975, *The Tibetan Medical Manual*, a conceptually and epistemologically Tibetan medical work, was published. The style and content of this work shows increased confidence in the wake of official relegitimization of Tibetan medicine at the time of publication. This is one of the earliest expressions of the sweeping changes in policy that ushered in the full legitimization of and efforts to revitalize Tibetan medicine over subsequent years, including a reintegration of Buddhist elements. There was, however, no way to return to the ways Tibetan medicine had been practiced, made, or classified in medical books before the Revolution. Later textbooks, and especially recent works in Tibetan medical pharmacology, still reflect the way knowledge of single and compounded Tibetan medicines was restructured, reclassified, and reinterpreted in the early 1970s.

While almost all Tibetan medical work came to an end at the Mentsikhang between 1966 and 1973–74, in the midst of the greatest contraction of Tibetan medical practice, a few doctors in a rural part of Tsang kept up their work and, in some exceptional cases, did so even within government facilities. The numbers of Tibetan *amchi* and the place of Tibetan medicine in the barefoot doctor campaign in areas like Ngamring were, however, limited. Only a few *amchi* mustered the right "class labels" or were accomplished in working the rhetoric of the regime. The situation in other Tibetan areas awaits future research, not least in Amdo, where several Socialist Realist revolutionary propaganda posters depicting male and female Tibetan barefoot doctors have emerged. In one poster, youths proudly ride horses through snow-covered Tibet, with their iconic leather medical kits worn over their *chuba*; another poster depicts a young pastoral woman as a barefoot doctor applying acupuncture on a soldier (see figures C.1 and 4.2). In Tsang, the barefoot doctors and later village health workers used fewer Tibetan remedies than biomedical drugs and diagnostic and therapeutic methods. The barefoot doctor campaign in Tibet therefore marked a key moment, for the first time spreading and firmly establishing the hegemony of biomedical injections and pills in remote rural areas. Earlier contact with British biomedical health care had been limited to people living in or traveling to larger towns. As in China proper, biomedicines have since become the dominant form of medical treatment in both rural and urban areas of Tibet, owing to a combination of cost, state subsidies, patient choice, and importantly, perceptions of modernity and efficacy among patients, doctors, and the wider society.

Most scholarship holds that a full-scale revival of Tibetan culture, Tibetan Buddhism in particular, started after 1978, following the Third Plenum of the National Party Congress in Beijing. Rulings from that gathering were fully translated into locally understandable (trustworthy) formulations and policies during and following Hu Yaobang's visit to Tibet in 1981. The revitalization of Tibetan medicine, much like that of Chinese medicine, began significantly earlier, however. Chinese state interests ensured that Tibetan medicine became a means through which the central government could convey overt respect, at the same time using these traditions for primary health care in rural areas. Yet many interest groups

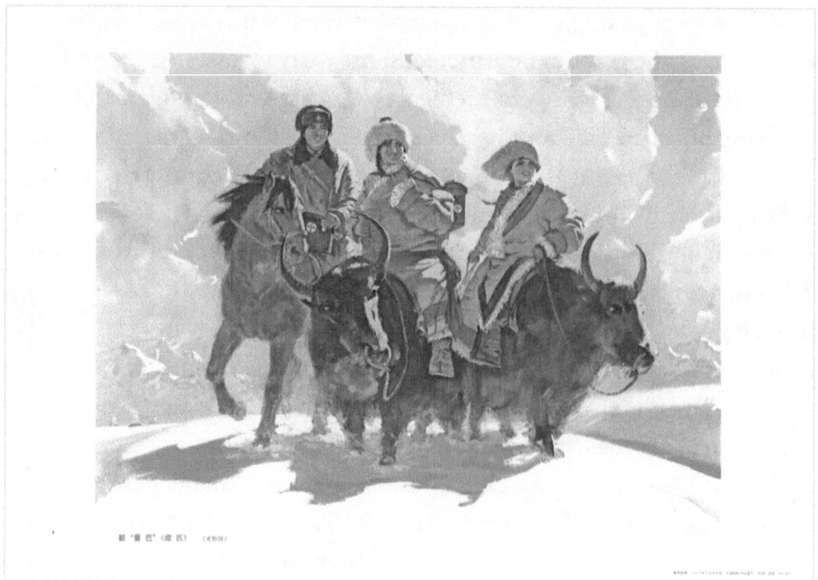

FIGURE C.1. *The New "Manba"* by artist Zhu Naizheng, early 1970s (38 × 54 cm). Courtesy of the International Institute of Social History, University of Leiden, Stefan R. Landsberger Collection, BG E15.

and approaches went beyond such political aims. During the 1990s, as the first privatizing reforms were implemented in the governmental health system, senior *amchi* in clinics and hospitals often wielded sufficient influence to negotiate concessions to keep Tibetan medicine in the government primary care plans. Private schools and clinics funded by international NGOs came on the scene. When new health care reforms, most notably the NCMS, began, many senior doctors were near retirement, and Tibetan medicine was no longer an integral part of health care for rural areas. Biomedical diagnostic and therapeutic techniques had become by far the dominant medical modality.

We have seen how a contemporary retired practitioner and a group of medicine producers continue to work within a distinct moral economy, which is primarily concerned with fostering the physical survival and well-being of poor patients via Tibetan medical treatment. This moral economy is also relevant to the industrialization and commercialization of Tibetan medicine production.

The ways Tibetan medicine is now taught—who has access and the kinds of clinical pathways that Tibetan medical graduates follow—have changed dramatically, and the socioeconomic and rural/urban makeup of Tibetan *amchi* students and practitioners is quite different. In line with a Communist egalitarian agenda, they now include many students and doctors from outside the traditional Medical Houses and monastic backgrounds. The reforms have also led to larger numbers of women *amchi* in Tibet, although there are still very few working in county hospitals and township clinics in rural Shigatse Prefecture. History is not just about the past, nor is it always about change; it may be equally about duration, about patterns persisting over long periods of time (Ortner 2006: 10–11). This holds true with regard to a continuing scarcity of female doctors in rural Tsang today.

Such differences between developments in rural and urban areas, centers and margins, point to the wider relevance of studying medicine in marginal areas and among marginal peoples. With a few exceptions (Fang 2012; Lora-Wainwright 2005), we lack studies in this regard—also for Chinese and Indian classical medicine—and for other forms of partly centralized and institutionalized cultural practices in Tibet. Recent work in the field of Tibetan medicine has begun to address this gap, including more marginal people and perspectives[1] and other aspects of Tibetan culture, such as Ache Lhamo and the performing and fine arts more widely (Henrion-Dourcy 2017; Tsewang Tashi 2014).

How, then, should we go forward in studying broader cultural transformations and continuities in Tibet involving the people at its geographical, social, and political centers and margins? Can we distill methodological implications from this study that are useful to the wider field of Tibetan and modern Chinese studies? And if so, how can these be undertaken in the increasingly limited and precarious circumstances for foreign and local researchers and people in Tibet?

ANTHROPOLOGY AND HISTORICITIES

What is considered short, middle, or long term in history from a Tibetan perspective probably differs from Chinese or European viewpoints, as expressed in the epigraph to this final chapter. By the sixth decade after the occupation of Tibet in 1950–51, I thought the long term had been reached and that the time had come to see if the official historiography was still intact and working to maintain its political purposes. At that time, I was working with Tibetan *amchi* in Tsang, with a focus on their references to and embodiment of the often-violent events of preceding years. Following analysis of my findings under the broad analytical frameworks of historicity and agency, I endeavored to make visible the *Historie* of the apparent "losers" in order to show up its fault lines with the *Geschichte* of the "winners," to paraphrase anthropologist James Scott's adaptation of "history according to winners and losers," where *Historie* is theorized as a "weapon of the weak" (1985). How does looking at the history of the losers reflect on the history of the winners?

People's references to the past pose one of the most crucial and difficult challenges to anthropologists—still insufficiently accounted for in much current work in the field (Fassin 2004: 319). Trouillot (1995) has been a forerunner and inspiration to many in the field willing to face this challenge, inspiring also my approach by embracing the study of "sociohistorical processes" and the "narrative construction about that process." At the same time, I have heeded the call of anthropologists Eric Hirsch and Charles Steward for "ethnographies of historicity" to "address the diverse modes through which people form their presents in world societies" (2005: 261). Rather than focus exclusively on the current moments of "looking at illness," the "doctor-patient relationship," or health inequity between margins and centers, as many works in medical anthropology do, I wanted these situations, events, and protagonists and their analysis to be situated within historical processes. This book attempts to meet a major challenge in anthropology through analysis of how the past, present, and future are made and remade in the everyday lives of my informants and in conversations with others and myself. It also offers a methodological and empirical contribution to modern Tibetan studies.

Much of Tibetan political history has relied on centralized government Tibetan or Chinese records, documents, memoires, oral history interviews, and accounts by those who occupied government political positions. A "history from below" (Thompson 1968) is only beginning to emerge, for instance in work on the social history of Tibet (Ramble, Schwieger, and Travers 2013). Other recent anthropological research looks beyond the limitations that elite government sources naturally pose, adding crucial dimensions to the documentation of how current sociopolitical contexts and everyday practices influence people's and institutions' relations with the past. One chapter in *Taming Tibet* by anthropologist Emily Yeh (2013), for instance, juxtaposes oral history interviews with official accounts of the creation of new farmland in and around Lhasa during the 1950s, emulating the early "agricultural model communes" in China. Charlene Makley's (2005, 2007) work on memory and the history of Maoist reforms is also exemplary and has been an inspiration. Reflecting on the work of these and other colleagues, Robert Barnett, a historian of modern Tibet, suggests that anthropologists in Tibetan studies "reclaim the field of modern Tibetan history-writing from historians, as well as claiming political analysis from political scientists, insisting on the insertion of culture into that discussion" (2010: 75).

McGranahan's (2010) work on the Khampa resistance fighters' *Historie*, researched with elderly veterans in exile, has been particularly noteworthy and inspiring for my research. She argues that in the context of exile and the Dalai Lama's advocacy of nonviolent resistance, the history of the Tibetans' violent resistance and contestation of the Chinese occupation has been to a large degree "arrested." It is now slowly emerging as an openly addressed topic. Similarly, but for different reasons, writing about the impact and reception of Communist reforms among Tibetan medical practitioners has been "hijacked," or perhaps "arrested," by central government institutions, such as the Lhasa Mentsikhang and the Dharamsala Men-Tsee-Khang. The voices of *amchi* in rural and marginal Tibetan areas, such as Ngamring and Tsang more broadly, have so far been neglected in the academic literature. Recording and reflecting on the memories and experiences of a group of people from marginal areas therefore offers a new space for thinking about the conditions under which Tibetans in central Tibet find "meaning in memory" (Kansteiner 2002)—and where and how they can express these today.

Speaking to Barnett's (2010) observations on China's oral history regime in Tibet, I found that the state was still more or less present in the encounters recorded for this book. We would have to acknowledge that we are therefore not yet beyond the conquerors' writing of history and that the ongoing vigilance of the state regarding Tibetans' engagements with each other when discussing the past is still present and influential.

TIBETAN STATES OF EMERGENCY

In March 2008 a protest by Tibetan Buddhist monks against the detention of a fellow monk and the state-police responses to that protest led to an outburst of violence from ordinary Tibetans, targeting primarily Chinese businesses in the central Barkor area of the old town of Lhasa. The several-day incident brought in its wake over 150 reported protests across the Tibetan plateau (Barnett 2009), several months of curfew and police searches in Tibetan homes in Lhasa, imprisonments, and greatly increased surveillance across the city and in Tibet at large. These trends were at first accompanied by a short-lived resurgence of critical writings, artwork, and songs by Tibetans in the PRC. In August of that same year the Olympic Games were held in Beijing, and the world's eyes fixed on how well China was doing with its human rights record, its reputation in this domain having suffered badly due to the state reaction to the Tibetan protests in March. Prior to the opening, the Olympic torch relay had encountered street protests throughout the Western world challenging China's hosting of the games, citing among other issues the violent crackdown on the Tibetan protests in March and afterward. When the Olympic flame passed through the TAR shortly before the games, there were no more protesters to contend with, as a violent state apparatus had successfully paralyzed and numbed Tibetans in the city.

In October 2008, I briefly visited Lhasa, where I experienced in and around the Barkor and much of the city a silence very different from my earlier stays and memories of the Barkor's bustling and noisy joie de vivre, characterized by Buddhist devotion mixed with shopping and socializing. Walking the *kora*, I had to step aside every fifty meters as fully uniformed soldiers with machine guns and shields patrolled the street in a counterclockwise direction, against the movement of Tibetan Buddhist worshippers and locals using the area. The roofs of most surrounding buildings held armed soldiers, and an evidently increased number of security cameras were affixed to buildings, both adding to a sense of profound unease. Since then, with few exceptions (Yeh 2013), few researchers have been able to report on events in Lhasa and elsewhere in the TAR, let alone do substantial, long-term anthropological research there. A further sad development has been that by May 2016 over 145 Tibetans had immolated themselves across the Tibetan areas of the PRC, in addition to eight in exile (see McGranahan and Litzinger 2012).

Since 2008 almost all international NGOs previously engaged in the TAR have ceased work, as they are no longer permitted to renew their contracts and agreements. One apparent exception is the Swiss Red

Cross, the only international NGO working mainly in Shigatse Prefecture. However, while working on a draft of this book, in April 2015, I was notified that even this internationally acclaimed humanitarian organization has been forced to leave, after almost thirty years of work in Tsang, after its contract was not renewed, despite the backing and close collaboration of its local partner, the Shigatse Red Cross. This trend has spread to Amdo and Kham in eastern Tibet, which had been more liberally administered. Many of the international NGOs supported rural health care and aspects of Tibetan medical practice as part of primary health care in the TAR. The ways in which national and international politics can adversely affect health care provision at a local level on the margins have been featured throughout the book. They have also been experienced firsthand, as I carried out research there, and as we can see all too clearly, they persist up to the present day.

The senior Tibetan *amchi*, Yonten Tsering, two students from his home village, and I discussed renovating the Térap Medical House and reinstalling a Tibetan medical clinic there. The two students, one a Pelshung graduate and both at that time in the last year of BA degrees from the Lhasa Tibetan Medical College, planned to learn practical skills from the elderly doctor, especially in diagnosis, external therapies, and medicine preparation. The aim was that after some months they would take full charge of the clinic, working independently from the senior doctor, their monthly income paid by small medical fees, a foreign sponsor, and donations from affluent Tibetans. The clinic would serve the immediate population of the valley (approximately two thousand people), as well as those from adjacent areas. My job was to raise the funds, in which I had succeeded by early 2010. As the renovations were about to begin and plans were made for the *amchi*'s stay in the village and the clinic and some related health outreach activities, the two students backed out of the project. This was perhaps coincidental, perhaps not. The state was discouraging Tibetans from working for the handful of international NGOs that had remained in central Tibet after the protests, and it is likely that the young doctors-in-training realized that future involvement of foreigners in Tibet was uncertain. And from all we know, they were right. This may even have been the advice of Yonten Tsering, himself a retired government employee. Whatever the reasons, after our initial disappointment, we were happy to hear that both graduates had found government positions, one in a county hospital and the other in a township clinic. This will ensure they receive a steady income, associated pay raises, and health care and social benefits.

BEGINNINGS, ENDS, AND HOPES

This latest chapter in the biography of Térap House and its medical work could be seen as contradicting an argument pertaining to local marginal *amchis*' agency. Wider pressures and concerns direct and limit the course of Tibetan medical practice. The two young doctors work instead in government clinics, no doubt relying mainly on whatever biomedical knowledge they have gained; they employ some Tibetan medical diagnosis but predominantly prescribe biomedical treatments: tablets and the famous cure-all of the *chutam*, intravenous drips with a range of antibiotics, hormones, and vitamins, popular across Tibetan areas and the PRC. No Tibetan medical pills are available there for their use, excluded as these medications are from the government insurance scheme and otherwise unaffordable for most local people. In 2014–15, however, there has been a slight shift in official policy so that some Tibetan medicines are now eligible for reimbursement via the NCMS, some even having been declared essential medicines, although the kinds and numbers vary across different provinces.

Yonten Tsering died in the summer of 2012, at age seventy-three. He did not manage to pass on his comprehensive medical knowledge and skill, even though he kept teaching Tibetan medicine modules at Shigatse Vocational Health School until shortly before his death. These classes certainly inspired an interest in further Tibetan medical studies for some but hardly provided students with the ability to apply Tibetan medical diagnostic and therapeutic skills. Yonten Tsering had written a handbook for rural doctors and health workers, and although it has yet to be published, as he kept saying, this will remain beyond his physical death. Also remaining in his Shigatse house, on the side of the altar in a statue of Chenresik, the Bodhisattva of Compassion, are the ashes from his cremation. The Medicine Buddha statue that had been the center of the altar during all the years I visited the house, however, was donated to be interred in the newly built stupa in Gye Village. Perhaps Yontan Tsering and his family thought his home village, which still lacks a clinic, is where the Medicine Buddha's powers to heal would be most in demand.

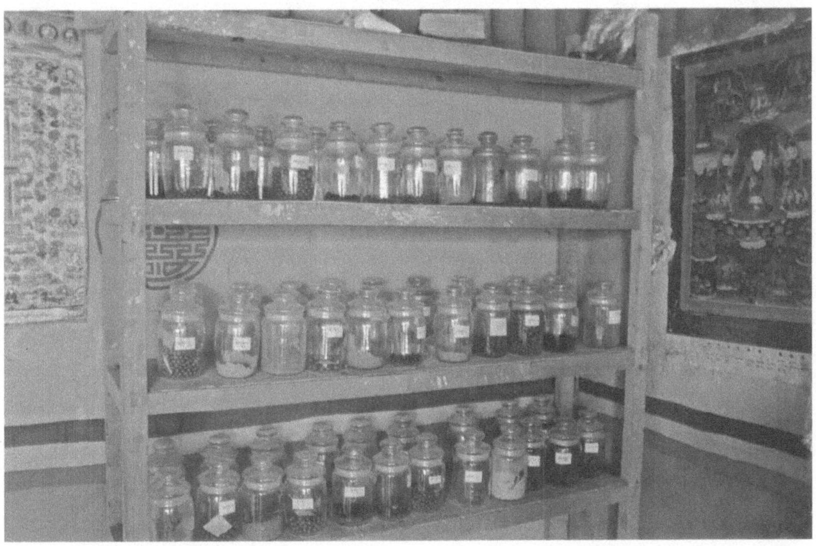

FIGURE C.2. Medicines in the home of an *amchi* in Sangsang who works in the local township clinic as well as from home, 2007. Photo by the author.

In common with earlier policies restricting Tibetan cultural expression, the restrictions that followed the March 2008 events will fail to completely determine how Tibetans provide health care of one kind or another, or how they are able to otherwise express their agency and obtain health care. The last I heard from Tashilhunpo Clinic was that they were still making Tibetan medicines, in a practice that runs parallel to GMP-accorded factories and that is now understood by Tibetans to fall within a PRC-wide law that regulates the so-called medicine preparation houses (C. *yiyuan zhiji shi*)—that is, the on-site production of medicines that are sold only by the associated doctors and not marketed elsewhere. Moreover, even large commercial factories have returned medical production for their noncommercially used medicines to the older, non-GMP-compliant buildings as the costs of production there are much lower (Saxer 2013).

Several Pelshung graduates have since earned the Tibetan Medical College's *kachupa* degree, thereby legitimizing their medical work. Jampa Trinlé, the highly respected retired director of the Mentsikhang, has also died. His many writings, especially the biographical *Recollections*, are now important sources for rethinking both the trajectory of the Lhasa Menstikhang as well as the writing of biographies and life writing on and by leading Tibetan government cadres (cf. Henrion-Dourcy 2013; Hofer 2013).

A knowledgeable *amchi* in his fifties resides in the township where one of Yonten Tsering's students, Tashi Tsering, now works. He makes his own medicines and practices Sowa Rigpa at home (figure C.2), his main employment being as a biomedical township clinic health worker. I am curious to see whether Tashi Tsering will take up study with the older *amchi*, to benefit from his skills. Will this doctor's expertise die with him, or live on—who knows—in some of the future work of the new township doctor?

How much I will continue to hear of that young doctor's future work and life remains to be seen. The many political changes over the past years have had profound effects on previously active and fruitful research collaborations of European and US universities with Tibetan institutions. It is yet unknown and will perhaps remain unknowable whether I or others will be allowed to return to rural Tsang, to have the chance to again spend extended periods of time with the practitioners and their associates who helped me learn and convey the substance of this book. Yet one thing is certain. As long as Yeshe Lhamo, Yontan Tsering's wife, is physically able to, she will go on her morning *kora* around Tashilhunpo Monastery, take a break in a local teahouse, and then do a second *kora* before heading home by midday.

NOTES

NOTE ON TERMINOLOGY AND ROMANIZATION

1 David Germano and Nicolas Tounadre, "THL's Simplified Phonetic Transcription of Standard Tibetan," Tibet and Himalayan Library, 2003, www.thlib.org/reference/transliteration/#essay=/thl/phonetics.

INTRODUCTION

1 *Amchi*, originally a Mongolian term for doctor, is used frequently, along with *menpa*, in contemporary Tibet. *Amchi* and *menpa* denote both medical and biomedical doctors. Although a division in clinical practice between Tibetan medicine and biomedicine can no longer be upheld, for clarity's sake I use *amchi* only for those mainly trained as Tibetan medical doctors, except in chapter 4.

2 Many Tibetans consider Ü-Tsang, together with Kham and Amdo (in far eastern Tibet), as the three parts of pre-1950s Tibet. Yet, the sociocultural and political diversity and internal divisions of this region make this a difficult proposition. For clarification, see Note on Terminology and Romanization.

3 For an in-depth analysis of the terms *Sowa Rigpa* and *Tibetan medicine* in the academic literature to date, see Craig and Gerke (2016).

4 On the humors in classical and contemporary Indian, Chinese, and Greco-Arabic medicine in South Asia, see Van Alphen and Aris (1995), Attewell (2007), and Langford (2002).

5 For example, the *Blue Beryl* and the *Supplement* by Desi Sangyé Gyatso and the *Transmission of the Elders* by Zurkar Lodrö Gyelpo.

6 Parfionovitch, Dorje, and Meyer 1992; Trinlé and Lei 1988; Gyatso 2015.

7 For a full review, see Hofer (2011d), chapter 4.

8 Cf. Mullaney 2010.

9 For example, Millard writes that after 1955 "the following decades presented great challenges" (2013: 365). Similarly, Soktsang and Millard summarize Janes (1995): "Although in the early period of Chinese rule Tibetan medicine had been supported

by the Chinese government, with the beginning of the Cultural Revolution in 1966 Tibetan medicine went into serious decline and was virtually non-existent by the mid-1970s" (Soktsang and Millard 2013: 3). Schrempf (2007), describing the transmission of medical knowledge among Bonpo practitioners in Nagchu, includes little information on the impact of the Maoist reforms on the group of practitioners with whom she worked.

10 Chatterjee 1993; Dirks 1996; Duara 1995; Prakash 1990; Spivak 1988.

11 Fjeld 2006; Jinba 2013; McGranahan 2010; Naktsang 2014; Roche 2017.

12 This research has resulted in a number of publications where the methods are discussed in more detail (Hofer 2012).

13 David Germano, discussant response on the panel "Applied Scholarship in Tibet" at the 12th International Association for Tibetan Studies Seminar, Vancouver, August 2010.

CHAPTER 1

1 Craig 2007, 2012; Garrett 2014; Hofer 2012; Schrempf 2007.

2 Attewell 2006, 2007; Barth 1990; Hsu 1999; Scheid 2007.

3 Hofer 2012: 21–25; Trinlé 2000; Kelsang Trinlé 1997; Rechung 1973; Sangyé Gyatso ([1703] 1994; 2010).

4 Aziz 1978; Childs 2004; Diemberger 1993; Levine 1981, 1988.

5 There are two Tibetan spellings: *sman grong*, meaning "Medical House" or "hamlet of doctors," and *sman 'khrungs*, "being born into medicine." In this context they mean more or less the same, but given the wider use of the Tibetan term *trong* (*grong*) for households with a corporate character in the Tibet kinship literature (Aziz 1978; Levine 1988) and how this term is spelled in Tibetan medical literature (for instance, the "Sakya Mentrong," Hofer 2012: 74), the first spelling, *sman grong*, and its meaning of "household of doctors" are more relevant here.

6 See Hofer 2012.

7 Parfionovich, Dorje, and Meyer 1992: 156.

8 *A mchi rgyud chad pa red*

9 Yonten Tsering's brother married outside as a *magpa*, one of his older sisters was ordained as a Buddhist nun at Jonang nunnery in the early 1950s, and another married into another taxpayer household of the village.

10 Khang dkar po (Khang Karpo).

11 None of the four thus ranked households in Gye was polyandrous, as was often the case among *trelpa* in other parts of Tsang, for instance Panam (Fjeld 2006).

12 As a so-called *grong sgags dmag mi*.

13 Taube 1981. The Gongmen continued the medical work of the nearby Sakya Medical House (Sakya Mentrong), where successive members of the Drangti medical family had played a major role up to the fifteenth century.

14 It was quite common for Buddhist monks who worked as physicians to create or propagate a lay Medical House, as in the case of Dramang Lharje, father to doctor Derge Purpa Dolma (Hofer 2015).

15 Whether members of other Medical Houses were students at the Lhünding Mentrong when the Fifth Dalai Lama sent financial allowances to Lhünding Dutsi

Gyurme and his students (Hofer 2012: 108), we cannot ascertain from current records or living memory.

16 For example, in the *Menghe* medical currents in Jiangsu and Shanghai (Scheid 2007) and at Medical Houses in contemporary Xin'an, Anhui Province, discussed by Hsu (2010).

17 Hsu 1998; Mueggler 2001; Wellens 2010.

18 I follow the US conventions here, taking the ground floor as the first floor.

19 See Carrasco 1959; Fjeld 2005; Goldstein 1989; Petech 1973; Childs 2004.

20 In Ngamring, although all land technically belonged to the Dalai Lama and the Lhasa Tibetan government, this was locally administered by monastic estates, such as Drepung, the Panchen Lama's Labrang, as well as other local, usually larger monasteries, or nobility from whom the *trelpa* families rented their land and to whose local administrators, or *ponpo*, they paid their taxes.

21 *Chos mdzad khyim tshang*

22 This tripartite social division also crops up in the history of Ngamring's main Gelugpa Ngamring Monastery, Ngamring Choede (Sherab Dorjé 1994).

23 When members of households of these three ranks entered monastic institutions, they made a substantial donation of money or goods to the monastery (for example, tea offerings to the assembly), and subsequently were spared from manual labor within the monastery, allowing them to concentrate solely on their religious studies.

24 On these groups in Tsang, see Fjeld (2008). An occurrence during Kim Gutschow's fieldwork in Ladakh is also interesting: she reports that some *amchi*, to keep the potency of medicines intact, kept their medicines away from "death pollution," that is, a place where someone was dying (Gutschow 2011: 202).

25 For details of the exact titles and authors, see Hofer (2011d: 357).

26 For digital copies of some works in this collection, see the Tibetan Buddhist Resource Centre website, under catalog numbers W4CZ20860–W4CZ20873. For images of selected manuscripts, see Hofer (2014a: 86, 181, 182, 185, 193).

27 Gongmen Konchog Pandar (Gong sman dkon mchog phan dar) n.d. In this work we also find details on surgical techniques and practices that he was famous for; see Arya (2014: 85–86).

28 A detailed study of these medical collections would enable a better appraisal of how conditions were diagnosed and treated, what recipes were like, and the differences among Medical Houses and traditions. It would also allow us to make some judicious remarks on the scope of medicine, in particular, its intersections with Buddhism at a time when this relationship had not been troubled through the socialist materialist logic promoted by the Chinese Communist Party (CCP) in Tibet. On earlier debates over the role and place of Buddhism within medicine, see Gyatso (2015).

29 There are only few studies of the work of private *amchi* outside of Lhasa during the 1940s and 1950s. Snellgrove and Richardson (1968: 262) hold that although healing did not play such an important role in Tibetan Buddhism as in Christianity, one was just as likely to find a layman or a monk medical practitioner. They write that in villages and the countryside, there were "no medical practitioners available," and "for most illnesses Tibetans put more faith in prayers, charms and amulets, than in medicine." This representation is filtered through the common

layer of British colonial perceptions of Tibet in the sphere of medicine and health care, most explicitly expressed in the memoires by a British Indian Indian Medical Services surgeon who served in Lhasa in the 1930s (Morgan 2007; cf. McKay 2007; and Hofer 2011d). Fosco Maraini, photographer on one of Guiseppe Tucci's expeditions, reported that a physician in Gyantse "wears the hat of a scientist with a large gold frieze and turquoises." Note in his caption to a b/w print and negative in Series T.37, No 2012, Archival Number: FFM99N551, Marini Photographic Collection, Gabinetto Scientifico Letterario G. P. Vieusseux, Palazzo Strozzi, Florence, Italy. A print of this photo can be found in Maraini (1952: plate 22).

Cassinelli and Ekvall (1969) report that at Sakya there were "at least three families of hereditary medical practitioners," one of which provided the "official" doctors for the K'ön (Akhon) family (324). They had clinic-like establishments where people went to get "purgatives, febrifuges and remedies for headaches and indigestion, to be bled, to have sores lanced and wounds cauterized, and to have broken bones set." The practitioners received payments for their services and gifts upon the recovery of their patients. They had the status of *Jo Lags*, "thus being recognized as performing government function." In Tibetan there are more accounts, also of the practical work, of five generations of the Dopta and Surkhang *amchi* (Amchi Tashi Namgyal 1999) and of the Khankar medical tradition in Kyirong (Norbu Chöphel and Tashi Tsering 2008).

30 *Chos sman gnyis 'brel*

31 The title of the manuscript is *Man ngag gyud 'bum dkar las byis pa dang mo nad gso ba'i sdeb bzhugs so.*

32 For a historic photograph of an *amchi* reading a patient's pulse, foregrounded by his medical bag and instruments on a low table, see Hofer (2014d: 60).

CHAPTER 2

1 The ten sciences comprised five major sciences (the inner science, *nang rikpa*; epistemology and logic, *tentsik rikpa*; grammar, *tra rikpa*; medicine, *sowa rigpa*; and the arts and crafts, *zorikpa*) in addition to the five minor sciences of poetry (*nyenag*), astrology (*tsi*), lexicography (*debjor*), the performing arts (*dögar*), and language (*ngöndzö*) (see Seyfort Ruegg 1995).

2 Bell 1925; Goldstein 1989; Kapstein 2006; McKay 2003; Shakabpa 1967; Shakabpa and Mahler 2009.

3 *Byis pa nyer spyod*

4 Studies of smallpox eradication in India reveal a complex mixture of decision making, unequal power relations and diverging understandings of success and acceptance of the vaccines by local people, as well as considerable local resistance (cf. McKay 2007: 134–42; Bhattacharya 2005). It is difficult to judge Cassinelli and Ekvall's assessment that the campaign met no resistance without knowing more about its reception. Smallpox was a disease that at least some Tibetan doctors are reported to have known how to cure, including the members of the Tsarong medical lineage, who had close historical ties with the Sakya medical establishment (Trinlé 2000: 255–65; Sangyé Gyatso [1703] 2010). One cannot, therefore, assume that there was no precursor to Western medical vaccines for dealing with the disease;

moreover, at least practitioners and recipients would receive the new methods used in the Sakya area.

5 Such surveys were carried out in many places in China, either during the Republican period or in the 1950s by the Communists; see Fang (2012: 21–23).

6 I interviewed them in 2003 during a two-day political meeting and followed up on these initial conversations with personal visits to many of their monasteries.

7 *Kun rtags gdon kyi nad*

8 *Gzhan dbang sngon gyi nad*

9 *Yongs grub tshe gi nad*

10 *Lhar snang phral kyi nad*

11 *Gdon*. These illnesses are dealt with in chapters 79–81 of the third volume of the *Four Treatises* and feature prominently in Tibetan medical pediatrics; see Jäger (1999).

12 These were Shershig (Sher shig dgon pa), Yartsen (Yar tzen dgon pa), Yülngön (Yul ngon dgon pa), and Ombo ('Om bo dgon pa).

13 Dpal ldan tshul khrims rin po che (1904–1972).

14 Thanks to Khyungtrul Rinpoche's initiative, Bonpo texts, including medical texts, were reprinted in the 1950s using modern printing techniques in India (Kvaerne 1998) and brought back to Tibet as part of a brief revival of Bon and Bonpo medical scholarship in northern and western Tibet (Millard 2013).

15 I would like to thank Ravenna Michalsen for sharing her translation of this biography and her unpublished MA thesis with me.

16 Skye med Rin po che

17 In 2007 one *dotsé* (*rdo tshad*) equaled ¥2.5, bringing the cost of one *rinchen rilbu* to about ¥250 in today's money.

18 A brief reference in the biography of the Lhasa-based physician Tenzin Chödrak (1924–2001) mentions that he met Ani Ngawang at the Mentsikhang after the end of the Cultural Revolution in the 1970s, having heard that she knew how to make *tsotel*. He and Khenpo Troru Tsenam tried to purify mercury for the first time after the reforms in Kongpo and were looking for instructions. Interestingly, no details are given on whether she gave him instructions. See Gerke 2015a.

19 On ideas about differential merit gained from offerings to Tibetan Buddhist monks and nuns in Ladakh, see Gutschow (2004) and in Tibet, see Schneider (2013).

20 This was the *Sman sbyor gyi nus pa phyogs bsdus phan bde'i legs bśad*, printed at the Mentsikhang in Lhasa in 1949.

21 This was also the case with the Bon lama and doctor Khyungtrul, who taught medicine to several nuns unrelated to him, including an elderly nun still resident at Gurgyam Monastery in western Tibet in 2009 (personal communication with Colin Millard in June, 2011; and Millard 2013: 13).

22 The Mentsikhang's eye surgery division was then run by two male physicians, while the number of cataract surgeries carried out by the biomedically trained Chinese eye surgeons at People's Hospital #1 in Lhasa increased dramatically.

23 For a history of Ngamring Chöde, see Sherab Dorjé (1994). Dowman gives a figure of four thousand monks, immediately before the start of reforms in the early 1960s (1988: 273).

24 On earlier activities and references to medical work at Tashilhunpo, see Carnahan and Rinpoche (1995: 38, 80–82), Gerke (2015b), Hofer (2012), Markham (1876), Turner (1800 [2006]), and Tsarong (2000: 87–88).

25 Skyid skyid nad ka

26 The full name of the school was Menlop Shi(ga)tse Dralhün Kyinak Drangsong Déling Menkhang (Sman slob gzhis rtze bgra lhun skyid nags drang srong bde gling sman khang) (Trinlé 2000: 557).

27 Lamenpa Kewang Solpön Dawa (Blas man Mkhan dbang gsol dpon zla ba), Tashilhunpo Dharpa Khamtsen's monk Kachen Lobsang Tashi (Dka' chen blo bzang bkra shis, a fifth-rank official) and Taygon Chakpo Khamchen's Trung Penpa are named personal physicians to the Ninth Panchen Lama, Thubten Chökyi Nyima (Thub bstan chos kyi nyi ma, 1883–1937; Trinlé 2000: 558). These doctors might also be mentioned in the autobiography of the Ninth Panchen Lama (Lobsang Tupten Chökyi Nyima 1944), but I was not able to obtain a copy. See Jagou 2011. All three teachers were also remembered by the graduates of Kikinaka whom I interviewed.

28 Interestingly, the majority of students had already left in 1958, well before the March 1959 uprising in Lhasa and the subsequent start of Democratic Reforms. One reason might have been rising tensions between the Tenth Panchen Lama and the Communist administration as the former gave refuge to several monks from his home region, Amdo, where attacks on religion had already started. There was no reduction in the number of monks in central Tibet in the 1950s; the loss of economic support for monastic landholdings would start in 1960–61 with the second stage of Democratic Reforms and other campaigns. Perhaps by 1958 there were increased local counterrevolutionary incidences and the closure was a preemptive measure to minimize opposition to the Communist presence in Shigatse.

29 "After Chakpori was established, the Regent declared that every main monastery would henceforth have a lama-doctor from there. This marked the beginning of 'public health' in Tibet" (Clifford 1994: 61).

CHAPTER 3

1 Goldstein 1997, 2007, 2013; Shakya 1999; Shakabpa 1967; Shakabpa and Mahler 2009; Smith 1996; Yeh 2013.

2 These autobiographies were partly ghostwritten and have been translated into several languages. On Tenzin Chödrak's biographies in the context of mercury purification, see Gerke (2015b).

3 Epa Sonam Rinchen 2009; Pasang Yonten 1987. For a fuller review of these often conflicting views, see Hofer (2011d: 101–35).

4 Makley's informants referred to these in Tibetan as *sdug ngal bshad pa/dran pa*.

5 See also Su Wenming (1983) and Chang Wei (1978).

6 See Strong (1959) for photographs of Chinese medical workers tending to those wounded by rebels during the March 1959 uprising. See also Epstein (1983) and Han (1977).

7 *sngon ma*

8 *gral rim gyi 'thab rtsod*

9 *gzhon nu gsang ba'i rkrig 'dzuks*

10 *bco brgyad drug bcu*

11 *lo rgyus kyu gnya' gnon shu zhog ki bdak po*

12 *lo rgyus sha mo*

13 *mi ngan sha mo*

14 The Tibetan term *mangtso* (the people) was coined by Tibetan translators in the 1950s to replace earlier terms such as *miser* (commoners, subjects) in an effort to render into Tibetan the Chinese term *ren min*, meaning "common folk," equivalent to the German *Volk* (Willock 2010).

15 *nang chen po*

CHAPTER 4

1 Contrary to widespread official claims (China Tibet Information Centre 2005; Epstein 1983: 386–400; Hsi and Kao 1977) and the situation in eastern Tibet (Weiner 2012: 200–209), there were no concerted CCP efforts during the 1950s to establish a permanent health care infrastructure in villages or nomadic areas of central Tibet. Communist medical activities remained largely restricted to Lhasa and prefectural capitals. When Communist cadres arrived in the villages in 1959–60, they did not regularly bring with them medical personnel or set up government clinics. Ngamring's first biomedical health post was established in the county seat in 1961, employing one Han doctor and two Tibetan health workers, and only occasionally treating Tibetans in nearby villages.

2 Fang 2012; Taylor 2005; Scheid 2002, 2007.

3 The ingredients listed for this medicine were various kinds of *gzi*, *pu shel*, *mrgta*, turquoise, and corals, which were donated to the Mentsikhang. In addition, three doctors went out to collect other ingredients, including "seven-rebirth flesh, the *ststsha* of the lords of the three families, *sbra tshal* and white mustard of *rgyal ba gya' bzang pa* and *chos rgyal bya pa*, as well as brain pills of *rgyal ba klong chen pa* (Trinlé 2006: 32).

4 The Norbulinka was renamed the People's Park, and Chakpori Hill became Victory Peak. On the Cultural Revolution in Lhasa, see Goldstein, Jiao, and Lhundrup 2009; Woeser 2006; Tubten Khétsun 2009; Barnett 2006.

5 *Sbyor med rig gnas gsar brched chen po*

6 It is rare that Tibetan writers describe their hardships in officially published works in the PRC. There is still pressure to present almost everything as uniformly better in the new society. The Cultural Revolution is a rare exception, the only period of modern Tibetan (or Chinese) history for which official concessions have been made to the CCP's otherwise tight censorship. This also varies between regions and over time, however, and has to be understood in the context of post-Mao official explanations for the Cultural Revolution. The official line is that the many acts of destruction and attacks on learning, religion, and culture were misguided, the actions of "ultra-leftists" for which the Gang of Four was duly sentenced and punished in 1981 (Barnett 2009: 9–10). The subsequent leadership apologized to the nation and to the Tibetans specifically in 1980 (Wang Yao 1996). According to Barnett, "Followers of this view speak as if a new Party and next Chinese government emerged in 1979 or 1980, with no responsibility for the previous era" (2006: 9–10).

7 Note that this marked the second time since the Communist takeover that the Tibetan medicine paintings were saved just as they were about to be destroyed,

most likely in both cases due to the favorable connections Jampa Trinlé had with leading CCP officials.

8 For another account of the June 7 massacre, see Goldstein, Jiao, and Lhundrup (2009: 45–58).

9 Tubten Khétsun 2009; Pema Konchok 2002; Goldstein, Jiao, and Lhundrup 2009; Woeser 2006; and others.

10 For comparison see Fjeld (2006: 74–77) and Ben Jiao (2001) for details in Panam.

11 Ngawang Dorjé was one of the *bumrampa* graduates from Tashilhunpo's Kikinaka Medical School, having been sent there from the local Samdrub Ganden Monastery. He had to leave the order in the early 1960s.

12 In his words, a *zing cha chen po*. This uprising is discussed in oral history accounts in Goldstein, Jiao, and Lhundren (2009: 172–82). On the Cultural Revolution in nearby Phala, also see Goldstein and Beal (1990).

13 This is not to be confused with 西医, or *xi yi* in Pinyin, meaning "Western medicine." Yet these two terms for biomedicine sound very similar.

14 See, for example, Yeh (2013: 60–91) for model agricultural communities that were emulated in the vicinity of Lhasa.

15 There were two main versions of *The Barefoot Doctor's Manual* in China, one for southern and one for northern parts of the country. These were updated over the years, complemented by regional additions and translations, as well as journals and magazines for barefoot doctors (see Fang 2012: 58–60).

16 Sidel 1972; Sidel and Sidel 1973; Chang 1978.

17 Konchok 2002: 48–50; Shakya 1999: 316–17; Pema Bhum 2001.

18 The preface acknowledges collaboration with the Institute of Botany of the Chinese Academy of Science and the Pharmacy Research Institute of the Academy of Chinese Medicine (RCTARHB 1973a, 1973b: 3). This makes it plausible that the editors continued or even reedited the work that Jampa Trinlé and his Mentsikhang colleagues had carried out prior to their demise in 1966, in preparation for the *First Study on Tibetan Medicine and Medical Materials* (1965). For this work they collaborated with Shao Wanggan of the Institute of Botany at the Beijing Academy, as well as one Chinese and three Western medical doctors from the Lhasa People's Hospital (Trinlé 2006: 35). Janes also refers to several United Front collaborations in the 1950s in the field of pharmacology, but without further details (1995: 16).

19 I found a copy of the Chinese edition in Lhasa through a book dealer, but not in Ngamring or in *amchis*' homes.

20 The full title in Tibetan is *Bod ljong rgyun spyo krung dbyi'i sman rigs*. Tibetan for Chinese is here spelled *krung dbyi*.

21 *sman rigs*

22 On the genre of illustrated Tibetan materia medica works, see Hofer (2014c).

23 For a discussion on Tibetan terms and classification of medical simples, or *trungpe*, see Hofer (2014b and 2014c).

24 *Gso rig dang sman rigs*

25 *Krung go'i gso rig dang sman rigs ni rlabs chen gi nor mdzod cig yin pas 'bad brtson chen pos sngog 'don byas te yar rgyas gtong dgos.* Literal translation: "The Chinese science of healing and pharmaceuticals is a marvelous treasury, so work hard to explore and develop it further." I follow the standard translation from Chinese, but add "pharmaceuticals" to highlight the new focus on material dimensions:

"Chinese medicine and pharmaceuticals are a great treasure house, they should be diligently explored and developed."

26 Liu Shaoqi had been a key figure during the early Cultural Revolution. He wanted to restrain the students and masses and retain a greater degree of government control in exposing counterrevolutionaries. He was later exposed as a "capitalist roader" and became one of the many official enemies and targets of the revolution. For details, see Dittmer (1998).

27 *Rang bzhin*: hot, cold, warming, and cooling.

28 *ro lnga*: sour, bitter, sweet, pungent, and salty.

29 *ro ba*

30 *phan nus*

31 *'gos nad*

32 *gnod 'bu*

33 *Srin 'bu*. These are my translations from Tibetan into English, including "contagious," "viruses," and "bacteria," all of which came up with a bilingual Tibetan/Chinese speaker looking at the same sections of the work in the Chinese version (1973b).

34 The concept of *chuser* in Tibetan medical works is otherwise intimately linked to this system's conception of the body's distilling and digesting of food and its transformation into the seven bodily constituents, where *chuser* is one of the waste products.

35 On the dire consequences of using and accessing Tibetan works, see Pema Bhum (2001).

36 This work was widely used among exiled Tibetan doctors into the 1990s (personal communications with Pasang Yonten, July 2014, and Barbara Gerke, September 2014). The copies of the work routinely circulating there had the introductory pages with Mao's quotations ripped out. The prime role of *The Sino-Tibetan Herbal* was rivaled only in 1995, when Gawo Dorjé's seminal work on Tibetan materia medica (1995), published in Beijing, was distributed in India. This work again used the Tibetan medical term *trungpé* for "simple" but no longer made any references to Mao.

37 *cha shas*

38 *snying bcud*

39 *phyi phyogs*

40 *bod gso rig*

41 *'phrod bsten gsar brje*

42 *rang mgo rang*

43 *rnying gtor bcud len*

44 *gna' bzang deng spyod, phyi bzang krung spyod*

45 *Sngo sbyor*. This most likely refers to the work *Sman sbyor bdud rtsi's thig le*. For recent reprints in India, see Tashigang (1974: 125–200) and, in China, see Ju Mipham (2006: 357–79).

46 *rang bzhin*

47 The *Nyer mkho'i sman sbyor 'chi med bdud rtsi'i bum bzang* by Mkhyen rab nor bu (Khyenrap Norbu 1995) and the *Sman sbyor gyi nus pa phyogs bsdus phan bde'i legs bshad* (largely the work) of Khyenrap Norbu.

48 Men-Tsee-Khang 2008, 2011.

49 *A gar go snyon*, Cinchona sp.

50 Even the Buddhist scholar Ju Mipham Namgyal Gyatso's nineteenth-century instructions on compounding medicines (Ju Mipham 2006) on average use more ingredients. This work is seen in medical circles as a collection of uniquely simplified medical compounds. It is this work that the introduction probably refers to as a source.

51 China Tibet Information Centre 2005; Epstein 1983: 386–400; Hsi and Kao 1977.

52 This mention of "no details" was probably Trinlé's veiled way of saying that whatever was considered "religious" and "superstitious" needed to be left out.

53 Ngawang Chödrak was rehabilitated from his "crimes" and rejoined the Mentsikhang in 1980 but passed away the following year (Trinlé 2000: 456–57).

54 We lack, however, a year of publication or the publisher, and so far I have not seen a copy of this work. This work was studied as a substitute for the *Four Treatises* by the rural Amchi Pema in Ruthog, alongside a republished work by Kongtrul Yonten Gyatso (1976).

55 Trinlé 2000, 2004. Others, for example, were in Namling, Ali, and Gyantse.

56 For these early years we have no separate records for western and Tibetan medical treatments, but combined, the hospital is reported to have carried out between 1974 and 1992 a total of 125,038 treatments, for an average of over 10,000 patients per year.

57 The document notes that between 1974 and 1988 staff of the Ngamring's People's Hospital collected 21,858 half-kilos (*kjama*) of dried plants.

58 Especially from the early 1980s, these included the *rinchen rilbu*, which were never made at the county hospital due to the great expense.

59 *mo rigs bya gzhag*

60 The Tibetan medical revolutionary pharmacological project requires further study and should include other sources, such as a three-volume pharmacopeia from Qinghai on Tibetan plants, published in Chinese: Qinghai Sheng sheng wu yan jiu suo, *The Clear Mirror of Materia Medica on the Plateau of Ching-hai and Tibet* (Qing Zang gao yuan yao wu tu jian), 2 vols. (Sining: Qinghai ren min chu ban she, 1975–78).

61 Cf. Lora-Wainwright 2005.

CHAPTER 5

1 Goldstein 1997; Goldstein and Kapstein 1998; Wang Yao 1994: 287–88.

2 Trinlé 2004, 2006; Chen Hua 2008.

3 Chinese Minority Medicine Committee Secretary 2007; Huang 2007.

4 On Tibetans leading the revival and renovation of Buddhist monasteries in Tsang, see Diemberger (2010).

5 Goldstein, Jiao, and Lhundrup (2009) hold that this was simply local factional fighting and not "protests."

6 In Panam, for example, a household received an average of 2.4 *mu* of farmland per person for administration and cultivation (Fjeld 2006: 85–89).

7 *Gdung rgyud shul 'dzin*

8 *Zhing pa 'bring pa*

9 *Nga dag'i dug rtsa*

10 Cf. Pema Bhum 2001.

11 *Tang gyi rgyud bzhi*

12 His dates are 1813–1899/1900.

13 The introduction to this reprint acknowledges by name classical sources (*gzhung lugs*) such as the *Four Treatises* as a basis for the reprint.

14 Some of these had been restored to the family. They regained the wooden materia medica box (which was empty) and the medical bags from fellow villagers, as well as some preserved Indian materia medica, all of which were installed in the altar room of the house.

15 For a more complete account of the Ruthog *amchi*'s work and history, see Hofer (2012), and on the family's medical compounding, Hofer (2011d).

16 *sger gyi A mchi*

17 This was similar to the situation of the famous *amchi* and Rinpoche Tenzin Wangdrak of western Tibet; Trinlé 2000: 554–56; Millard 2013.

18 Spel gzhung slob gra

19 Given that the TDF was partly financed by the United Front Work Department, it might be better characterized as a nonparty, charity, or welfare organization rather than nongovernmental.

20 For a documentary film on early SRC work in Shigatse, see Neuenschwander (1989).

21 After supporting the training of seven hundred health workers, this project was discontinued in 2003. There had been long-standing discrepancies between the approaches of the SRC and the local Health Bureau to rural primary health care provision and promotion, especially regarding the use of essential drugs (see Hofer 2011a). Subsequently, SRC activities shifted toward preventive rather than curative measures. To this end, a new collaboration began with the Tibetan Women's Federation.

The SRC also steered away from the rural health care system, moving toward a community-oriented strategy, including health promotion, the prevention of the spread of sexually transmitted diseases (STDs), and the building of green houses and distribution of solar water heaters. Only the cataract eye surgery camps remained as a curative project.

22 Personal communication with Frances Howland and Phillipe Dufourg, August 2003, and personal observations in October 2002, August 2003, and throughout 2006–7.

23 The *Lus thig zla ba nor bu'i me long* by Zurkar Nyamnyi Dorjé.

24 See Khyenrap Norbu 1995.

25 Moxibustion, bloodletting, cupping, and golden needle treatment.

26 In fact, some have never replenished their stocks of medicines since graduating. Similar problems are faced by graduates of the Kailash Medical Project school; personal communication with its director, Lhasa, November 2006.

27 Meyer 1998: 11.

28 Heimsath 2003: 3–5.

29 Three out of the twenty-one graduates from the first intake whom I interviewed in 2006 worked in a governmental clinic, as well as nine of the twenty-eight graduates from the second cohort whom I interviewed in 2007 (see Hofer 2007a, 2007b).

30 Shigatse Vocational Health School provides a three-year health worker training course. It includes only few Tibetan medical modules, which are insufficient to qualify anyone to practice Tibetan medicine.

31 Swiss Red Cross 2005. Note that this reflects one individual's opinion about the

reasons for the closure of the school, and not those of SRC, its International Cooperation Department, or subsequent SRC delegates to Tibet.

32 This document is based on senior doctors' accounts, official statistics, and Health Bureau and policy documents. The text thus sheds light on how doctors negotiated and organized their work in relation to wider local, regional, and national demands highlighted here. In contrast to Jampa Trinlé (2004) and to some extent Janes (1995, 2002), who emphasize the role of the central Mentsikhang-related medical bureaucracy, the *Short History* focuses on local developments at the county level and was meant for consumption by Health Bureau and other government employees.

33 Ngamring was the only one of five county capitals (out of seventy-five in the TAR), to gain a full, structurally independent Tibetan medical hospital (Trinlé 2004: 138–39).

CHAPTER 6

1 October 7, 2006: 8,198 patients; August 7, 2007: 10,631 patients; September 19, 2007: 10,831 patients. In less than a year Yonten Tsering saw 2,632 patients.

2 Hofer 2007a, 2007b, 2008b.

3 Craig 2012; Adams and Craig 2008; Blaikie et al. 2015.

4 Bloom and Jing 2003; Lora-Wainwright 2005; Farquhar 1996.

5 Ngamring Health Report 2002; Hofer 2008a, 2008b.

6 Janes et al. 2006; Nguyen and Peschard 2003; Farmer 2015.

7 Adams and Craig 2008; Craig 2014; Hofer 2011a.

8 Hofer 2008a, 2008b, 2011d, 2012.

9 Janes 1999a, 2002; Craig 2012; Saxer 2013.

10 Adams 2001; Adams and Li 2008; Adams, Dhondup, and Le 2011.

11 On case record writing and keeping, see Hofer 2012.

12 *khog pa*, literally, "inside, the trunk of the body."

13 Originally part of the Mentsikhang, it later became an independent institution. Its relatively short history notwithstanding, the bag attested to the factory's history going back to 1696, the founding year of the long-destroyed Chakpori Medical College.

14 *Dribgyön* is a multifaceted illness category I often encountered in Ngamring. Its etiology was variously understood and addressed through different techniques that involved monks and nuns chanting and saying prayers, patients making offerings to deities, ingestion of Tibetan medicines (*rinchen rilbu*), and the application of golden needle therapy (*ser khab*), as well as oracles to suck out the disease.

15 Although I have collected and analyzed several illness narratives from Yonten Tsering's patients, constraints of space did not permit inclusion.

16 For details of production, see Hofer 2012, 2014b.

CONCLUSION

1 Blaikie 2013a; Craig 2012; Millard 2013; Soktsang and Millard 2013; Blaikie et al. 2015.

GLOSSARY

Phonetic spelling is followed, in parentheses, by the Wylie (1959) transliteration. Terms are Tibetan unless otherwise indicated: (C) Chinese, (Skt) Sanskrit.

ach a (a ce) older sister; wife; respectful term for a woman in Tsang
agar gonyön (A gar go snyon) *Cinchona* sp.
amchi (a mchi) Mongolian-derived word for medical doctors widely used in Tibet and across the Himalayas
amchi kangjenma (a mchi [sman pa] rkang rjen ma) barefoot doctor
arak (a rag) distilled grain alcohol
arura (a ru ra) "king of medicines"; Terminalia chebula

barché (bar che) obstacles
bardo (bar rdo) realm between death and rebirth
béken (bad kan) "phlegm"; one of the three *nyépa* or "humors" in Tibetan medicine
Bö (Bod) Tibet
bömen (bod sman) Tibetan medicine
Bon (Bon chos) collective term for pre-Buddhist religious traditions in Tibet; today acknowledged as one of the main schools of Tibetan Buddhism
bongkar (bong dkar) *Aconitum* spp.
Bonpo (bon po) a practitioner of the Bon religion
bu (bu') bug, microorganism, insect

Bumshi *(Bum bzhi)* Bon medical text, equivalent to the Buddhist *Gyüshi*

cham ('cham) Tibetan religious dance form
chang (chang) fermented barley beer
chijiao yisheng 赤脚医生 (C) barefoot doctor
Chijiao yisheng shouce 赤脚医生手册 (C) *The Barefoot Doctor's Manual*
chikgyel (phyi rgyal) foreigner; stranger; outsider
Chikhyap Khenpo (spyi khyab mkhan po) "chief abbot"; head of the ecclesiastical branch of the Tibetan government in Lhasa
Chimagyü *(Phyi ma rgyud)* *Last Treatise*, the fourth volume of the *Four Treatises*
chimen (phyi sman) "outsider medicine"; Chinese-style biomedicine; also called *tangmen*, *gyamen/jermen*
chitsok nyingpa (spyi tshogs rnying pa) "Old Society"; term introduced by the Communists to refer to pre-1950/59 Tibetan society and way of life
chiyi (phyi dbyi) "outsider medicine"; combining "foreign" in Tibetan with the phonetic pronunciation of *yi* 艺 for "medicine" in Chinese
chö (chos) religion; Buddhism; Skt. *Dharma*
chödzé (chos mdzad) member of a family of medical practitioners; one of the tripartite social and professional categorization of *chödzé shabdrung jedrung* in Tsang, prior to 1959
chödzé household (chos mdzad khyim tshang) term used in pre-1959 Tibetan society to denote a medical family
chökhang (chos khang) Buddhist chapel; altar room
chökyi khorlo (chos kyi 'khor lo) Dharma wheel; Skt. *Dharma cakra*
chöten (chos rten) Buddhist reliquary; Skt. *stupa*
chöyon (mchod yon) patron and recipient
chu (chu) water; river; one of the five elements
chuba (phyu pa) Tibetan style dress
chuser (chu gser) "yellow water"; term used to denote various fluids in Tibetan medical ideas about the body; a waste product from the transformation of nutrition into the seven bodily constituents

dépa (dad pa) faith
dikpa (sdig pa) sin

dön (gdon) nefarious spirit

döndre (gdon dre) nefarious spirit

dotsé (rdo tshad) traditional currency of Tibet

drelpa ('grel pa) commentary; explanation

drelrimgyi taptsö (gral rim gyi 'thab rtsod) class struggle

drib (grib) "shadow"; spiritual defilement and pollution

drö (drod) medicine with warming character

drumbu ('grum bu) joint pain and condition, often associated with rheumatoid arthritis

drumné ('brum nad) smallpox

duksum (dug gsum) "three poisons"; the *nyépa sum*; Skt. *kleśa*; attachment/desire (*'dod chags*), hatred/aversion (*zhe sdang*), and ignorance (*gti mug*)

dunggyü (gdung rgyud) bone lineage; family transmission; descent

dürapa (bsdus ra pa) degree in Tibetan medicine; comparable to a bachelor's degree in the modern Tibetan medical education system

dütsi (bdud rtsi) nectar; divine nectar; associated with production of medicine

dzong (rdzong) district capital; fortress; citadel

gangla métok (gangs lha me tog) Saussurea medusa/laniceps

Gelug (Dge lugs) "the virtuous ones"; one of the main schools in Tibetan Buddhism, founded by Tsongkhapa Lobsang Drakpa

gen/gen la (rgan lags) "sir/madam" or "teacher"; honorific form of personal address

gerpa (sger pa) a category of former Tibetan nobility

guanxi 关系 (C) connections, relations, social networks

gyamen (rgya sman) Chinese medicine; synonym for *biomedicine* and *Western medicine*

Gyenlok (gyen log) "rebels"; one of two major political groups that formed in Tibet during the Cultural Revolution

gyü (rgyud) tantric treatise; thread; string; character; consciousness and life; continuity, connection, lineage

Gyüshi (*Rgyud bzhi*) *Four Treatises*; core texts of Tibetan medicine

hormen (hor sman) "Mongolian medicine"; a remedy in Tibetan medicine made up of a small cotton bag filled with spices and *tsampa* that is warmed and applied to specified points on the body

Janglug (byang lugs) school of medicine that originated in [La-stod] Byang, also known as the Northern School or Northern Tradition
jedrung (rje drung) members of aristocratic families in pre-1959 central Tibet
jindak (sbyin bdag) master of the gift; patron; sponsor
jinlap (sbyin slab) ritual blessing
jungwa nga (byung ba lnga) "five elements"; earth, water, air/wind, fire, and space

kachupa (bka' bcu pa) a degree in Tibetan medicine, comparable to a master's degree in the modern Tibetan medical education system
Kagyü (Bka' brgyud) one of the schools in Tibetan Buddhism
kathag (kha btags) offering scarf
khandro (mkha' 'gro) sky dancer; Skt. *dakini*, female tantric deity; personal name
khuwa (khu ba) white and red reproductive substances
khyimgyü (khyim rgyud) a lineage of the household; a family lineage; short for *kyimtsang gyü* (khyim tshang rgyud)
kjama (rgya ma) half kilogram, equivalent to the Chinese *jin* measure
kora (skor ba) circumambulation
kutra (sku drag) lay Tibetan nobility

ladzi (gla rdzi) musk
laklén (lag lan) practice; experience
lama (bla ma) spiritual teacher or mentor; Skt. *Guru*
lamenpa (bla sman / bla sman pa) personal physician
lé (las) "action"; the law of cause and effect; Skt. *karma*
lha (lha) god; deity
lha jé (lha rje) honorific term for Tibetan medical doctor
lobgyü (slob gryud) teaching lineage
logyü (lo rgyus) "the running of the years"; history
lokchöpa (log spyod pa) reactionary
lu (klu) serpent spirit; Skt. *naga*
lü (lus) the physical body

lum (lums) medicinal bath
lung (rlung) air; wind; one of the "five elements"; one of the three *nyépa*; oral instruction
lungné (rlung nad) wind disorder

magpa (mag pa) a husband who moves into his wife's family home and resides there
mangdag (dmangs bdag) "owner of many"; Communist term for "exploiters" and land owners
Mangtso Chögyur (dmangs gtso bcos bsgyur) Democratic Reforms; a series of reforms implemented in central Tibet after the Dalai Lama escaped to India, crucially including the redistribution of land, which began in Tsang in 1960
mani rilbu (ma ni ril bu) pills empowered by prayers
marsuma (dmar srung dmag) Red Guard army; Red Guards
mé (me) fire; flame; one of the five elements
métsa (me btsa') cauterization therapy; moxibustion
men (*sman*) medicine
mendrup (sman grub) medical empowerment ritual
Menngakgyü (*Man ngag rgyud*) *Oral Instruction Treatise*, the third volume of the *Four Treatises*
mengyü / menpé gyü (sman rgyud / sman pa'i rgyud) doctor's lineage; medical lineage
menjor (sman sbyor) compounding medicines
menkhang (sman khang) medical house; clinic, hospital, or pharmacy; a named medical house; room in a medical house where medicines are kept
Menla (Sman bla) Medicine Buddha
menngak (man ngag) "secret oral" knowledge and transmission thereof
menpa (sman pa) physician, doctor; equivalent to *amchi*
menrampa (sman ra ba) medical degree awarded at Chakpori Medical College after nine years of study
Mentrong (sman grong) village or hamlet of doctors/medicine; medical house
Mentrong (sman 'khrungs) honorific term for a place where a doctor is born

Mentsikhang (Sman rtsi khang) Institute of Medicine and Astrology; the original building of this institution is in Lhasa dating to 1916; Men-Tsee-Khang is the roman spelling of the 1961 foundation in Dharamsala, North India; used in general for Tibetan medicine hospitals in Tibet

mimang künhré (mi dmangs kun hre) people's communes (term derived from Chinese)

minzu 民族 (C) minority nationality; ethnic group in the PRC

miser (mi ser) common people; used widely in Tibet's pre-1959 society to refer to people of low social class; still sometimes used to refer to rural Tibetans

mo (mo) divination; prophecy

moné (mo nad) women's illness

namkha (nam mkha') sky; space; one of the five elements

namthar (rnam thar) hagiography; biography

natsa taya (na tsha bltas) "look at illness"; to examine and review an illness

nepa taya (na pa bltas) seeing patients

ngakpa (sngags pa) "someone practicing mantra"; tantric practitioner

ngojor (sngo sbyor) medical compounding of herbs

ngomen (sngo sman) simple herbal medicines

ngönma (sngon ma) before; earlier; in the past

nüpa (nus pa) potency, effect; sometimes a gloss for the strength of a medicine

Nyamdre (mnyam 'brel) one of two major political groups formed in Tibet during the Cultural Revolution

nyelwa (dmyal ba) underworld; hell

nyépa / nyépa sum (nyes pa gsum) commonly translated as three humors; the three faults or dynamics corresponding to wind, bile, and phlegm; three forces

nying (snying) heart

nyingjé (snying rje) compassion

Nyingma (rnying ma) School of the Elders; one of the schools of Tibetan Buddhism

nyingné (snying nad) disease/illness of the heart; heart distress

nyom (snyoms) medicine of neutral character
nyomba (snyom ba) crazy; mentally unstable

peja (dpe cha) Tibetan-style book in which loose pages are held together between two boards made of wood or paper, wrapped in a piece of cloth
pennü (phan nus) benefit
pentok (phen thogs) benefit
Pökar 10 (pos dkar 10) name of a Tibetan medicine
polha (pho lha) deity of the patrilateral kin group
putsé (pu tse) quality

rangzhin (rang bzhin) inherently existing; natural; spontaneous
rapjampa (rabs 'byams pa) an advanced degree in Tibetan medicine
rigné chu (rig gnas bcu) tenfold system of the Tibetan sciences derived from the Indian system of the (Skt) *vidyāsthāna*
rik (rigs) kind, category, hereditary social status
rik thopo (rigs mtho po) high rank
rikgyü dzinpa (rigs rgyud 'dzin pa) lineage holder
rilbu (ril bu) Tibetan medical pill
rinchen rilbu (rin chen ril bu) precious pills
Rinchen Tsotru Dashel (Rin chen btso bkru zla shel) a particular type of "precious jewel" pill
rinpoche (rin po che) precious jewel; honorific title given to religious teachers; precious and semiprecious gems used in Tibetan medicinal compounds
ro druk (ro drug) six tastes
rogré (rogs res) mutual aid teams
rü (rus) bone; the father's side of one's lineage or biological inheritance
rügyü (rus rgyud) patrilineage

sa (sa) earth; soil; land; a categories of ingredients used in Tibetan medical compounds; one of the "five elements"
Sakya (Sa skya) one of the schools of Tibetan Buddhism; a place in central Tibet
sang (srang) 1 ounce (28.35 grams)

sangbo druk / sang druk (bzang po drug / bzang drug) "six excellent ones"; six medicines, including bamboo pith, saffron/safflower, green and black cardamom, cloves, and nutmeg

Sangyé Menla (Sangs rgyas sman bla) "master of remedies"; Medicine Buddha; Skt. *Bhaisajyaguru*

Seljé 25 (gsal byad 25) name of a Tibetan medicine

sem (sems) heart/mind

sem sangpo (sems bzang po) a pure heart/mind

Sendu nyikhyil (sendu nyi kyil) name of a Tibetan medicine

ser khab (gser khab) Tibetan medical golden needle therapy

sha (sha) flesh

shabden (zhabs rten) longlife prayer; blessing

shabdrung (zhabs drung) a type of lay tantric family in Tsang

Shégyü (*Bshad rgyud*) *Explanatory Treatise*, the second volume of the *Four Treatises*

sil (bsil) medicine of cooling character

sok lung (srog rlung) "life-force wind"; a type of disease in Tibetan medicine

solo marpo (sro lo dmar po) *rhodiola crenulata*

sorig dang menrig (gso rig dang sman rigs) "healing and types of medicines/pharmaceuticals"; Tibetan translation of *yiyao* 医药 (C) "medicine and pharmacology"

Sowa Rigpa (gso ba rig pa) "science or art of healing"; one of the five "major Tibetan sciences"; Tibetan medicine

suku 诉苦 (C) "speaking of bitterness" (the hardship in pre-Communist China)

ta rek dri (bltas reg dris) the main three Tibetan medical diagnostic methods: visual observation, feeling the pulse, and questioning the patient

tangmen (tang sman) Communist medicines; Chinese-style biomedicine; the term combines the Chinese term for "Communist [Party]" with the Tibetan word for "medicine"

terma (gter ma) "treasure"; hidden texts that are revealed at later times and under more favorable conditions

thamzing ('thab 'dzing) struggle sessions; fighting

thanka (thang kha) Tibetan Buddhist scroll painting

thob wang (thob dbang) rights; sovereignty
torma (tor ma) ritual barley cake offering
trak (khrag) blood, female reproductive substance
trakshé thopo (khrag tshad mtho po) high blood pressure
trelpa (khral pa) "taxpayer"; landholders in the pre-1959 Tibetan sociopolitical organization
trenpa (dren pa) memory
Trinsel 25 (mgril tshal 25) a medicine to treat *drumbu*
tripa (mkhris pa) bile; one of the three *nyépas* or humors
trungpé ('khrungs dpe) medical simple; single medical raw ingredient
trungyi (khrung dbyi) Tibetanized compound word rendering the Chinese term *zhong yi* 中医 (Chinese medicine). *Trung* was the new, politically correct term for the PRC, in contrast to *Gyanag* (China), while *yi* was imported from Chinese and spelled phonetically as *dbyi* (*yi*) in Tibetan
tsa̤ (rtsa) channels; roots; often translated as veins, arteries, and nerves, depending on context
tsab (mtshabs) substitute; used to refer to medical materials that replace an original in a recipe or formula
tsadrum (rtsa 'grum) medical condition that affects bodily channels; conventionally translated as "rheumatism" or "arthritis"
Tsagyü (*Rtsa rgyud*) *Root Treatise*, the first volume of the *Four Treatises*
tsakar (rtsa dkar) white channels in the body
tsampa (tsam pa) roasted barley flour; Tibetan staple food
tsatsa (tsa tsa) small clay icon of a deity
tshek (tsheg) intersyllabic punctuation mark in written Tibetan
tsön, ken, chak (mtshon kan chag) three points at the radial arteries where the pulse is felt in a Tibetan medical diagnosis, when the index, middle, and ring fingers are pressed at different levels and at three points; the general pulse qualities, specific organs pulses, and the upper, middle and lower parts of the body are examined through palpation by the different fingers
tsotel (btso thal) mercury-sulfide powder; purified mercury for use in medicines
tulku (sprul sku) reincarnated lama
tursel lung (thur sel rlung) downward cleansing wind; a physiological function in the body

uchen (dbu can) Tibetan print letters

Ü-Tsang (Dbus gtsang) central Tibet

wang (dbang) empowerment; consecration

xiang 乡 (C) township

Xizang 西藏 (C) "western treasure"; Tibet

yartsa gunbu (dbyar rtswa dgun 'bu) "summer grass-winter insect"; *Ophiocordyceps sinensis*; valuable medicinal plant exported from the Tibetan plateau to China proper

yenlak dün (yan lag bdun) seven-limb procedure for preparing medicines, described in the *Four Treatises*

yiku sitian 忆苦思甜 (C) recalling of bitterness (of the past) and thinking of sweetness (of the present)

yiyao 医药 (C) medicine and pharmacology

yokpo (gyog po) servants; landless laborer; in Communist parlance, "serf"

yonten (yȯn tan) good qualities; aptitude; virtue; a personal Tibetan name

zang yi 藏医 (C) Tibetan medicine

Zhijé 6 or Zhijé 11 (Zhi byed 6 or 11) two kinds of Tibetan medical formulas

zhong yi 中医 (C) Chinese medicine

zukpo (gzugs po) the corporeal body

Zurlug (zur lugs) major medical tradition, the Southern School, founded by Zurkhar Nyamnyi Dorjé (fifteenth century)

BIBLIOGRAPHY

Adams, Vincanne. 1992. "The Production of Self and Body in Sherpa-Tibetan Society." In *Anthropological Approaches to the Study of Ethnomedicine*, ed. M. Nichter, 149–90. Yverdon: Gordon and Breach.

———. 1998. "Suffering the Winds of Lhasa: Politicized Bodies, Human Rights, Cultural Difference, and Humanism in Tibet." *Medical Anthropology Quarterly* 12: 74–102.

———. 2000. "Particularizing Modernity: Tibetan Medical Theorizing of Women's Health in Lhasa, Tibet." In *Healing Powers and Modernity: Traditional Medicine, Shamanism and Science in Asian Societies*, ed. L. H. Connor and G. Samuel, 222–46. Westport, CT: Bergin & Harvey.

———. 2001. "The Sacred in the Scientific: Ambiguous Practices of Science in Tibetan Medicine." *Cultural Anthropology* 16 (4): 542–75.

Adams, Vincanne, and Sienna R. Craig. 2008. "Global Pharma in the Land of Snows." *Asian Medicine: Tradition and Modernity* 2 (1): 1–28.

Adams, Vincanne, Renchen Dhondup, and Phuoc V. Le. 2011. "A Tibetan Way of Science: Revisioning Biomedicine as Tibetan Practice." In *Between Science and Religion: Explorations on Tibetan Grounds*. ed. V. Adams, M. Schrempf, and S. R. Craig, 107–26. Oxford: Berghahn.

Adams, Vincanne, and Dashima Dovchin 2001. "Women's Health in Tibetan Medicine and Tibet's 'First' Female Doctor." In *Women's Buddhism, Buddhism's Women: Tradition, Revision, Renewal*, ed. E. B. Findly, 433–50. Boston: Wisdom Publications.

Adams, Vincanne, and Fei Fei Li. 2008. "Integration or Erasure? Modernizing Medicine at Lhasa's Mentsikhang." In *Exploring Tibetan Medicine in Contemporary*

Context: Perspectives in Social Sciences, ed. L. Pordié, 105–31. London: Routledge.

Adams, Vincanne, Mona Schrempf, and Sienna R. Craig. 2010. *Between Science and Religion: Explorations on Tibetan Grounds*. Oxford: Berghahn.

Ahmad, Z., trans. 1999. *Sangs-rgyas Rgya-mtsho: Life of the Fifth Dali Lama*. New Delhi: International Academy of Indian Culture and Aditya Prakashan.

Alexander, André. Forthcoming. *The Lhasa House: Typology of an Endangered Species*. Chicago: Serindia.

Amchi Tashi Namgyal (Mdo phra spor rtsa zur khang Em chi Bkra shis rnam rgyal). 1999. *Zur khang gi mi rgyud dang sman pa rim byung mdo phra'i yul ljongs bcas kyi lo rgyus mdo bsdus*. Gangtok, Sikkim: TransHimalaya.

Anagnost, Ann. 1994. *National Past-Times: Narrative, Representation, and Power in Modern China*. Durham, NC: Duke University Press.

Arnold, David. 1993. *Colonizing the Body: State Medicine and Epidemic Disease in Nineteenth-Century India*. Berkeley: University of California Press.

Arya, Pasang Yonten. 2014. "External Therapies in Tibetan Medicine: The Four Tantras, Contemporary Practice and a Prelimininary History of Surgery." In *Bodies in Balance: The Art of Tibetan Medicine*, ed. T. Hofer, 64–89. New York: Rubin Museum of Art (in association with University of Washington Press).

Attewell, Guy. 2006. "The End of the Line? The Fracturing of Authoritative Tibbi Knowledge in Twentieth-Century India." *Asian Medicine: Tradition and Modernity* 1 (2): 387–419.

———. 2007. *Refiguring Unani Tibb: Plural Healing in Late Colonial India*. Hyderabad: Orient Longman.

Aziz, Barbara. 1978. *Tibetan Frontier Families*. New Delhi: Vikas.

Barefoot Doctor's Manual. See QTMCRCWTG 1972.

Barnett, Robert. 1994. "Symbols and Protest: The Iconography of Demonstrations in Tibet, 1987–1990." In *Resistance and Reform in Tibet*, ed. R. Barnett and S. Akiner, 238–58. London: Hurst.

———. 1997. "Preface." In *A Poisoned Arrow: The Secret Report of the 10th Panchen Lama: The Full Text of the Panchen Lama's 70,000 Character Petition of 1962*, ed. TIN, 238–58. London: TIN.

———. 2003. "Chen Kuiyan and the Marketisation of Policy". In *Tibet and Her Neighbours: A History*, ed. A. McKay, 229–39. London: Hansjörg Mayer.

———. 2006. "Beyond the Collaborator-Martyr Model: Strategies of Compliance, Opportunism, and Opposition within Tibet." In *Contemporary Tibet: Politics, Development, and Society in a Disputed Region*, ed. S. A. Dreyer, 25–66. New York: M. E. Sharpe.

———. 2007. *Lhasa: Streets with Memories*. New York: Columbia University Press.

———. 2009a. "Introduction." In Tsering Shakya and Wang Luixong, *The Struggle for Tibet*, 1–33. London: Verso.

———. 2009b. "The Tibet Protests of Spring 2008." *China Perspectives* 3: 6–23.

———. 2010. "Understated Legacies: Uses of Oral History and Tibetan Studies." *Inner Asia* 12 (1): 63–93.

Barth, Frederik. 1990. "The Guru and the Conjurer: Transactions in Knowledge and the Shaping of Culture in Southeast Asia and Melanesia." *MAN*, n.s., 25 (4): 640–53.

Bell, Charles. 1925. *Tibet Past and Present*. Oxford: Clarendon Press.

Bellezza, John V. 2005. *Spirit-Mediums, Sacred Mountains and Related Bon Textual Traditions in Upper Tibet*. Leiden: Brill.

Ben Jiao. 2001. "Socio-economic and Cultural Factors Underlying the Contemporary Revival of Fraternal Polyandry." PhD diss., Case Western Reserve University.

Bhattacharya, Sanjoy. 2005. *Expunging Variola: The Control and Eradication of Smallpox in India, 1947–1977*. London: Sangam.

Blaikie, Calum. 2013a. "Currents of Tradition in Sowa Rigpa Pharmacy." *East Asian Science, Technology and Society: An International Journal* 7 (3): 1–27.

———. 2013b. "Making Medicine: Materia Medica, Pharmacy and the Production of Sowa Rigpa in Ladakh." PhD diss., University of Kent.

Blaikie, Calum, S. Craig, B. Gerke, and T. Hofer. 2015. "(Co)Producing Efficacious Medicines: Collaborative Event Ethnography with Tibetan Medicine Practitioners in Kathmandu, Nepal." *Current Anthropology* 56 (2): 178–204.

Blondeau, A.-M., and E. Steinkellner, eds. 1996. *Reflections of the Mountain: Essays on the History and Social Meaning of the Mountain Cult in Tibet and the Himalaya*. Vienna: Verlag der Österreichischen Akademie der Wissenschaften.

Bloom, Gerald, and F. Jing. 2003. *China's Rural Health System in a Changing Institutional Context*. IDS Working Paper 194. Brighton: Institute of Development Studies, University of Sussex.

Bolsokhoyeva, Natalia. 2007. "Tibetan Medical Schools of the Aga Area (Chita Region)." *Asian Medicine: Tradition and Modernity* 3 (2): 334–46.

Bourdieu, Pierre. 1977. *Outline of a Theory of Practice*. Cambridge: Cambridge University Press.

Bulag, Uradyn. 2010a. "Alter/Native Mongolian Identity: From Nationality to Ethnic Group." In *Chinese Society: Change, Conflict and Resistance*, ed. E. J. Perry and M. Selden, 261–87. London: Routledge.

———. 2010b. "Can the Subalterns Not Speak? On the Regimes of Oral History in Socialist China." *Inner Asia* 12 (1): 95–111.

Cameron, Mary. 2010. "Feminization and Marginalization? Women Ayurvedic Doctors and Modernizing Health Care in Nepal." *Medical Anthropology Quarterly* 24 (1): 42–63.

Carnahan, Sumner, and Lama Kunga Rinpoche. 1995. *In the Presence of My Enemies: Memoirs of Tibetan Nobleman Tsipon Shuguba*. Santa Fe, NM: Clear Light.

Carrasco, Pedro. 1959. *Land and Polity in Tibet*. Seattle: University of Washington Press.

Carrin, Guy, Ron Aviva, Yang Hui, Wang Hong, Zhang Tuohong, Zhang Licheng, Zhang Shuo, et al. 1999. "The Reform of the Rural Cooperative Medical System in the People's Republic of China: Interim Experience in 14 Pilot Counties." *Social Science and Medicine* 48: 961–72.

Carsten, J., and S. Hugh-Jones. 1995. *About the House: Lévi-Strauss and Beyond*. Cambridge: Cambridge University Press.

Cassinelli, Charles. W., and Robert B. Ekvall. 1969. *A Tibetan Principality: The Political System of Sa sKya*. Ithaca, NY: Cornell University Press.

Castro, Arachu, and Merill Singer. 2004. *Unhealthy Health Policy: A Critical Anthropological Examination*. Walnut Creek, CA: Altamira Press.

Chang Wei. 1978. *Co-operative Medical Services Is Fine*. Beijing: Foreign Languages Press.

Chatterjee, Partha. 1993. *The Nation and Its Fragments: Colonial and Postcolonial Histories*. Princeton, NJ: Princeton University Press.

Chen, Nancy N. 2003. *Breathing Spaces: Qigong, Psychiatry, and Healing in China*. New York: Columbia University Press.

Chen Hua. 2008. "The Diffusion of Tibetan Medicine in China: A Descriptive Panorama." In *Tibetan Medicine in the Contemporary World: Global Politics of Medical Knowledge and Practice*, ed. L. Pordié, 91–102. London: Routledge.

Chie, Nakane. 1970. *Japanese Society*. London: Weidenfeld & Nicolson.

Childs, Geoff. 2004. *Tibetan Diary: From Birth to Death and Beyond in a Himalayan Valley in Nepal*. Berkeley: University of California Press.

China Tibet Information Centre. 2005. "The Change of Medicare Situation in Tibet." http://eng.tibet.cn/lifestyle/health/200801/t20080117_357502.htm (accessed March 2010)

Chinese Minority Medicine Committee Secretary. 2007. *Report on Chinese Minority Medicine* 3 (105).

Clark, Barry. 1995. *The Quintessence Tantras of Tibetan Medicine*. Ithaca, NY: Snow Lion.

Clifford, Terry. 1994. *Tibetan Buddhist Medicine and Psychiatry: The Diamond Healing*. Wellingborough: Crucible.

Cooper, F., and A. Stoler, eds. 1996. *Tensions of Empire: Colonial Cultures in a Bourgeois World*. Berkeley: University of California Press.

Craig, Sienna R. 2007. "A Crisis in Confidence: A Comparison between Shifts in Tibetan Medical Education in Nepal and Tibet." In *Soundings in Tibetan Medicine—Anthropological and Historical Perspectives: Proceedings of the 10th Seminar of the International Association for Tibetan Studies, Oxford 2003*, ed. M. Schrempf, 127–54. Leiden: Brill.

———. 2008. "Place and Professionalisation: Navigating *amchi* Identity in Nepal." In *Tibetan Medicine in the Contemporary World: Global Politics of Medical Knowledge and Practice*, ed. L. Pordié, 62–90. London: Routledge.

———. 2009. "Pregnancy and Childbirth in Tibet: Knowledge, Perspectives, and Practices." In *Childbirth across Cultures*, ed. H. Selin, 145–60. New York: Springer.

———. 2012. *Healing Elements: Efficacy and the Social Ecologies of Tibetan Medicine*. Berkeley: University of California Press.

Craig, Sienna R., Mingji Cuomo, Frances Garrett, and Mona Schrempf, eds. 2010. *Studies of Medical Pluralism in Tibetan History and Society: Proceedings of the 11th Seminar of the International Association for Tibetan Studies*. Bonn: Institute for Tibetan and Buddhist Studies.

Craig, Sienna R., and Barbara Gerke. 2016. "Naming and Forgetting Sowa Rigpa and the Territory of Asian Medical Systems." *Medicine Anthropology Theory* 3 (2): 87–122.

Craig, Sienna R., and Denise Glover, eds. 2009. "Cultivating the Wilds: Idioms of Potency, Protection and Profit in the Sustainable Use of *Materia Medica* in Transnational Asian Medicine." *Asian Medicine: Tradition and Modernity* 5 (2).

Cuomo, Mingji. 2015. Response to "(Co)Producing Efficacious Medicines: Collaborative Event Ethnography with Tibetan Medicine Practitioners in Kathmandu, Nepal." *Current Anthropology* 56 (2): 195–96.

Das, Veena, and Deborah Poole. 2004. *Anthropology in the Margins of the State*. Santa Fe, NM: School for Advanced Research Press.

Dawa Ridak. 2003. *Bod kyi gso ba rig pa las sman rdzas sbyor bzo'i lag len gsang sgo byed pa'i lde mig*. Delhi: Rig Drag.

Dhondub Chödon. 1978. *Life in the Red Flag People's Commune*. Dharamsala: Information Office of His Holiness the Dalai Lama.

Diemberger, Hildegard. 1993. "Blood, Sperm, Soul and the Mountain: Gender Relations, Kinship and Cosmovision among the Khumbo (N.E. Nepal)." In *Gendered Anthropology*, ed. T. del Valle, 88–127. London: Routledge.

———. 2005. “Female Oracles in Modern Tibet.” In *Women in Tibet*, ed. Janet Gyatso and Hanna Havnevik, 113–68. London: Hurst.

———. 2007. *When a Woman Becomes a Religious Dynasty: The Samding Dorje Phagmo of Tibet*. New York: Columbia University Press.

———. 2010. “Life Histories of Forgotten Heroes? Transgression of Boundaries and the Reconstruction of Tibet in the Post-Mao Era.” *Inner Asia* 12 (1): 113–25.

Dirks, Nicholas. 1996. “Is Vice Versa? Historical Anthropologies and Anthropological Histories.” In *The Historic Turn in the Human Sciences*, ed. T. McDonald, 17–51. Ann Arbor: University of Michigan Press.

Dittmer, Lowell. 1998. *Liu Shaoqi and the Chinese Cultural Revolution*. Armonk, NY: M. E. Sharpe.

Dorjé, Gawo (Dga’ ba’i rdo rjes). 1995. *’Khrungs dpe dri med shel gyi me long (Crystal Mirror of Medical Simples)*. Pe cin: Mi rigs dpe skrun khang.

Dorje, Gyurme. 2010. “Introduction.” In *Jokhang: Tibet’s Most Sacred Buddhist Temple*, ed. Gyurme Dorje et al. London: Hansjörg Mayer.

———. 2014. “The Buddhas of Medicine.” In *Bodies in Balance: The Art of Tibetan Medicine*, ed. T. Hofer, 127–53. New York: Rubin Museum of Art (in association with University of Washington Press).

Dowman, Keith. 1988. *The Power-Places of Central Tibet: The Pilgrim’s Guide*. New Delhi: Timeless.

Duara, Prasenjit. 1995. *Rescuing History from the Nation: Questioning Narratives of Modern China*. Chicago: Chicago University Press.

Eck, Diana L. 1998. *Darśan: Seeing the Divine Image in India*. New York: Columbia University Press.

Emwall, Joakim. 2014. “China’s Minority Language Policy: Perspectives from Inner Mongolia.” Presentation given at Uppsala University, November 3–4.

Epa Sonam Rinchen. 2009. “Sman rtsis bstan pa’i srog shing dge ba’i bshes gnyen chen mo mkhyen rab nor bu’i mdzad rjes rnam thar rjes su dran pa skal ldan ’tsho mdzad dgyes pa’i mchod sprin.” In *Bod kyi srol rgyun sman rtsis rig pa’i dpyad yig mu tig phren mdzes (stod cha)*. Dharamsala: Library of Tibetan Works and Archives.

Epstein, Israel. 1983. *Tibet Transformed*. Beijing: New World Press.

Fang, Xiaoping. 2012. *Barefoot Doctors and Western Medicine in China*. Rochester, NY: Rochester University Press.

Farmer, Paul. 2004. “An Anthropology of Structural Violence.” *Current Anthropology* 45 (3): 305–25.

———. 2015. “Who Lives and Who Dies: Paul Farmer on the Iniquities of Healthcare Funding.” *London Review of Books* 37 (3): 17–20.

Farquhar, Judith. 1994. *Knowing Practice: The Clinical Encounter of Chinese Medicine*. Boulder, CO: Westview Press

———. 1996. "Marketing Magic: Getting Rich and Getting Personal in Medicine after Mao." *American Ethnologist* 23: 239–57.

Fassin, Didier. 2004. Response to "An Anthropology of Structural Violence." *Current Anthropology* 45 (3): 318–19.

Fisher, Andrew. 2002. *Poverty by Design: The Economics of Discrimination in Tibet*. Montreal: Canada Tibet Committee.

———. 2005. *State Growth and Social Exclusion in Tibet: Challenges of Recent Growth*. Copenhagen: NIAS.

———. 2013. *The Disempowered Development of Tibet in China*. Lanham, MD: Lexington Books.

Fjeld, Heidi E. 2005. *Commoners and Nobles: Hereditary Divisions in Tibet*. Copenhagen: Northern Institute of Asian Studies.

———. 2006. "The Rise of the Polyandrous House: Marriage, Kinship and Social Mobility in Rural Tsang, Tibet." PhD diss., University of Oslo.

———. 2008. "Pollution and Social Networks in Contemporary Rural Tibet." In *Tibetan Modernities*, ed. R. Barnett and R. Schwartz, 113–37. Leiden: Brill.

Fjeld, Heidi E., and Theresia Hofer. 2010/11. "Introduction: Women and Gender in Tibetan Medicine." *Asian Medicine: Tradition and Modernity* 6 (2): 175–216.

Foucault, Michel. 1973. *The Order of Things: An Archeology of the Human Sciences*. New York: Vintage.

———. 1977. *Discipline and Punish: The Birth of the Prison*. London: Penguin.

———. 1980. *Power/Knowledge*. Brighton: C. Gordon.

———. 1981. *The History of Sexuality*. Vol. 1. London: Penguin.

Furth, Charlotte, and Angela Leung, eds. 2010. *Health and Hygiene in Chinese East Asia: Politics and Publics in the Long Twentieth Century*. Durham, NC: Duke University Press.

Garrett, Frances. 2008. *Religion, Medicine and the Human Embryo in Tibet*. London: Routledge.

———. 2009. "The Alchemy of Accomplishing Medicine (*sman sgrub*): Situating the *Yuthok Heart Essence* (*G.yu thog snying thig*) in Literature and History." *Journal for Indian Philosophy* 37: 207–30.

———. 2014. "The Making of Medical History: Twelfth to Seventeenth Century." In *Bodies in Balance: The Art of Tibetan Medicine*, ed. T. Hofer, 178–97. New York: Rubin Museum of Art (in association with University of Washington Press).

Garrett, Frances, and Vincanne Adams. 2008. "The Three Channels in Tibetan Medicine, with a Translation of Tsultrim Gyaltsen's *A Clear Explanation of the*

Principal Structure and Location of the Circulatory Channels as Illustrated in the Medical Paintings." *Traditional South Asian Medicine* 8: 86–115.

Gerke, Barbara. 2012. *Long Lives and Untimely Deaths: Life-Span Concepts and Longevity Practices among Tibetans in the Darjeeling Hills, India*. Leiden: Brill.

———. 2015a. "Biographies and Knowledge Transmission of Mercury Processing in 20th Century Central and South Tibet." *Asiatische Studien—Études Asiatiques* 69 (4): 867–99.

———. 2015b. "The Poison of Touch: Tracing Mercurial Treatments of Venereal Diseases in Tibet." *Social History of Medicine* 28 (3): 532–54.

———. In preparation. *Taming the Poisonous: Mercury, Toxicity, and Safety in Tibetan Medical Practice.*

Gerl, Robert, and Jürgen Aschoff. 2005. *Die Medizinhochschule Tschagpori (lCag-po-ri) auf dem Eisenberg in Lhasa—Geschichte, Fakten, Zeitzeugen.* Ulm: Fabri.

Glover, Denise. 2005. "Up from the Roots: Contextualizing Medicinal Plant Classification of Tibetan Doctors in Rgyalthang, PRC." PhD diss., University of Washington.

Goldstein, Melvyn C. 1989. *A History of Modern Tibet, 1913–1951: The Demise of the Lamaist State*. New Delhi: Munishiram Manoharlal.

———. 1994. "Change, Conflict and Continuity among a Community of Nomadic Pastoralists: A Case Study from Western Tibet, 1950–1990." In *Resistance and Reform in Tibet*, ed. R. Barnett and S. Akiner, 76–111. London: Hurst.

———. 1997. *The Snow Lion and the Dragon: China, Tibet and the Dalai Lama.* Berkeley: University of California Press.

———. 2007. *A History of Modern Tibet: The Calm before the Storm, 1951–1955.* Berkeley: University of California Press.

———. 2013. *A History of Modern Tibet: The Storm Clouds Descend*, 1955–1957. Berkeley: University of California Press.

Goldstein, Melvyn C., and Cynthia Beall. 1990. *Nomads of Western Tibet: The Survival of a Way of Life*. Hong Kong: Odyssey.

Goldstein, Melvyn C., Ben Jiao, and Tanzen Lhundrup. 2009. *On the Cultural Revolution in Tibet: The Nyemo Incident of 1969*. Berkeley: University of California Press.

Goldstein, Melvyn C., and Matthew Kapstein, eds. 1998. *Buddhism in Contemporary Tibet: Religious Revival and Cultural Identity.* Berkeley: University of California Press.

Gongmen Konchog Pandar (Gong sman Dkon mchog phan dar). n.d. *Nyams yig brgya rtsa* (A hundred verses written from experience). Unpublished document.

Good, Byron. 1977. "The Heart of What's the Matter: The Semantics of Illness in Iran." *Culture, Medicine and Psychiatry* 1 (1): 25–58.

Gutschow, Kim. 2004. *Being a Buddhist Nun: The Struggle for Enlightenment in the Himalayas.* Cambridge, MA: Harvard University Press.

———. 2011. "From Home to Hospital: The Extension of Obstetrics in Ladakh." In *Medicine between Science and Religion: Explorations on Tibetan Grounds*, ed. V. Adams, M. Schrempf, and S. Craig, 185–213. Oxford: Berghahn.

Gyatso, Janet. 2015. *Being Human in a Buddhist World: An Intellectual History of Medicine in Early Modern Tibet.* New York: Columbia University Press.

Gyatso, Janet, and Hanna Havnevik, eds. 2005. *Women in Tibet.* London: Hurst.

Gyatso, Yonten. 2005/6. "Nyes pa: A Brief Review of its English Translation." *Tibet Journal* 4: 109–18.

Han, Suyin. 1977. *Lhasa, the Open City: A Journey to Tibet.* London: J. Cape.

Hansen, Mette H. 2006. "In the Footsteps of the Communist Party: Dilemmas and Strategies." In *Doing Fieldwork in China*, ed. Maria Heimer and Stig Thøgersen, 81–95. Honolulu: University of Hawai'i University Press.

Hansen, Peter H. 2003. "Why Is There No Subaltern Studies for Tibet." *Tibet Journal* 28 (4): 23–38.

Harris, Clare. 1999. *In the Image of Tibet: Tibetan Painting after 1959.* London: Reaktion Books.

Heimsath, Kabir. 2003. "Traditional Tibetan Medicine in Rural Tibet: Evaluation of the 1996 Graduates of Pelshong, Shigatse." Unpublished report, SRC.

Henrion-Dourcy, Isabelle. 2005. "Women in the Performing Arts: Portraits of Six Contemporary Singers." In J. Gyatso and H. Havnevik, *Women in Tibet*, 195–258. London: Hurst.

———. 2013. "Easier in Exile? Comparative Observations on Doing Research among Tibetans in Lhasa and Dharamsala." In *Red Stamps and Gold Stars: Fieldwork Dilemmas in Upland Socialist Asia*, ed. Sarah Turner, 201–19. New York: University of Columbia Press.

———. 2017. *Le théâtre "Ache Lhamo": Jeux et enjeux d'une tradition tibétaine.* Leuven: Peeters.

Hillier, Sheila M., and J. A. Jewell. 1983. *Health Care and Traditional Medicine in China, 1800–1982.* London: Routledge.

Hirsch, Eric, and Charles Steward. 2005. "Introduction: Ethnographies of Historicity." *History and Anthropology* 16 (3): 261–74.

Hobsbawm, Eric, and Terence Ranger. 1983. *The Invention of Tradition.* Cambridge: Cambridge University Press.

Hofer, Theresia. 2007a. "Evaluation and Needs Assessment I: The 1996 Graduates from the Tibetan Medical School, Shigatse, Tibet Autonomous Region." Unpublished report, SRC.

———. 2007b. "Evaluation and Needs Assessment II: The 2003 Graduates from the Tibetan Medical School, Shigatse, Tibet Autonomous Region." Unpublished report, SRC.

———. 2007c. "Preliminary Investigations into New Oral and Textual Sources on *Byang lugs*—the "Northern School" of Tibetan Medicine." In *Soundings in Tibetan Medicine—Anthropological and Historical Perspectives: Proceedings of the 10th Seminar of the International Association for Tibetan Studies, Oxford 2003*, ed. M. Schrempf, 373–410. Leiden: Brill.

———. 2008a. "Socio-Economic Dimensions of Tibetan Medicine in the Tibet Autonomous Region, China: Part One." *Asian Medicine: Tradition and Modernity* 4 (1): 174–200.

———. 2008b. "Socio-Economic Dimensions of Tibetan Medicine in the Tibet Autonomous Region, China: Part Two." *Asian Medicine: Tradition and Modernity* 4 (2): 492–514.

———. 2011a. "Changing Representations of the Female Tibetan Medical Doctor Khandro Yangkar (1907–1973)." In *Buddhist Himalayas: Studies in Religion, History and Culture. Proceedings of the Golden Jubilee Conference of the Namgyal Institute of Tibetology Gangtok, 2008*, vol. 1, ed. Alex McKay and Anna Balicki-Dengjongpa, 99–122. Gangtok: Namgyal Institute of Tibetology.

———. 2011b. "Making Nationality Medicine 'Ethnic': Re-invention and Loss of Tibetan Medicine at Centers and Margins." Paper presented at the annual meeting of the American Anthropological Association (AAA), Montreal, November.

———. 2011c. "*The Mirror of the Moon*—Khyenrap Norbu's Text on Tibetan Medical Methods for Assisting Births." Presentation at the Medical Texts in Translation Series, University College, London, May 10.

———. 2011d. "Tibetan Medicine on the Margins: Twentieth Century Transformations of the Traditions of Sowa Rigpa in Central Tibet." PhD diss., University College, London.

———. 2012. *The Inheritance of Change: Transmission and Practice of Tibetan Medicine in Ngamring*. Vienna: Wiener Studien zur Tibetologie und Buddhismuskunde.

———. 2013. "Encounters and Engagements of the Scholar-Physician Jampa Trinlé with Chinese Communists during the 1950s and early 1960s." Paper presented at the International Association for Tibetan Studies (IATS) Conference, Ulaan Batoor, Mongolia, July 21, 2013.

———, ed. 2014a. *Bodies in Balance: The Art of Tibetan Medicine*. New York: Rubin Museum of Art (in association with University of Washington Press).

———. 2014b. "Foundations of Tibetan Pharmacology and the Compounding of Tibetan Medicines." In *Bodies in Balance: The Art of Tibetan Medicine*, ed. T. Hofer, 46–63. New York: Rubin Museum of Art (in association with University of Washington Press).

———. 2014c. "Illustrated *Materia Medica* Prints, Manuscripts and Modern Books." In *Bodies in Balance: The Art of Tibetan Medicine*, ed. T. Hofer, 226–45. New York: Rubin Museum of Art (in association with University of Washington Press).

———. 2015. "Gender and Medicine in Kham: An Analysis of the Medical Work and Life of Derge Phurpa Dolma." *Revue d'études tibetaines*, no. 34 (Décembre): 53–77.

Hofer, Theresia, and Knud Larsen. 2014. "Pillars of Tibetan Medicine: History and Architecture of the Chagpori and Mentsikhang Medical Institutes in Lhasa." In *Bodies in Balance: The Art of Tibetan Medicine*, ed. T. Hofer, 257–67. New York: Rubin Museum of Art (in association with University of Washington Press).

Hsi Changhao and Kao Yuanmei. 1977. *Tibet Leaps Forward*. Beijing: Foreign Languages Press.

Hsu, Elisabeth. 1998. "Moso and Naxi: The House." In *Naxi and Moso Ethnography: Kin, Rites, Pictographs*, ed. Michael Oppitz and Elisabeth Hsu, 47–80. Zürich: Völkerkundemuseum Zürich.

———. 1999. *The Transmission of Chinese Medicine*. Cambridge: Cambridge University Press.

———. 2006. "Reflections on the 'Discovery' of the Antimalarial Qinghao." *British Journal of Clinical Pharmacology* 61 (6): 666–70.

———. 2008. "Medicine as Business: Chinese Medicine in Tanzania." In *China Returns to Africa: A Rising Power and a Continent Embrace*, ed. C. Alden, D. Large, and R. Soares de Oliveira, 221–36. London: Hurst.

———. 2009. "The History of Chinese Medicine in the People's Republic of China and Its Globalization." *East Asian Science, Technology and Society: An International Journal* 2 (4): 465–84.

———. 2010. "The Authority of the Chinese Medical 'House' in Contemporary Xin'an Yixie." Paper presented at University of Westminster, August 20.

Huber, Toni, ed. 2007. *Nomads of Eastern Tibet: Social Organisation and Economy of a Pastoral Estate in the Kingdom of Dege*. By Rinzin Thargyal. Leiden: Brill.

Inhorn, Marcia. 2006. "Defining Women's Health: A Dozen Messages from More Than 150 Ethnographies." *Medical Anthropology Quarterly* 20 (3): 345–78.

Ingold, Tim. 2000. *The Perception of the Environment: Essays in Livelihood, Dwelling and Skill*. London: Routledge.

———. 2011. *Being Alive: Essays on Movement, Knowledge and Description*. London: Routledge.

Jacoby, Sarah. 2014. *Love and Liberation: Autobiographical Writings of the Tibetan Buddhist Visionary Sera Khandro*. New York: Columbia University Press.

Jäger, Katrin. 1999. *"Nektar der Unsterblichkeit" Zwei Kapitel der Tibetischen Kinderheilkunde*. Engelsbach: Verlag Dr. Hänsel-Hohenhausen.

Jagou, Fabienne. 2011. *The Ninth Panchen Lama (1883–1937): A Life at the Crossroads of Sino-Tibetan Relations*. Translated by R. B. Buechel. Paris: École Française d'Extrême-Orient.

Janes, Craig. 1995. "The Transformation of Tibetan Medicine." *Medical Anthropology Quarterly* 9 (1): 6–39.

———. 1999a. "The Health Transition, Global Modernity and the Crisis of Traditional Medicine: The Tibetan Case." *Social Science and Medicine* 48 (12): 1803–20.

———. 1999b. "Imagined Lives, Suffering, and the Work of Culture: The Embodied Discourses of Conflict in Modern Tibet." *Medical Anthropology Quarterly* 13 (4): 391–412.

———. 2002. "Buddhism, Science, and the Market: The Globalisation of Tibetan Medicine." *Anthropology and Medicine* 9 (3): 268–89.

Janes, Craig, and O. Chuluundorj. 2004. "Free Markets and Dead Mothers: The Social Ecology of Maternal Mortality in Post-Socialist Mongolia." *Medical Anthropology Quarterly* 18 (2): 230–57.

Janes, Craig, O. Chuluundorj, C. E. Hilliard, K. Rak, and K. Janchiv. 2006. "Poor Medicine for Poor People? Assessing the Impact of Neoliberal Reform on Health Care Equity in a Post-Socialist Context." *Global Public Health* 1 (1): 5–30.

Janes, Craig, and C. Hilliard. 2008. "Inventing Traditions: Tibetan Medicine in the Post-Socialist Contexts of China and Mongolia." In *Tibetan Medicine in the Contemporary World: Global Politics of Medical Knowledge and Practice*, ed. L. Pordié, 35–61, London: Routledge.

Jinba, Tenzin. 2013. *In the Land of the Eastern Queendom: The Politics of Gender and Ethnicity on the Sino-Tibetan Border*. Seattle: University of Washington Press.

Ju Mipham ('Ju Mi pham). 2006. *'Ju Mi pham gyi sman yig gces btus*. Pe cin: Mi rig dpe skrun khang.

Kansteiner, Wulf. 2002. "Finding Meaning in Memory: A Methodological Critique of Collective Memory Studies." *History and Theory* 41 (2): 179–97.

Kapstein, Matthew. 2006. *The Tibetans*. Oxford: Blackwell.

Kelsang Trinlé (Skal bzang 'phrin las). 1997. *Bod kyi gso rig byung 'phel gyi lo rgyus* (The origin and development of Tibetan medicine). Shan xi: Krung go'i bod kyi shes rig dpe skrun khang.

Khyenrap Norbu (Mkhyen rab Nor bu). 1924. *Byis pa btsa' thabs kun phan zla ba'i me long zhes bya ba.* (Mirror of the moon: Methods for giving birth helpful to all). Lhasa: Lhasa Mentsikhang.

———. 1995. *Sman sbyor nus pa phyogs bsdus phan bde legs bshad.* Dharamsala: Men-Tsee-Khang.

Kleinman, Arthur. 1980. *Patients and Healers in the Context of Culture.* Berkeley: University of California Press.

Kloos, Stephan. 2004. *Tibetan Medicine among the Buddhist Dards of Ladakh.* Vienna: Arbeitskreis für Tibetologie und Buddhistische Studien der Universität Wien.

———. 2008. "The History and Development of Tibetan Medicine in Exile." *Tibet Journal* 33 (3): 15–49.

———. 2010. "Tibetan Medicine in Exile: The Ethics, Politics, and Science of Cultural Survival." PhD diss., University of California, Berkeley.

Kolås, Åshild, and Monika P. Thowsen. 2005. *On the Margins of Tibet: Cultural Survival on the Sino-Tibetan Frontier.* Seattle: University of Washington Press.

Konchok, Pema. 2002. "Buddhism as a Focus of Iconoclash in Asia." In *Iconoclash: Beyond the Image Wars in Science, Religion, and Art*, ed. Bruno Latour and Peter Weibel, 40–59. Cambridge, MA: MIT Press.

Kværne, Per. 1998. "Khyung-sprul 'Jigs-med nam-'mkha'i rdo-rje: An Early Twentieth-Century Pilgrim in India." In *Pilgrimage in Tibet*, ed. A. McKay, 71–84. Surrey: Curzon.

Lamphere, Louise. 2003. "The Perils and Prospects for an Engaged Anthropology: A View from the United States." *Social Anthropology* 11 (2): 153–68.

———. 2004. "The Convergence of Applied, Practicing, and Public Anthropology in the 21st Century." *Human Organization* 63 (4): 431–43.

Langford, J. M. 2002. *Fluent Bodies: Ayurvedic Remedies for Postcolonial Imbalance.* Durham, NC: Duke University Press.

Larsen, Knud, and Amund Sinding-Larsen. 2001. *The Lhasa Atlas: Traditional Tibetan Architecture and Townscape.* Boulder, CO: Shambala.

Levine, Nancy. 1981. "The Theory of *Rü* Kinship, Descent and Status in a Tibetan Society." In *Asian Highland Societies in Anthropological Perspective*, ed. C. Fürer-Haimendorf, 52–78. Paris: Presses Universitaires de France.

———. 1988. *The Dynamics of Polyandry. Kinship, Domesticity, and Population on the Tibetan Border.* Chicago: University of Chicago Press.

Lévi-Strauss, Claude. (1982) 1987. *The Way of the Masks.* London: Jonathan Cape.

———. 1991. "Maison." In *Dictionnaire de l'ethnologie et de l'anthropologie*, ed. P. Bonte and M. Izard, 434–36, Paris: Presses Universitaires de France.

Lhasa City Mentsikhang [Grong khyer lHa sa sman rtsis khang, LCM]. 1975.

Sman pa rkang rjen ma'i bod sman sbyor sde gsar bsgrigs (Barefoot doctor's new Tibetan medical compounding manual). Lhasa: Bod ljongs mi dmangs dpe skrun khang.

Lindskog, Benedikte V. 2014. "Natural Calamities and 'the Big Migration': Challenges to the Mongolian Health System in 'the Age of the Market.'" *Global Public Health* 9 (8): 880–93. DOI:10.1080/17441692.2014.940361.

Liu, X., and W. Hsiao. 1995. "The Cost Escalation of Social Health Insurance Plans in China: Its Implication for Public Policy." *Social Science and Medicine* 41 (8): 1095–1101.

Lobsang Dolma Khangkar. 1998. *Lectures on Tibetan Medicine*. Dharamsala: Library of Tibetan Works and Archives.

Lobsang Tupten Chökyi Nyima (Blo bzang Thub bstan chos kyi nyi ma). 1944. *Skyabs mgon thams cad mkhyen pa blo bzang thub bstan chos kyi nyi ma dge legs rnam rgyal bzang po'i zhal snga nas kyi thun mong pa'i rnam bar thar pa rin chen dbang gi rgyal po'i phreng ba* (The autobiography of the Sixth [Ninth] Panchen Lama Blo-bzang thub-bstan chos-kyi nyi-ma). Shigatse: Tashilhunpo Monastery.

Lobsang Wangyal. 2007. *My Life, My Culture: Autobiography and Lectures on the Relationship between Tibetan Medicine, Buddhist Philosophy and Tibetan Astrology and Astronomy*. Dharamsala: Dawa Ridak.

Lora-Wainwright, Anna. 2005. "Using Local Resources: Barefoot Doctors and Bone Manipulation in Rural Langzhong, Sichuan Province, PRC." *Asian Medicine: Tradition and Modernity* 1 (2): 470–89.

Maas, Philipp A. 2007/8. "The Concepts of the Human Body and Disease in Classical Yoga and Āyurveda." *Wiener Zeitschrift für die Kunde Südasiens* (Vienna Journal of South Asian Studies) 51: 125–62.

Makley, Charlene. 2005. "'Speaking Bitterness': Autobiography, History, and Mnemonic Politics on the Sino-Tibetan Frontier." *Comparative Studies in Society and History* 47 (1): 40–78.

———. 2007. *The Violence of Liberation: Gender and Tibetan Buddhist Revival in Post-Mao China*. Berkeley: University of California Press.

Maraini, Fosco. 1952. *Secret Tibet*. London: Hutchinson.

Markham, Clements R., ed. 1876. *Narratives of the Mission of George Bogle to Tibet and of the Journey of Thomas Manning to Lhasa*. London: Trubner.

McGranahan, Carole. 2010. *Arrested Histories: Tibet, the CIA, and Memories of a Forgotten War*. Durham, NC: Duke University Press.

McGranahan, Carole, and Ralph Litzinger. 2012. "Self-Immolation as Protest in Tibet." Hot Spots, *Cultural Anthropology* website, April 9. https://culanth.org/fieldsights/93-self-immolation-as-protest-in-tibet.

McKay, Alex. 2003. *The History of Tibet*. London: Routledge Curzon.

———. 2007. *Their Footprints Remain: Biomedical Beginnings across the Indo-Tibetan Frontier*. Amsterdam: Amsterdam University Press.

———. 2011. "Biomedicine at the Edge of Modernity" In *Medicine between Science and Religion: Explorations on Tibetan Grounds*, ed. V. Adams, M. Schrempf, and S. R. Craig, 33–55. Oxford: Berghahn.

McKhann, Charles F. 1989. "Fleshing Out the Bones: The Cosmic and Social Dimensions of Space in Naxi Architecture." In *Ethnicity and Ethnic Groups in China*, ed. Chien Chiao and Nicholas Tapp, 157–77. Hong Kong: Chinese University.

Men-Tsee-Khang. 2008. *The Basic Tantra and the Explanatory Tantra from the Secret Quintessential Instructions on the Eight Branches of Ambrosia Essence Tantra*. Dharamsala: Men-Tsee-Khang.

———. 2011. *The Subsequent Tantra from the Four Tantras of Tibetan Medicine*. Dharamsala: Men-Tsee-Khang.

Meyer, Fernand. 1995. "Theory and Practice of Tibetan Medicine." In *Oriental Medicine: An Illustrated Guide to the Asian Arts of Healing*, ed. J. van Alphen and A. Aris, 109–41. London: Serindia.

———. 1998. *Report of the Missions in Tibet for the Swiss Red Cross, September, October 1998*. Paris: SRC.

Michalson, Ravenna N. 2012. "Daughter of Self-Liberation: Lineage Position and Transmission in the Namthar of Do Dasel Wangmo." MA thesis, University of Colorado, Boulder.

Millard, Colin. 2002. "Learning Processes in a Tibetan Medical School." PhD diss., University of Edinburgh.

———. 2009. "The Life and Medical Legacy of Khyung sprul 'Jig med Nam-mkha'i rDo rje (1897–1955)." *East and West* 2 (59): 1–4.

———. 2013. "Bon Medical Practitioners in Contemporary Tibet: The Continuity of a Tradition." *East Asian Science, Technology and Society: An International Journal* 7 (3): 353–79.

Morgan, William S. 2007. *Amchi Sahib: A British Doctor in Tibet 1936–1937*. Charlestown, MA: Acme Bookbinding.

Mueggler, Eric. 2001. *The Age of Wild Ghosts: Memory, Violence, and Place in Southwest China*. Berkeley: University of California Press.

Mullaney, Thomas S. 2010. *Coming to Terms with the Nation: Ethnic Classification in Modern China*. Berkeley: University of California Press.

Naktsang, Nulo. 2014. *My Tibetan Childhood: When Ice Shattered Stone*. Durham, NC: Duke University Press.

Neuenschwander, Jürg. 1989. *Shigatse: One Injection Asks for More*. Documentary film, 90 minutes. Berne: Container Film AG.

Ngyuyen, Vinh-Kim, and Karine Peschard. 2003. "Anthropology, Inequality, and Diseases: A Review." *Annual Review of Anthropology* 32: 447–74.

Nianggajia. 2011. "Local Health Seeking Strategies and the New Cooperative Medical Scheme in Contemporary Phyed ri Village, Amdo." MA thesis, University of Oslo.

Norbu, Dawa. 1997. "Historical Introduction." In *A Poisoned Arrow: The Secret Report of the 10th Panchen Lama: The Full Text of the Panchen Lama's 70,000 Character Petition of 1962*, ed. TIN, xxv–xxxiv. London: TIN.

———. 1999. *Tibet: The Road Ahead*. London: Rider.

Norbu Chöphel and Tashi Tsering (Nor-bu Chos-'phel and bKra-shis Tshe-ring). 2008. *Mnga' ris smad yul skyid grong rgya dgu'i lo rgyus dang brel ba'i skyid grong grwa khang dkar ba'i sman pa mkhas grags can blo bzang sgrol ma'i nang mi'i lo rgyus nor bu'i me long* (A brief account of the famous Tibetan lady doctor Lobsang Dolma Khangkar [1935–1989] and her family, including historical materials on Kyirong, South West Tibet). Dharamsala: Amnye Machen Institute.

Ortner, Sherry. 2006. *Anthropology and Social Theory: Culture, Power, and the Acting Subject*. Durham, NC: Duke University Press.

Paljor, Kunsang. 1977. *Tibet: The Undying Flame*. Dharamsala: Information & Publicity Office of His Holiness the Dalai Lama.

Palmer, David. 2007. *Qigong Fever: Body, Science, and Utopia in China*. London: Hurst.

Parfionovich, Yuri, Gyurme Dorje, and Fernand Meyer, eds. 1992. *Tibetan Medical Paintings: Illustrations to the Blue Beryl Treatise of Sangye Gyamtso*. London: Serindia.

Pasang Yontan. 1987. *Bod kyi gso ba rig pa'i lo rgyus kyi bang mdzod g.yu thog bla ma dran pa'i pho nya*, Leh: Yuthok Institute of Tibetan Medicine.

Pema Bhum. 2001. *Dran tho smin drug ske 'khyog. Six Stars with a Crooked Neck: Tibetan Memoirs of the Cultural Revolution*. Translated by Lauren Hartley. Dharamsala: Bod kyi dus (Tibetan times).

Penpa Tsering. 2013. *Ngamring rdzong gi dgon sde'i lo rgyus dang da lta'i gnas babs* (History and today's situation of temples and monasteries in Ngamring). Lhasa: Bod ljongs bod yig dpe rnyin dpe skrun khang.

Petech, Luciano. 1973. *Aristocracy and Government in Tibet 1728–1959*. Roma: ISMEO.

Prakash, Gyan. 1990. "Writing Post-Orientalist Histories of the Third World: Perspectives from Indian Historiography." *Comparative Studies in Society and History* 32 (2): 383–408.

Prost, Audrey. 2008. *Precious Pills: Medicine and Social Change among Tibetan Refugees in India*. Oxford: Berghahn.

Qian, Jiwei. 2010. *Regional Inequality in Healthcare in China*. Singapore: East Asian Institute, National University of Singapore.

Qian, Jiwei, and Åke Blomqvist. 2014. *Health Policy Reforms in China: A Comparative Perspective*. Hackensack, NJ: World Scientific.

QTMCRCWTG (Qinghai Tibetan Medical College Revolutionary Committee Writing and Translation Group). 1972. *Chijiao yisheng shouce: "Rkang rjen sman pa'i" slob deb* (The barefoot doctor's manual). Chinese-Tibetan bilingual edition (*Rgya bod shan sbyar*). Xining: Mtso sngon gso rig slob grwa chen mo'i gsar brje u yon ltan khang.

Ramble, Charles, Peter Schwieger, and Alice Travers. 2013. *Tibetan Who Fell through the Historian's Net: Studies in the Social History of Tibetan Societies*. Kathmandu: Vajra Books.

RCTARHB (Revolutionary Committee of the TAR Health Bureau). 1973a. *Bod ljong rgyun spyo krung dbyi'i sman rigs* (Chinese herbal medicines common in Tibet). Lhasa: Bod ljong mi dmangs dpe skrun khang.

———. 1973b. *Xizang changyong zhong caoyao* (Chinese herbal medicines common in Tibet). Lhasa: Xizang Renmin Chubanshe.

Rechung, Rinpoche. 1973. *Tibetan Medicine: Illustrated in Original Texts*. London: Wellcome Institute of the History of Medicine.

Reichle, Franz. 1995. *Das Wissen vom Heilen*. Documentary film, 93 minutes. Zürich: T&C Film.

Roche, Gerald. 2017. "Introduction: The Transformation of Tibet's Language Ecology in the Twenty-First Century." *International Journal of the Sociology of Language* 245: 1–35.

Rogasky, Ruth. 2004. *Hygienic Modernity: Meanings of Health and Disease in Treaty-Port China*. Berkeley: University of California Press.

Sabernig, Katharina. 2007. *Kalte Kräuter und heisse Bäder: Die Anwendung der Tibetischen Medizin in den Klöstern Amdos*. Vienna: LIT Verlag.

———. 2014. "The Tree Murals of Labrang Monastery's Medical College, Eastern Tibet." In *Bodies in Balance: The Art of Tibetan Medicine*, ed. T. Hofer, 221–25. New York: Rubin Museum of Art (in association with University of Washington Press).

Sagli, Gry, Jinming Zhang, Benedicte Ingstad, and Heidi E. Fjeld. 2012. "Poverty and Disabled Households in the People's Republic of China: Experiences with a New Rural Health Insurance Scheme." *Disability & Society* 28 (2): 218–23.

Samuel, Geoffrey. 1993. *Civilized Shamans: Buddhism in Tibetan Societies*. Kathmandu: Mandala Book Point.

———. 2010. "Epilogue: Towards a Sowa Rigpa Sensibility." In *Between Science and Religion: Explorations on Tibetan Grounds*, ed. V. Adams, M. Schrempf, and S. R. Craig, 319–36. Oxford: Berghahn.

———. 2012. *Introducing Tibetan Buddhism*. New York: Routledge.

———. 2013. "Introduction: Medicine and Healing in Tibetan Societies." *East Asian Science, Technology and Society: An International Journal* 7: 1–17.

Sangyé Gyatso, Desi (Sangs-rgyas rgya-mtsho). (1703) 1994. *Gso rig sman gyi khog 'bugs* (Interior analysis of medicine). Dharamsala: Bod gzhung sman rtsi khang.

———. (1703) 2010. *Mirror of Beryl: A Historical Introduction to Tibetan Medicine*. Translated by Gavin Kilty. Boston: Wisdom Publications.

Saxer, Martin 2006. "Journeys with Tibetan Medicine." Documentary film, 136 minutes. Zürich: ANYMA Film.

———. 2012. "A Goat's Head on a Sheep's Body? Manufacturing Good Practices for Tibetan Medicine." *Medical Anthropology* 31 (6): 497–513. DOI:10.1080/01459740.2011.631958.

———. 2013. *Manufacturing Tibetan Medicine and the Moral Economy of Tibetanness*. Oxford: Berghahn.

Schaeffer, Kurtis R. 2003. "Textual Scholarship, Medical Tradition, and Mahayana Buddhist Ideals in Tibet." *Journal of Indian Philosophy* 31: 621–41.

Scheid, Volker. 2002. *Chinese Medicine in Contemporary China: Plurality and Synthesis*. Durham, NC: Duke University Press.

———. 2007. *Currents of Tradition in Chinese Medicine, 1626–2006*. Seattle: Eastland Press.

Schneider, Nicola. 2013. *Le renoncement au féminine: Couvents et nonnes dans le Bouddhisme Tibétain*. Nanterre: Presses Universitaires de Paris Ouest.

Schrempf, Mona. 2007. "Bon Lineage Doctors and the Local Transmission of Knowing Medical Practice in Nagchu." In *Soundings in Tibetan Medicine: Anthropological and Historical Perspectives*, ed. M. Schrempf, 91–126. Leiden: Brill.

———. 2011. "Between Mantra and Syringe: Healing and Health-Seeking Behaviour in Contemporary Amdo." In *Between Science and Religion: Explorations on Tibetan Grounds*, ed. V. Adams, M. Schrempf, and S. R. Craig, 157–83. Oxford: Berghahn.

SCMC, ZCMC, and ZCMRI (Shanghai Chinese Medical College, Zhejiang Chinese Medical College, and Zhejiang Chinese Medicine Research Institute [Shanghaishi zhongyi xueyuan, Zhejiangshen zhingyi xueyuan, Zhejiangsheng zhongyi yanjiuyuan]). 1969. *Chijiao yisheng shouce* (The barefoot doctor's manual). Shanghai: Shanghai kexue jishu chubanshe.

Scott, James C. 1976. *The Moral Economy of the Peasant: Rebellion and Subsistence in Southeast Asia*. New Haven, CT: Yale University Press.

———. 1985. *Weapons of the Weak: Everyday Forms of Peasant Resistance*. New Haven, CT: Yale University Press.

Seyfort Ruegg, D. 1995. *Ordre spirituel et ordre temporel dans la pensée bouddhique de l'Inde et du Tibet*. Paris: Collège de France.

Shakabpa, W. D. 1967. *Tibet: A Political History*. New Haven, CT: Yale University Press.

Shakabpa, Tsepon W. D., and D. Mahler. 2009. *One Hundred Thousand Moons: An Advanced Political History of Tibet*. 2 vols. Leiden: Brill.

Shakya, Tsering. 1999. *The Dragon in the Land of Snow: A History of Modern Tibet since 1947*. London: Pimlico.

Sherab Dorjé (Shes-rab rdo-rje). 1994. *Mkhas dbang grub pa'i 'byung gnas byang ngam ring chos sde chen po'i chos 'byung rna ba'i bdud rtsi'i snying po ngam ring chos sde'i lo rgyus* (History of Ngamring Chöde Monastery). Lhasa: Bod ljong mi dmangs dpe skrun khang.

Sidel, Ruth. 1972. *Women and Child Care in China: A Firsthand Report*. New York: Penguin.

Sidel, Victor W., and Ruth Sidel. 1973. *Serve the People: Observations on Medicine in the People's Republic of China*. New York: Josiah Macy, Jr. Foundation.

Sino-Tibetan Herbal. See RCTARHB 1973a.

Smith, Warren. 1996. *Tibetan Nation: The History of Tibetan Nationalism and Sino-Tibetan Relations*. Boulder, CO: Westview Press.

Snellgrove, David L., and Hugh Richardson. 1968. *A Cultural History of Tibet*. Boston: Shambhala.

Sochong. 2009. "'Long Distance Medical Treatment' in Old Tibet." Dictated by Ngawang Dorje and recorded by Sochung. *China's Tibet* 20: 24–26.

Soktsang, Lobsang Dhonden, and Colin Millard. 2013. "Diversity in Unity: The Changing Forms of Tibetan Medicine." *East Asian Science, Technology and Society: An International Journal* 7 (3): 1–20.

Spivak, Gayatri C. 1988. "Can the Subaltern Speak?" In *Marxism and the Interpretation of Culture*, ed. C. Nelson and L. Grossberg, 271–31. Basingstoke: Macmillan.

Stoddard, Heather. 1994. "Tibetan Publications and National Identity." In *Resistance and Reform in Tibet*, ed. R. Barnett and S. Akiner, 121–56. London: Hurst.

Strong, Anna L. 1959. *Tibetan Interviews*. Beijing: Foreign Languages Press.

Su Qiong (Sonam Tsering). 2008. *Niangrongxia sishu de chuangban ren: Renzeng Lunzhu Banjue* (Rinchen Lhundrub Paljor: The founder of the Nyerongsha's private school). Lhasa: Xizang Renmin Chubanshe (Tibet People's Publishing House).

Su Wenming, ed. 1983. *Tibet: Today and Yesterday*. Beijing: Beijing Review.

Swiss Red Cross. 1998. "Médicine traditionelle: Engagement de la Coix-Rouge Suisse (CRS) par example en Bolivie, au Tchad et au Tibet." Berne: International Cooperation Department.

———. 2001. "Médicin d'un village universel." In *Nouvelles de la Croix-Rouge Suisse*. Berne: International Cooperation Department.

———. 2003. *Introduction to Programs & Activities*. Shigatse: Swiss Red Cross Tibet Delegation.

———. 2005. *Swiss Red Cross—Tibet—China Delegation at Xigaze, 1998–2005*. Shigatse: Swiss Red Cross Tibet Delegation.

Tambiah, Stanley Jeyaraja. 1976. *World Conqueror and World Renouncer: A Study of Buddhism and Polity in Thailand against a Historical Background*. Cambridge: Cambridge University Press.

———. 1985. *Culture, Thought and Social Action: An Anthropological Perspective*. Cambridge, MA: Harvard University Press.

Tashi Tsering. 2005. "Outstanding Women in Tibetan Medicine." In *Women in Tibet*, ed. J. Gyatso and H. Havnevik, 169–94. London: Hurst.

Tashigang, Tashi 1974. *Fundamentals of Tibetan Medical Practice: Lha-sa Sman-rtsis-khang Prints of Works of Mkhen-rabs-nor-bu, 'Ju Mi-pham, Chos-grags rgya-mtsho, and 'Jam-mgon Kon-sprul*. Vol. 49. Leh: Sman rtsis Shes rig Spen dzod.

Taube, Manfred. 1981. *Beiträge zur Geschichte der Medizinischen Literatur Tibets*. (Contributions to the history of Tibetan medical literature). St. Augustin: VGH Wissenschaftsverlag.

Taylor, Kim. 2004. "Divergent Interests and Cultivated Misunderstandings: The Influence of the West on Modern Chinese Medicine." *Social History of Medicine* 17: 93–111.

———. 2005. *Chinese Medicine in Early Communist China, 1945–1963: A Medicine of Revolution*. London: Routledge.

Tenzin Chödrak. 2000. *The Rainbow Palace*. London: Bantam .

Thompson, Edward P. 1968. *The Making of the English Working Class*. New York: Vintage.

———. 1971. "The Moral Economy of the English Crowd in the Eighteenth Century." *Past and Present* 50: 76–136.

Tibet Information Network (TIN). 2000. *China's Great Leap West*. London: TIN.

———. 2002. *Delivery and Deficiency: Health and Healthcare in Tibet*. London: TIN.

———. 2004. *Tibetan Medicine in Contemporary Tibet: Health and Health Care in Tibet II*. London: TIN.

Tibetan Medical Manual. See Lhasa City Mentsikhang 1975.

Trinlé, Jampa (Byams pa 'phrin las). 2000. *Gangs ljongs gso rig bstan pa'i nyin byed rim byong gyi rnam thar phyogs bsrigs* (Namthar of famous doctors in the transmission of the Tibetan Sowa Rigpa). Pe cin: Mi rigs dpe skrun khang.

———. 2004. *Gso rig lo rgyus*. Pe jin: Mi rigs dpe skrun khang.

———. 2006. *Mkhas dbang byams pa 'phrin las mchog gi bod lugs gso rig gi dran gsos gtam rna ba'i bcud len* (Essence of the learned Jampa Trinlé's recollected stories on the great Tibetan science of healing [Recollections]). Edited by Tseten Jigmé (Tshe brtan 'jigs med). Pe cin: Mi dmangs dpe skrun khang.

Trinlé, Jampa, and Wang Lei. 1988. *Tibetan Medical Thankas of the Four Medical Tantras*. Translated by Cai Jingfeng. Lhasa: People's Publishing House.

Trouillot, Michel-Rolph. 1995. *Silencing the Past: Power and the Production of History*. Boston: Beacon Press.

———. 2003. *Global Transformations: Anthropology and the Modern World*. New York: Palgrave.

Tsarong, Dasang D. 2000. *In Service of His Country: The Biography of Dasang Damdul Tsarong, Commander General of Tibet*. Ithaca, NY: Snow Lion.

Tsewang Tashi. 2014. "Modernism in Tibetan Art: The Creative Journey of Four Artists." PhD diss., Norwegian University of Science and Technology, Trondheim.

Tubten Khétsun. 2009. *Memories of Life in Lhasa under Chinese Rule*. Translated by Matthew Akester. New Delhi: Penguin.

Tupten Chödar (Thub bstan Chos dar). 2008. "Mdo zla gsal dbang mo'i rnam thar." In *Mdo mkhyen brtse ye shes rdo rje'i gdung rgyud rim byon gyi rnam thar* (Namthar of the family lineage of Do Khyentse Yeshe Dorje). Mi Nyag: Tibetological Publishing House of China.

Turner, Samuel. (1800) 2006. *An Account of an Embassy to the Court of the Teshoo Lama in Tibet: Containing a Narrative of a Journey through Bootan, and part of Tibet*. Uckfield: Rediscovery.

Union Research Institute (URI). 1968. *Tibet 1950–1967*. Hong Kong: Union Research Institute.

Van Alphen, J., and A. Aris. 1995. *Oriental Medicine: An Illustrated Guide to the Asian Arts of Healing*. London: Serindia.

Van Vleet, Stacey. 2010/11. "Children's Healthcare and Astrology in the Nurturing of a Central Tibetan Nation-State, 1916–24." *Asian Medicine: Tradition and Modernity* 6 (2): 348–86.

———. 2014. "Medicine, Monasteries and Empire: Rethinking Tibetan Buddhism in Qing China." Ph.D. diss., Columbia University, New York.

Wagstaff, A., M. Lindelow, G. Jun, X. Lin, and Q. Juncheng. 2008. "Extending Health Insurance to the Rural Population: An Impact Evaluation of China's New Cooperative Medical Scheme." *Journal of Health Economics* 28 (1): 1–19.

Wang Yao. 1994. "Hu Yaobang's Visit to Tibet, May 22–31, 1980: An Important

Development in the Chinese Government's Tibet Policy." In *Resistance and Reform in Tibet*, ed. R. Barnett and S. Akiner, 285–95. London: Hurst.

Wangnam. 1999. *Short History of Ngamring Dzong Tibetan Medical Hospital.* Unpublished document.

Ward, Martha. 1998. "Women's Health, Women's Lives." *Medical Anthropology Quarterly* 12 (3): 384–90.

Wei, Chang. 1978. *Co-operative Medical Services Is Fine: How the Rural Co-operative Medical System Works in Changwei Prefecture, Shantung Province.* Beijing: Foreign Languages Press.

Weiner, Benno R. 2012. "The Chinese Revolution on the Tibetan Frontier: State Building, National Integration and Socialist Transformation, Zeku (Tsekhok) County, 1953–1958." PhD diss., Columbia University, New York.

Wellens, Koen. 2010. *Religious Revival in Tibetan Borderlands: The Premi of Southwest China.* Seattle: University of Washington Press.

Whitehead, M., G. Dahlgren, and T. Evans. 2001. "Equity and Health Sector Reforms: Can Low-Income Countries Escape the Medical Poverty Trap?" *Lancet* 358: 833–36.

Willock, Nicole D. 2010. "A Tibetan Buddhist Polymath in Modern China." PhD diss., Indiana University.

Woeser, Tsering. 2000. *Gsar brje* (Revolution). Oslo: Nor lbe bod don lhan tshogs nas par bskrun zhus (Norwegian Tibet Committee).

———. 2006. *Sha jie: Si shi nian de ji yi jin qu, jing tou xia de Xizang wen ge* (Forbidden memory: Tibet during the Cultural Revolution). Taipei: Locus Publishing.

Wylie, Tyrell V. 1959. "A Standard System of Tibetan Transcription." *Harvard Journal of Asiatic Studies* 22: 261–76.

Xu, Judy, and Yue Yang. 2009. "Traditional Chinese Medicine in the Chinese Health Care System." *Health Policy* 90: 133–39.

Yang Ga. 2014. "The Origins of the Four Tantras and an Account of Its Author, Yuthog Yonten Gonpo." In *Bodies in Balance: The Art of Tibetan Medicine*, ed. Theresia Hofer, 154–77. New York: Rubin Museum of Art (in association with University of Washington Press).

Yeh, Emily T. 2006. "'An Open Lhasa Welcomes You': Disciplining the Researcher in Tibet." In *Doing Fieldwork in China*, ed. Maria Heimer and Stig Thøgersen, 96–109. Honolulu: University of Hawai'i Press.

———. 2013. *Taming Tibet: Landscape Transformation and the Gift of Chinese Development.* Ithaca, NY: Cornell University Press.

Yinba. 2008. *Qinrenuobu yu zangyi tianwen lisuan* (The great teacher Khyenrap

Norbu and Tibetan medicine, astrology, calendar science). Lhasa: Xizang Renmin Chubanshe (Tibet People's Publishing House).

Yonten Gyatso, Jamgon Kongtrul ('jam mgon kong sprul yon tan rgya mtsho). 1976. *Gso rig zin tig.* Qinghai: Tsongon Tibetan Medical Hospital.

Zhang Xiaoming, ed. 2009. "Pacification and Democratic Reforms of TAR." Special issue, *China's Tibet.*

Zhen, Yan, and Cai Jingfeng. 2005. *China's Tibetan Medicine.* Beijing: Foreign Languages Press.

Zheng. 1997. "Maoism, Feminism, and the UN Conference on Women: Women's Studies Research in Contemporary China." *Journal of Women's History* 8 (4): 126–52.

INDEX

STUDIES ON ETHNIC GROUPS IN CHINA

Stevan Harrell, Editor

Cultural Encounters on China's Ethnic Frontiers, edited by Stevan Harrell

Guest People: Hakka Identity in China and Abroad
edited by Nicole Constable

Familiar Strangers: A History of Muslims in Northwest China
by Jonathan N. Lipman

Lessons in Being Chinese: Minority Education and Ethnic Identity in Southwest China, by Mette Halskov Hansen

Manchus and Han: Ethnic Relations and Political Power in Late Qing and Early Republican China, 1861–1928, by Edward J. M. Rhoads

Ways of Being Ethnic in Southwest China, by Stevan Harrell

Governing China's Multiethnic Frontiers, edited by Morris Rossabi

On the Margins of Tibet: Cultural Survival on the Sino-Tibetan Frontier
by Åshild Kolås and Monika P. Thowsen

The Art of Ethnography: A Chinese "Miao Album"
translation by David M. Deal and Laura Hostetler

Doing Business in Rural China: Liangshan's New Ethnic Entrepreneurs
by Thomas Heberer

Communist Multiculturalism: Ethnic Revival in Southwest China
by Susan K. McCarthy

Religious Revival in the Tibetan Borderlands: The Premi of Southwest China
by Koen Wellens

Lijiang Stories: Shamans, Taxi Drivers, and Runaway Brides in Reform-Era China
by Emily Chao

In the Land of the Eastern Queendom: The Politics of Gender and Ethnicity on the Sino-Tibetan Border, by Tenzin Jinba

Empire and Identity in Guizhou: Local Resistance to Qing Expansion
by Jodi L. Weinstein

China's New Socialist Countryside: Modernity Arrives in the Nu River Valley
by Russell Harwood

Mapping Shangrila: Contested Landscapes in the Sino-Tibetan Borderlands
edited by Emily T. Yeh and Chris Coggins

A Landscape of Travel: The Work of Tourism in Rural Ethnic China, by Jenny Chio

The Han: China's Diverse Majority, by Agnieszka Joniak-Lüthi

Xinjiang and the Modern Chinese State, by Justin M. Jacobs

In the Circle of White Stones: Moving through Seasons with Nomads of Eastern Tibet, by Gillian Tan

Medicine and Memory in Tibet: Amchi *Physicians in an Age of Reform,* by Theresia Hofer

www.ingramcontent.com/pod-product-compliance
Lightning Source LLC
LaVergne TN
LVHW041110090826
844660LV00056B/128

* 9 7 8 0 2 9 5 7 4 2 9 8 4 *